COLOUR ATLAS OF GYNAECOLOGY

Illustrations by

Photography   Joseph M. Schramp, L.A.S.(Leiden), F.M.P.I.A., A.I.A.P., M.I.P.T.
                                   Alison M. Scarfe, Dip. Art.
Layout   Alison M. Scarfe, Dip. Art.
Design   Dorothy M. Huffell

COLOUR ATLAS
OF
GYNAECOLOGY

NORMAN A. BEISCHER, M.D., B.S., M.G.O., F.R.C.S.(Edin.),
F.R.A.C.S., F.R.C.O.G., F.R.A.C.O.G.

*Professor of Obstetrics and Gynaecology, University of Melbourne, Senior
Gynaecologist Obstetrician, Mercy Maternity Hospital. Senior Gynaecologist
Austin Hospital and Repatriation General Hospital.*

ERIC V. MACKAY, M.B., B.S., M.G.O., F.R.C.S.(Edin.), F.R.A.C.S.,
F.R.C.O.G., F.R.A.C.O.G., F.A.C.O.G.(Hon.).

*Professor of Obstetrics and Gynaecology, University of Queensland. Senior
Gynaecologist Royal Brisbane Hospital and Queensland Radium Institute. Editor
of the Australian and New Zealand Journal of Obstetrics and Gynaecology.*

W. B. SAUNDERS COMPANY
Sydney Philadelphia London Toronto

W. B. Saunders
9 Waltham Street, Artarmon, NSW 2064, Australia

© 1981 Holt-Saunders Pty Limited

National Library of Australia
Cataloguing-in-Publication entry

Beischer, Norman A. (Norman Albert), 1930-
    Colour atlas of gynaecology.

    Includes index.
    ISBN 0 03 900238 1.

    1. Gynaecology. I. Mackay, Eric V. (Eric Vincent),
    1924-. II. Title.

618.1

---

*This atlas is gratefully dedicated
to our patients and colleagues who
have so willingly helped us in
its preparation.*

Contents

Preface

The focal point of obstetrics is the miracle of childbirth and the newborn infant. Gynaecology is a broader subject concerning the diseases peculiar to women. Previous atlases have concentrated on such special aspects as gynaecological surgery, laparoscopy, colposcopy, and cytology; in the present atlas we have provided a visual overview of the entire subject, including aspects of anatomy, embryology, pathology and diseases of the breast, as are seen in clinical practice.

The magic of gynaecology concerns the process of ovulation — the beginning of life, and its control. This is the basis of the endocrinology of reproduction and birth control. The sequelae of parturition and senescence provide the gynaecologist with the need to understand not only the mechanical problems of uterovaginal prolapse, but also the endocrinology of the postmenopause, where therapy includes the need for sexual counselling as well as the prescription of hormones. Of major importance in gynaecology, because of the relevance to almost all women at some time during the reproductive era, is the control of pain and abnormal bleeding associated with menstruation. The cervix, uterus and ovaries are the sites of origin of a wide range of benign and malignant tumours, so that there is necessarily a heavy emphasis on many aspects of gynaecological cancer.

The first chapter deals with terms and definitions, because the student must learn the language of gynaecology before an understanding of the subject can begin. It was included so that the atlas became a complete textbook within itself and allowed the beginner to find the information required to understand the diseases illustrated in the colour plates and the points raised in the legends.

The legends in most instances are case histories and our objective has been to extend the teaching message beyond the illustration itself. In writing the legends, we have stressed the importance of the patient as well as the disorder. We have avoided gruesome pictures that might upset the beginner and tried to select specimens not as trophies captured by an ambitious surgeon but for their intrinsic teaching message. Some illustrations showing advanced disease have been included when typical of a common mode of presentation, for this occurs in all communities, because of the patient's age, or social, geographic or cultural considerations. We offer no apologies for inclusion of some rarities, since they often kindle interest, capture the imagination, and provide insight.

The detailed section on questions and answers is included mainly as a teaching exercise, but also for the purposes of revision and to help the reader gain clinical perspective. There should be no secrets in teaching, or special 'clever' questions withheld for purely examination purposes. In the past 20 years we have spent many hours with our co-examiners in undergraduate and postgraduate nursing and medical examinations, and we have attempted to pass on to the reader the essence of this experience.

With the proliferation of specialist disciplines in medical schools, and their inclusion in the curriculum, there is now less time available to master the essentials of gynaecology. In many medical schools, access to clinical material is limited and this applies especially to the common 'minor' conditions which are, nevertheless, of considerable importance to the patient. It was with these considerations in mind that our decision to produce this colour atlas of gynaecology was born.

Acknowledgements

We wish to thank our colleagues at the Mercy Maternity Hospital, Queen Victoria Memorial Hospital, Royal Brisbane Hospital and Royal Women's Hospital for permission to reproduce photographs of patients. We also acknowledge our indebtedness to our patients who agreed to be photographed! Although we have systematically collected gynaecological illustrations for this Atlas, the acquisition of many of them could not have been planned. We are fortunate to have been granted access to the private collections of our colleagues: Dr David Abell (plates 31, 58, 59, 98-101, 116, 126, 157, 160, 195, 204, 228, 229, 245); Dr Neil Astill (plates 151, 159, 210); Dr William Chanen (plates 156, 242, 287-290, 294, 296, 298, 299); Dr Michael Drake (plates 259, 265-280); Professor William Hare (plates 79-81); Dr John Hueston (plates 63-73); and Dr Robert Zacharin (plates 33, 51-56, 60, 147, 177, 194, 196, 198, 199, 221, 227, 237-239, 422), whose generosity is greatly appreciated. Dr Susan A. Wheildon arranged access to the photographic files of the Queen Victoria Memorial Hospital (plates 120, 123, 136, 202, 205, 219, 235, 240) and Dr Denys W. Fortune to those of the Royal Women's Hospital (plates 6, 7, 9, 11-18, 21, 22, 84, 87, 95, 108, 110-112, 114, 115, 122, 124, 128, 135, 137, 138, 141, 150, 152-155, 158, 161, 162, 167, 169, 201, 203, 206, 209, 218, 225, 230-234, 243, 244, 246-250, 256, 257, 261-263, 281, 286, 300-306, 308, 313, 314, 317, 320-322, 338, 340, 344-355, 370, 372-379, 381). Dr John Hobbs provided the photographs shown in plates 23, 24, 27, 28, 32, 140, 260, 264, 334-337, 343. It is also a pleasant duty to acknowledge the sub-editorial assistance of Dr David Abell and the help received from our medical students, in particular Miss Patricia Crock.

Terms and Definitions

A means not or not having: hence amenorrhoea — not having periods.

Abortion. The expulsion or extraction of the products of conception from the uterus via the birth canal before 20 weeks' gestation (28 weeks in some communities) (plates 102-106).

(a) *Threatened.* Onset of vaginal bleeding before 20 weeks' gestation with or without uterine pain; the cervix (internal os) is closed.
(b) *Inevitable.* Bleeding and pain with dilatation of the cervix; uterine size equivalent to menstrual data.
(c) *Incomplete.* Bleeding and pain with dilatation of cervix and passage of placental tissue; uterus smaller than dates.
(d) *Missed.* The fetus has died, but the cervix remains closed; uterus smaller than dates. The conceptus may be entirely absorbed or shed piecemeal when spontaneous abortion eventually occurs. Missed abortion is usually preceded by an episode of bleeding (threatened abortion).
(e) *Septic.* When abortion is complicated by infection (offensive purulent discharge, pyrexia, local or generalized abdominal tenderness).
(f) *Habitual.* Three or more successive spontaneous abortions.
(g) *Therapeutic.* Deliberate induction of abortion before 20 weeks' gestation (28 weeks in some countries).

Adenomyosis (endometriosis interna). Occurs when the endometrial glands invade the myometrium. Sections of the uterus show a thickened myometrium with dark spots which indicate areas of ectopic endometrium with retained menstrual blood. Clinically it is associated with secondary dysmenorrhoea and regular uterine enlargement (plate 90).

Adenosis of the vagina. Presence of mucous glands in an organ that normally has none. Rare except in females exposed to stilboestrol in early intrauterine life, it warrants surveillance because of the possible development of clear cell adenocarcinoma (plate 245).

Adnexa (plural of adnexum — 'at the side of'). Structures at the side of the uterus (ovary, Fallopian tube, contents of the broad ligament) (plates 4, 8, 33).

Adolescence. The period of life during which a child becomes an adult; there is mental, physical and emotional adaptation to the onset of sexual maturity.

Adrenogenital syndrome. A familial disease with recessive inheritance due to an enzyme defect resulting in the interruption of cortisol production by the adrenal cortex. There is a resultant hypersecretion of adrenocorticotrophin by the pituitary and adrenal hyperplasia. Virilization results from increased secretion of androgenic precursors by the adrenal glands.

Anorexia nervosa. Loss of appetite due to psychogenic causes with resultant drastic weight loss, amenorrhoea and infertility.

Amenorrhoea.
(a) *Primary.* Failure of the onset of menstruation by the age of 18 years (plate 62).
(b) *Secondary.* Cessation of menstruation for 6 months or more. Causes can be physiological (pregnancy, lactation, menopause) or pathological (plates 127, 128).

Anteversion of the uterus. This describes the normal anatomical position in relation to the long axis of the body — held forwards.

Apareunia. The inability to practise coitus due to anatomical or psychological causes (plates 237-239).

Arcuate uterus. Minor degree of uterine malformation characterized by a depression in the uterine fundus.

Ascites. Accumulation of fluid in the peritoneal cavity due to congestive cardiac failure, hepatic or renal disease or carcinoma involving the peritoneum. Difficult to distinguish from a large ovarian cyst. Can be due to an ovarian fibroma (Meigs' syndrome) (plates 356-364).

Asherman's syndrome. Secondary amenorrhoea resulting from too vigorous curettage performed to control haemorrhage, usually in the presence of postpartum or postabortal infection. There are multiple intrauterine adhesions present. The endometrium often regenerates if the uterine walls are held apart by an intrauterine contraceptive device.

Atrophic (senile) vaginitis. Inflammation of the vaginal epithelium due to infection by pyogenic organisms after the menopause when oestrogen lack results in thinning of the epithelium and loss of glycogen, which in turn affects lactic acid production by Doderlein's bacilli (plates 92-95, 144).

Azoospermia. Absence of spermatozoa in seminal fluid.

Bartholin's cyst. Arises as a result of blockage of the duct draining the gland. There is an accumulation of glandular secretion with resultant swelling of the duct. If the contents become infected a Bartholin's abscess will result (plates 211-216).

Billings' method of natural birth control. This method is based on identification of the time of impending ovulation by noting the change in the nature of cervical mucus (becomes slippery like the white of an egg) due to the preovulation surge in oestrogen secretion by the Graafian follicle.

Bimanual examination. Clinical examination of the pelvic contents, usually with the patient in the dorsal position. The size, position, mobility, regularity of outline and tenderness of the uterus are noted. The presence of tubal or ovarian pathology is elicited.

Blighted ovum. Occurs in the early weeks of pregnancy when the fetus is either absent or has stopped developing. Placental tissue has chromosomal abnormalities in approximately 30% of cases. Spontaneous abortion occurs usually after 6-10 weeks' amenorrhoea.

Bonney's test. Elevation of the bladder neck (correction of the posterior urethrovesical angle) with fingers or open sponge forceps (without occluding the urethra) to see if stress incontinence of urine is controlled; if it is, the test indicates that buttressing of the bladder neck area at anterior colporrhaphy is likely to cure the symptom.

Brenner tumour. Solid, benign ovarian tumour resembling a fibroma except that it contains islands of clear transitional cells (plate 350).

Carcinoma. A malignant growth arising from and composed of epithelial cells (plates 224, 225, 244, 305, 333, 371, 381).

Carcinoma in situ (intraepithelial carcinoma). A lesion with atypical cells and nuclei, indistinguishable from those of an invasive growth, extending through the full thickness of the squamous epithelium, but not transgressing the basement membrane. Detectable by cytology or colposcopy and confirmed by biopsy (plates 243, 262-264, 267, 268, 287, 288, 290-292, 294, 295).

Carneous mole. A mass of tissue comprising blood clot, shrunken amniotic sac and chorionic tissue (placental tissue) found in the uterus after the embryo has died and been reabsorbed.

Cervical erosion. See erosion.

Cervicitis. Inflammation of the cervix. The infection can be either acute or chronic and is a common cause of vaginal discharge. In the acute phase, the cervix appears reddened and congested (plates 141, 145).

Cervix. Means neck by derivation — the lower part of the uterus. It is about 4 cm long and extends from the isthmus into the vagina. The attachment of the vagina to the cervix divides it into the supravaginal portion and the vaginal portion. The endocervical canal is lined by columnar epithelium and normally this changes to squamous epithelium at the level of the external os (the squamocolumnar junction) (plates 2, 3, 47).

Chancre. The primary lesion of syphilis. It usually occurs on the vulva, vagina, cervix, lip or anus. It is a hard, red papule which breaks down to form the classic punched-out ulcer with wash-leather base (plate 156).

Chancroid. A venereal infection caused by Haemophilus ducreyi. It presents as multiple painful ulcers on the vulva. Oral tetracycline therapy is the treatment of choice. It is wise to perform serology to exclude syphilis.

Chiari-Frommel syndrome. Persistent postpartum lactation, amenorrhoea and superinvolution of the uterus due to disorder of the hypothalamus, often associated with excessive secretion of prolactin.

Choriocarcinoma. Malignant disease of the trophoblast involving both syncytial and cytotrophoblastic cells, causing haemorrhagic necrosis of invaded tissue. Incidence about 1 in 20,000 pregnancies; 40% follow a hydatidiform mole, 40% an abortion and 20% a normal pregnancy. Metastasizes to lung, liver, brain and vagina, but responds to cytotoxic drug therapy (methotrexate; actinomycin D) (plates 116, 124, 125, 126).

Cleisis means to obliterate, e.g., colpocleisis.

Climacteric. The phase of waning ovarian function (3-5 years or more) in women making the transition from the reproductive to the nonreproductive era; it includes the event of the menopause (permanent cessation of menses). Irregular or heavy menstruation at this time should not be regarded as physiological and should always be investigated.

Clitoris. Homologue of the male penis but not containing the urethra, this 2-3 cm long organ is composed of erectile tissue and lies directly below the symphysis pubis. The labia minora fuse anteriorly to form its prepuce and frenulum (plate 1).

Colpocleisis. Surgical obliteration of the vagina performed as a last resort (no more coitus) to cure genital prolapse or vesicovaginal/rectovaginal fistula (plate 245).

Colporrhaphy. Repair of the vagina.
(a) *Anterior.* Repair of a cystocele (and urethrocele if present) by excision of redundant vaginal epithelium and correction of the bulging bladder and urethra by plication of the pubocervical fascia (plates 175, 184-192, 387-389).
(b) *Posterior.* Repair of a rectocele and/or enterocele and deficient perineal body. The lower part of the pouch of Douglas is obliterated by excision of peritoneum (enterocele) and the rectovaginal septum is reconstituted by suturing the uterosacral ligaments, rectovaginal fascia and levatores ani muscles in the midline posteriorly. Redundant vaginal epithelium is excised and the introitus restored to normal dimensions by reconstruction of the perineal body (perineorrhaphy) (plates 179, 390-392, 410-416).

Colpos means vagina.

Colposcopy. A technique for visualizing the cervix using an optical instrument (colposcope) under conditions of good lighting and magnification 12-20 times normal. The cellular and vascular patterns of the epithelium allow prediction of the diagnosis of neoplastic conditions (dysplasia, intraepithelial carcinoma, invasive carcinoma), assessment of the extent of the lesion, and site for target biopsy for histological diagnosis. Colposcopy is indicated in the presence of abnormal cytology or a clinically suspicious cervical lesion (plates 281-300).

Condylomata acuminata. Multiple warty growths of various sizes on the vulva, perineum, vagina or cervix; due to the papilloma virus, but often associated with chronic vaginal discharge due to trichomonal or monilial infection (plates 146-149, 277, 299, 300).

Condylomata lata. Flat, raised skin lesions of secondary syphilis. They occur in groups on the vulva and perineum. They ulcerate and drain a seropurulent fluid that teems with spirochaetes (plates 159, 210).

Conization of the cervix. Excision of a cone of tissue, the base extending from the external os, sufficient to include the squamocolumnar junction, the apex being as high as possible in the endocervical canal. It is performed to exclude invasive carcinoma in the patient with a positive smear and abnormal lesion extending beyond the reach of the colposcope (plates 287-291, 422).

Cornual pregnancy. Ectopic pregnancy in a rudimentary horn of the uterus. Rupture occurs later (12-18 weeks) than with tubal pregnancies because the muscular wall is thicker. Treatment is excision of the rudimentary horn or hysterectomy.

Corpus means body.

Corpus luteum. Yellow body in the ovary that develops from the ovarian follicle after ovulation. It continues the secretion of oestrogen but also produces progesterone that prepares the endometrium for implantation of the fertilized ovum (plates 8-10, 18, 113, 114).

Corpus luteum cyst. A cyst due to haemorrhage into a corpus luteum or excessive serous fluid production by theca cells. It presents as a palpable ovarian tumour, or as a result of rupture causing haemorrhage and an acute abdomen simulating a ruptured ectopic pregnancy (plates 9, 114, 115).

Cryosurgery (kryos means cold). Freezing with probes cooled by liquid nitrogen, carbon dioxide or Freon gas. It is an alternative to electrocoagulation diathermy or laser in conservative treatment of intraepithelial cervical neoplasia (dysplasia, carcinoma in situ) (plate 294).

Cryptomenorrhoea means hidden menstruation. The menstrual flow is retained because of vaginal obstruction (imperforate hymen, transverse vaginal septum), absent vagina or cervical stenosis. Clinical presentations include primary amenorrhoea, urinary retention (large haematocolpos causing urethral obstruction), haematosalpinges, sterility (tubal inflam-

mation), endometriosis (due to retrograde menstruation) (plates 58, 59, 234-236).

Culdotomy (colpotomy). An opening in the posterior vaginal wall into the pouch of Douglas to inspect the contents of the peritoneal cavity (exclusion of cancer, tubal pathology, endometriosis), drain a pelvic abscess or to operate on the pelvic organs (tubal ligation, ovarian biopsy).

Cullen's sign. A rare periumbilical bluish discoloration indicative of retroperitoneal haemorrhage as seen with subacute ruptured ectopic pregnancy where blood enters the mesosalpinx (plate 111). Blood reaches the umbilical skin in lymphatics running along the obliterated umbilical arteries (lateral umbilical ligaments).

Cyst. An epithelial-lined space that grows by expansion, e.g., Bartholin's cyst, follicular cyst.

Cysto means the bladder or a cyst. Cystectomy is to cut out or remove a cyst or the bladder.

Cystadenocarcinoma. Serous and mucinous cystadenocarcinomas are common primary ovarian carcinomas that can arise from benign cystadenomas. The other common primary adenocarcinoma of the ovary is the endometrioid variety which is a solid tumour (plates 371, 373, 375).

Cystadenoma. Together with cystic teratomas comprise about 80% of all ovarian neoplasms.

(a) *Mucinous* cystadenomas are the commonest. They are usually unilateral, multilocular and are often enormous (plates 356-362).

(b) *Serous* cystadenomas are usually papilliferous and often bilateral. They have a greater tendency to malignant change than the mucinous variety (plate 374).

Cystic glandular hyperplasia. Proliferative overgrowth of the endometrium due to anovulation and persistence of the ovarian follicle; there is persistent, unopposed (no progesterone) exposure to oestrogen. If seen after the menopause this endometrial pattern is more frequently associated with more severe degrees of hyperplasia and frank carcinoma (plates 85-87, 91, 341-343).

Cystic teratoma (dermoid cyst). Common, benign ovarian neoplasm usually containing sebaceous material and hair, the cyst wall being lined by skin and its appendages. About 20% contain teeth and about 20% are bilateral. Treatment is ovarian cystectomy (plates 344, 345, 351).

Cystocele. Prolapse of upper half of the anterior vaginal wall. This is the commonest type of genital prolapse. It is often a prelude to, or associated with, uterine prolapse. It is due to tearing of the pubocervical fascia during distension of the vagina at childbirth. In about 30% of patients there is associated stress incontinence of urine (plates 3, 167-175, 184-186, 387).

Cytology. The study of cells. Main application is in the detection of cervical carcinoma and its precursors by the Papanicolaou stain of a smear taken from the cervix ± the endocervical canal and posterior fornix where desquamated cells collect. Also permits diagnosis of trichomonas, monilia, herpes simplex, wart virus disease and bacterial infections. Exfoliative cytology is used for detection of carcinomas of the lung, bladder and bowel, but its dominant application is in the discipline of gynaecology (plates 21-25, 30, 259, 262, 265-280, 313, 338).

Decidua. The exaggerated endometrial reaction to oestrogen and progesterone. The glands are tortuous and the stromal cells enlarge, becoming polyhedral and packed together. A decidual reaction in endometrial stroma is not histological proof of pregnancy; for this the presence of chorionic villi is required (plates 10, 17, 18).

Decidual cast. Decidua shed from the uterus as a single piece; a sign suggestive of ectopic pregnancy.

Decubitus ulceration. When there is extensive prolapse, the cervix is sat upon or abraded by clothing, causing ulceration with discharge and haemorrhage. Malignant ulceration must be excluded by biopsy if healing fails to occur after reduction of the prolapse (plate 171).

Dermoid cyst (cystic teratoma). A benign ovarian neoplasm comprising a combination of structures arising from ectoderm, mesoderm and endoderm. It has a smooth, thick capsule and so is readily enucleated with conservation of the ovary (ovarian cystectomy). It is the commonest ovarian tumour associated with pregnancy (plates 344, 345, 351).

Dilatation and curettage. The commonest gynaecological operation. The cervix is dilated to allow the passage of a polyp forceps and curette into the uterine cavity to sample the endometrial lining or terminate a pregnancy (plates 382-386).

Discharge. A vaginal discharge is considered to be abnormal if the patient's underclothes are consistently stained or if she needs to wear a pad. Physiological discharge is mucoid, without significant odour and is largely an oestrogenic effect, being more pronounced in pregnancy. If there is itching or the discharge is yellow or offensive then speculum examination is required to investigate the cause (plate 26, 29).

Dys means ill, bad, difficult (Greek). Dysuria is painful or difficult micturition.

Dysgerminoma. Solid ovarian neoplasm occurring in adolescents and young women. It exhibits malignancy in about 30% of cases. Histologically it is identical to the seminoma of the testes with cords of round, primitive cells arranged in tubules, and a connective tissue stroma containing many lymphocytes (plates 354, 355).

Dysmenorrhoea. Painful menstruation. It is impossible to exaggerate the importance of this symptom, so poorly understood by men. It is experienced, to a greater or lesser extent, by 70% of women during the reproductive years.

(a) *Primary* (spasmodic). Begins with the onset of ovulation 1-2 years after the menarche, and usually is not associated with organic disease. It tends to improve with age, sexual maturity and parturition.
(b) *Secondary* (congestive). Usually associated with organic disease (endometriosis, chronic pelvic inflammatory disease) and commonly the patient is aged 30 years or more. Unlike primary dysmenorrhoea, the pain persists throughout the menses.

Dyspareunia. Painful intercourse. Apart from pain due to an unyielding or intact hymen and recent episiotomy, psychological causes are more likely to cause superficial perineal pain (e.g., vaginismus with spasm of levatores ani muscles). Pain on deep penetration is suggestive of endometriosis or chronic pelvic inflammatory disease.

Dysplasia (cervix, vagina, vulva). Presence of atypical cells and nuclei in the deeper layers of squamous epithelium, but with normal maturation of the surface layers. Classified mild to severe according to degree, the latter being more likely to progress to carcinoma in situ. Dysplasia is detected by exfoliative cytology or colposcopy and is confirmed by biopsy (plates 259-261, 265, 266, 286, 301, 302).

Ectomy means to cut out; e. g. hysterectomy, ovarian cystectomy.

Ectopic pregnancy. Implantation of the fertilized ovum outside the normal uterine cavity (Fallopian tube, ovary, abdominal cavity, rudimentary uterine horn, cervix) (plates 107-112, 114-116).

Endocervix. The lining of the cervical canal from the internal os to the external os (plate 88, 89).

Endometrial hyperplasia. Excessive growth of endometrium due to prolonged oestrogenic stimulation unopposed by progesterone. Usually the histological pattern is proliferative (no ovulation so no progesterone effect), often cystic (cystic glandular hyperplasia or Swiss cheese pattern), and sometimes atypical, which when severe is difficult to distinguish from adenocarcinoma (plates 85-87, 91, 341-343).

Endometriosis. Presence of endometrial glands and stroma outside the uterus (ovaries, pelvic peritoneum, uterosacral ligaments, bowel) or within the uterine muscle wall (adenomyosis) (plates 129-135).

Endometrium. The lining of the uterus which responds to oestrogen and progesterone produced by the ovary and is shed cyclically during the reproductive era (plates 11-19).

Enterocele. Herniation of the pouch of Douglas into the vagina. It can occur as part of a uterovaginal prolapse or after hysterectomy due to failure of the vaginal vault supports. It bulges the upper one-third of the posterior vaginal wall. A finger in the rectum will usually help to differentiate a rectocele from an enterocele. Often a high rectocele cannot be distinguished from an enterocele until the pouch of Douglas is opened at operation (plates 177, 179).

Erosion (ectopy, ectropion). Erosion suggests ulceration, but the pinkish-red velvety appearance commonly seen on the ectocervix is due to the presence of columnar epithelium (single cell layer) that shows the underlying vessels. It is due to eversion of the cervix caused by hormonal changes at puberty, first pregnancy or use of the oral contraceptive pill. Eversion of the endocervix into the vagina gives the apparent effect of caudal migration of the squamocolumnar junction (plates 36, 38, 39, 284).

Exenteration. Total pelvic exenteration comprises radical hysterectomy with bilateral salpingo-oophorectomy, pelvic lymphadenectomy and removal of the bladder and rectum. It can be a curative procedure for advanced carcinoma (cervix, bladder, rectum) confined to the pelvis. The patient has a colostomy and ileal loop urinary conduit (plate 320). In anterior exenteration, the rectum and anal canal are spared; in posterior exenteration, the bladder and urethra are spared.

Fallopian tube (oviduct). Muscular tube with a lining of ciliated cells. The distal end is trumpet-shaped (ampulla) and has finger-like processes (fimbriae) that clasp the Graafian follicle at ovulation and capture the ovum, which is usually fertilized in the outer third of the tube during its journey to the uterine cavity (plates 4, 5, 8, 430).

Ferning. A term used to describe the fern-like pattern of cervical mucus dried on a glass slide. It is due to a certain ratio of sodium chloride to proteins in cervical secretion and is an oestrogenic effect (preovulation). Change to a cellular pattern without crystals indicates that ovulation has occurred (progesterone effect).

Fibromyoma (leiomyoma, fibroma, myoma, 'fibroid'). The commonest tumour in women (present in 30% of women aged 30 years or more) and with the mucinous cystadenoma of the ovary, the largest of them all. Fibromyomas are benign tumours arising in uterine muscle and microscopically show a whorled pattern of smooth muscle and connective tissue. There is a pseudocapsule of compressed muscle that permits ready enucleation (myomectomy). They are usually multiple and can be subserous, intramural, submucous or intraligamentary in position. They can be asymptomatic or associated with a number of symptoms, including menorrhagia and infertility. Pain is uncommon and is due to ischaemic necrosis (red degeneration); this complication typically occurs in pregnancy (plates 323-329, 331, 332).

Fimbriae. Finger-like projections at the end of the Fallopian tube. Their role appears to be the collection of the free ovum once it has been released from the Graafian follicle.

Flushes (flashes). These occur on the face and neck; together with attacks of sweating they are the clinical stigmata of the climacteric. They are due to oestrogen deficiency as a result of waning ovarian function. These symptoms sometimes occur when the patient is still menstruating.

Fourchette. Fold of skin below the hymen posteriorly, formed by fusion of labia minora and majora. There is also an anterior fourchette where the labia minora fuse to form the prepuce of the clitoris (plate 1).

Fractional curettage. Curettage of the endocervical canal, lower one-half of the uterine body, then the fundus of the uterus, with separate collection of curettings, performed in patients suspected of having carcinoma to determine if the growth extends to the lower half of uterus or to the cervix — in which case treatment involves radical rather than simple hysterectomy (plate 20).

Galactorrhoea. Secretion of milk in the absence of a recent pregnancy (inappropriate lactation).

Gartner's duct cyst. Single or multiple mucus-containing cysts formed in the remnants of the mesonephric duct. They are found in the anterolateral aspect of the vagina, usually in the upper half (plates 61, 167, 240).

Gene. The functional unit of heredity; large numbers are situated in each of the 46 chromosomes in the cell nucleus.

Genotype. The hereditary constitution of genes of an individual.

Gonorrhoea. A common venereal disease due to infection with the bacterium Neisseria gonorrhoeae which attacks columnar epithelium (not squamous). Sites of initial infection are urethra, paraurethral glands, Bartholin's duct and gland, endocervix, pharynx, anal canal. Spread then occurs to endometrium, Fallopian tubes and pelvic peritoneum (salpingitis, peritonitis). Tuboovarian abscesses result in chronic pelvic pain, tubal obstruction and sterility (plates 31, 32, 136-139).

Graafian follicle. An ovarian follicle at the final stage of development before rupture and release of the ovum (ovulation). The mean preovulatory diameter of the follicle (measured by ultrasound) is 2 cm (volume 5 ml) (plates 7, 9).

Granuloma inguinale. Venereal disease of the vulva due to the bacterium Donovania granulomatis. This infection produces ulceration and hypertrophic granulation tissue. Lymphatic obstruction can result in elephantiasis of the vulva (plate 151).

Granulosa cell tumour. An ovarian neoplasm which originates from granulosa cell nests. It produces oestrogen as do thecomas and luteomas; about 15% are malignant and 15% are associated with adenocarcinoma of the endometrium, presumably due to prolonged, unopposed stimulation by oestrogen (plates 341-343, 347-349, 353).

Gumma. The lesion of tertiary syphilis. Endarteritis causes necrosis and ulceration of nodules that appear in skin and other organs.

Haematocolpos. Distension of the vagina with retained menstrual blood usually due to a transverse vaginal septum or imperforate hymen (plates 58, 59, 234-236).

Haematometra. Retention of blood in the uterine cavity due to obstruction of the vagina or cervix (congenital, or due to surgery, electrocautery or irradiation).

Haematosalpinx. Distension of the Fallopian tube with blood as a result of obstruction of the vagina or cervix. It also occurs due to retrograde menstruation or at the time of abortion; for the same reason it is sometimes seen on the normal side when operating for ruptured tubal pregnancy (plates 107, 109, 110-112, 114).

Haemoperitoneum. Blood in the peritoneal cavity. The commonest cause is retrograde menstruation which is often asymptomatic and noted when laparotomy/laparoscopy is performed during the menses. Other causes are ruptured ectopic pregnancy, ovulatory haemorrhage, ruptured ovarian or endometriotic cyst, ruptured liver or spleen (plates 107-116).

Haemorrhage.

(a) *Primary* haemorrhage is that occurring during an operation.
(b) *Reactionary* postoperative haemorrhage occurs within 24 hours of an operation and is due to inadequate ligation of an artery.
(c) *Secondary* haemorrhage most commonly occurs 8-10 days after an operation and is due to infection.

Hegar's sign of pregnancy. Bimanual palpation of a soft uterine isthmus between the cervix below and the uterine body above. Used before modern urine tests for pregnancy became available; best avoided if the patient has a history of previous spontaneous abortions.

Hermaphrodite. Person having both male and female sexual organs (plates 98-101).

Herpes genitalis. Infection of the vulva, vagina or cervix due to herpes type 2 virus. It presents as an acute inflammation characterized by painful blisters which rupture to form superficial ulcers. It is a venereal disease of increasing prevalence. Often the patient suffers recurrent attacks. The cytological features of this infection are found in 1 in 1,000 asymptomatic patients having cervical smears (plates 150, 275, 276).

Hirsutism. A local or generalized excessive growth of hair. It is not a specific disease but a response of hair follicles to androgenic stimulation. Growth of hair is influenced by racial, genetic and hormonal factors. It can be constitutional or pathological, in which case there is excessive production of androgenic hormones (adrenogenital syndrome, Cushing's syndrome, Stein-Leventhal syndrome, masculinizing tumours of the ovary) (plates 82, 83, 127, 128).

Huhner's test. Postcoital smear from the endocervix and vaginal pool taken soon after coitus to detect the presence of motile spermatozoa. The test is performed to exclude cervical hostility (local inflammation, immunological reaction by cervical secretion) as a cause of sterility.

Hydatidiform mole. Partial or complete conversion of chorionic villi into grape-like vesicles. The villi are avascular and there is trophoblastic proliferation. The condition can result in malignant trophoblastic disease (invasive mole or choriocarcinoma). Clinically often presents as a threatened abortion and the diagnosis is made by ultrasonography or the passage of vesicles (plates 118-121).

Hydrosalpinx. Distension of the Fallopian tube with watery fluid as a result of occlusion of the fimbrial end. It is usually the end result of acute infection (pyosalpinx) (plates 137, 139).

Hymen. Membrane which partially or completely occludes the vaginal opening and is covered by squamous epithelium on upper and lower surfaces. If occlusion is complete, haematocolpos will occur when the menarche occurs (plates 58, 59, 217, 234-236).

Hymenectomy. Surgical excision of the hymen.

Hyster means uterus (Latin).

Hysterectomy. Removal of the uterus via the abdomen (plates 42-50) or vagina (plates 393-409).

(a) Total hysterectomy is removal of uterine body and cervix. In patients approaching the menopause or after, bilateral salpingo-oophorectomy is also performed.

(b) Subtotal hysterectomy is removal of the uterus above the level of the internal os; the cervix remains. The operation is seldom performed because the cervix has no menstrual or proven coital value and carries the risk of development of carcinoma.

(c) Radical (Wertheim's) hysterectomy is performed for carcinoma of the cervix and involves removal of the uterus, Fallopian tubes, ovaries, parametrium (uterosacral, transverse cervical ligaments), upper third of the vagina, and paravaginal tissue. Usually a pelvic lymphadenectomy is also performed.

Hysterosalpingography. Visualization of endo-cervical canal, uterine cavity and Fallopian tubes performed by injection of radio-opaque dye through the cervix in the first half of the menstrual cycle (to avoid possibility of disturbing an early pregnancy). Used in investigation of infertility and identifies congenital uterine abnormalities, intrauterine polyps, adhesions (Asherman's syndrome), tubal occlusion, cervical incompetence.

Hysteroscopy Inspection of intrauterine contents under direct vision through an endoscope. Useful in staging of endometrial carcinoma and detection of intrauterine polyps, adhesions and intrauterine devices with missing threads.

Hysterotomy. An incision through the uterine wall into the uterine cavity. It can be performed either vaginally or abdominally. Although infrequently used now as a method of midtrimester abortion, it is still performed during the conservative surgical treatment of fibromyomas.

Imperforate hymen. Hymen without an opening. After the first menstruation, haematocolpos will occur (plates 58, 59, 234-236).

Implantation. Penetration of the endometrium by the early fertilized ovum (blastocyst) which becomes completely surrounded by decidua. Occurs 6-8 days after ovulation (plate 10).

Inclusion cyst (inclusion dermoid). Occurs in the vagina due to squamous epithelium being buried during repair of a laceration or episiotomy. Content resembles pus, but is formed from cells desquamated from the squamous epithelium lining the cyst (plate 206).

Incompetent cervix. Results from damage to the cervix during dilatation (especially therapeutic abortion) or cone biopsy. As a result, the cervix dilates silently during the second trimester with the result that the membranes bulge and rupture and the fetus drops out. A curable cause of habitual abortion and prematurity (plates 422, 423).

Incontinence. Inability to hold in something — urine, faeces, words (plates 198, 199).

Infertility. Inability to conceive:
  (a) *Primary.* A patient unable to conceive for the first time (plates 62, 127, 128, 130-133, 135).
  (b) *Secondary.* A patient unable to conceive who has had a viable child or miscarriage in the past (plate 136). Strictly defined, infertile means not productive. Plasma beta-HCG assays late in the luteal phase have shown that infertility can be due to recurrent very early spontaneous abortion, without menstrual irregularity or other symptoms of pregnancy.

Infundibulopelvic ligament. The fold of broad ligament peritoneum running from where the infundibulum of the Fallopian tube embraces the ovary to the lateral pelvic wall. It contains the ovarian artery, veins and lymphatics and crosses the pelvic brim where the ureter passes anterior to the division of the common iliac artery and descends on the lateral pelvic wall, visible through the peritoneum to which it is attached (plates 4, 5, 43).

Introitus. Entrance to the vagina (plates 1-3, 216, 217).

Invasive mole. Malignant complication of hydatidiform mole. The trophoblast penetrates the uterine wall and can cause death from haemorrhage or infection. Although local spread is the rule, metastases to the lung and vagina sometimes occur (plates 122, 123).

Klinefelter's syndrome. A sex chromosome abnormality (XXY) in which there is development of male external genitalia, but the seminiferous tubules fail to develop and there is azoospermia or severe oligospermia. The individual is eunuchoid and tall and although not impotent he is sterile and often presents because of this.

Krauro means dry (Greek).

Kraurosis vulvae. Means shrunken vulva. This rare disorder occurs as an extreme form of postmenopausal atrophy in a patient not receiving oestrogen replacement therapy, and who has ceased having regular coitus. It can also follow leukoplakia or lichen sclerosis et atrophicus. The usual presentation is dyspareunia (plate 220).

Krukenberg tumour. Secondary ovarian tumour, usually bilateral and mobile, with microscopic features of signet ring cells and myxomatous stroma. The primary growth usually arises in the gastrointestinal tract or breast, and can be clinically silent at the time the ovarian lesion is diagnosed (plates 376, 377).

Labia majora. Longitudinal skin folds that form the lateral boundaries of the vulva. They contain hair follicles together with sebaceous and sweat glands. They meet posterior to the introitus, and together with the labia minora form the posterior fourchette (plate 1).

Labia minora. Bilateral skin folds medial to the labia majora. Superiorly they enclose the clitoris, forming the prepuce anteriorly and frenulum posteriorly (plate 1).

Labour. The process by which the products of conception are expelled from the uterus via the birth canal after 20 weeks' gestation (defined as 28 weeks in some countries).

Laparoscopy. Visualization of the abdominal and pelvic viscera with an endoscope inserted through the abdominal wall. Used for diagnosis (tubal adhesions or patency, ectopic pregnancy, inflammatory disease, endometriosis) and surgical procedures (tubal sterilization, ovarian biopsy, lysis of peritubal adhesions, aspiration of ova for in vitro fertilization).

Laparotomy. Approach to the abdominal contents through a surgical incision in the abdominal wall.

Leucorrhoea. An excessive amount of physiological vaginal discharge that is colourless (white) and is not associated with itch or odour. It is common before ovulation and during pregnancy and can cause the patient to believe she has a vaginal infection. It is an oestrogen effect and is often associated with an ectropion (plate 36).

Leukoderma. Depigmented areas of skin seen on the vulva and elsewhere.

Leukoplakia. Hyperkeratotic lesions of the vulva, vagina or cervix which appear as white patches on macroscopic inspection. They can be the end results of chronic vulval irritation and can be associated with intraepithelial or invasive carcinoma. Therefore, biopsy is required. This term should not be used to describe whitening of the cervix that appears after

8

application of acetic acid during colposcopy (plates 218, 219, 221, 298, 303, 420).

Libido. Psychic energy associated with the sex instinct. A measure of sexual excitability and ease of sexual arousal. It depends on personality, mood, age, environment, hormonal factors and alcohol. There is a marked individual variation and even variation in the same individual.

Lithopaedion. A calcified fetus. It is a rare, late complication of fetal death with prolonged retention and usually is associated with an extrauterine (abdominal) pregnancy.

Lochia. The discharge from the uterus during the puerperium; it is initially red (lochia rubra), then yellow (serosa), and finally white (alba).

Luteal cells. Granulosa cells of the ovary that form the corpus luteum after ovulation; responsible for the production of oestrogen and progesterone (plate 7).

Luteal phase defect. Shortening of the luteal phase of the menstrual cycle due to a defective corpus luteum; there is a reduced secretion of progesterone. Should be considered as a cause of infertility in patients with patent Fallopian tubes and ovulatory cycles (husband's seminal analysis normal). The condition can be diagnosed by endometrial biopsy (patchy secretory changes) in conjunction with a basal temperature chart failing to show a sustained rise in temperature after ovulation or a luteal phase duration of 10 days or less.

Lyphadenectomy. Removal of lymph nodes. Pelvic lymphadenectomy is removal of the pelvic lymph nodes including those of the obturator, internal and external iliac chains. The procedure is performed with a radical hysterectomy as the treatment of Stage 1 and Stage 2 carcinoma of the cervix.

Lymphogranuloma venereum. A venereal infection of viral origin which produces ulceration of the genitalia with inguinal lymphadenopathy and occasionally rectal strictures. Unlike granuloma inguinale (which spreads through the skin) the infection primarily involves the lymph vessels and nodes.

Mackenrodt's ligament (cardinal or transverse cervical ligament). Condensation of fascia at the base of the broad ligament extending from each side of the cervix and vagina to the lateral pelvic wall. It is the main ligamentous support of the cervix and vagina; laxity results in uterovaginal prolapse (plates 46, 47, 52, 186, 400, 401).

Mammography. Radiographic study of the breasts used to elucidate the nature of breast lumps detected at clinical examination or to detect subclinical carcinoma in high risk patients (strong family history raises risk from 7% to 25%) (plates 78-81).

Manchester repair (plates 184-193, 387-392). Devised by Fothergill and Donald from Manchester the operation consists of: —

(a) Dilatation and curettage to exclude endometrial

pathology and allow resuturing of vaginal epithelium to cervix after (b).
(b) Amputation of the cervix.
(c) Anterior colporrhaphy and suturing of transverse cervical (cardinal) ligaments anterior to the remaining cervical stump.
(d) Posterior colpoperineorrhaphy.

Marsupialization. Operation to convert a cyst to a pouch by opening the cyst and suturing its lining to the edges of the skin incision. In gynaecology it is used in the treatment of a Bartholin's cyst or abscess (plates 211-216).

Meigs' syndrome. Association of benign ovarian tumour, usually fibroma, with ascites and right-sided pleural effusion. The moral is that not all tumours associated with ascites are malignant; laparotomy is always warranted.

Menarche. Onset of menstruation, the average age being 13 years.

Menopause. The final menstruation occurring during the climacteric at an average age of 50 years. In developed countries 95% of women live to experience the menopause. The modern woman spends one-third of her life in the postmenopause.
(a) *Delayed menopause.* Menstruation continuing over 55 years of age. Curettage is indicated to exclude endometrial carcinoma. The presence of an oestrogen-producing tumour should also be suspected.
(b) *Premature menopause.* Cessation of menstruation before the age of 40 years due to spontaneous ovarian failure. Bilateral oophorectomy before this age also warrants oestrogen replacement therapy. In secondary amenorrhoea due to other causes (pituitary or hypothalamic disorders), the ovary still contains primary follicles as can be shown by biopsy via a laparoscope (plate 6).

Menses. Plural of mensis (Latin) meaning month. The monthly discharge from the uterus.

Menstrual disorders.

(a) *Menorrhagia.* Cyclical bleeding at normal intervals but with an increased amount or duration of bleeding. Defined as menstrual loss exceeding 80 ml (average 35-40 ml).
(b) *Hypomenorrhoea.* Scanty periods of normal frequency; the opposite of menorrhagia.
(c) *Metrorrhagia.* Irregular menstruation or intermenstrual bleeding; an example is *postcoital bleeding* that always raises the suspicion of cervical cancer.
(d) *Polymenorrhoea.* Cyclical bleeding normal in amount but occurring at intervals of less than 24 days; polymenorrhagia is abnormally heavy bleeding occurring at intervals of less than 24 days.
(e) *Oligomenorrhoea.* Infrequent periods; the opposite of polymenorrhoea. Usually the cycle is irregular, e.g., menses occurring every 6-12 weeks.

Metaplasia. Squamous metaplasia is replacement of columnar cells with squamous cells which occurs in the transformation zone of the cervix. It can result in Nabothian follicles (plates 40, 41, 89, 281-283, 285).

Metra means uterus, womb (Greek).

Metropathia haemorrhagica. Synonym for cystic glandular hyperplasia. Heavy, often irregular bleeding associated with anovulation (plates 85-87, 91, 341-343).

Microcarcinoma. Stage 1a. A term used to describe invasive squamous carcinoma that has penetrated less than 3-4 mm into the stroma beneath the basement membrane, without evidence of extension into lymphatic vessels. Treatment does not require radical surgery (plate 296).

Mittelschmerz. Midcycle pain probably due to irritation of the peritoneum by blood shed from the ovary at the site of ovulation. The pain is usually in the iliac fossa, often persists for 3-5 days and can cause major discomfort.

Monilial vaginitis. A common infection of the vagina with the fungus Candida albicans. Presenting symptoms are discharge and pruritus vulvae. The vaginal epithelium is oedematous and reddened and usually has white patches like curds of milk. The male partner often has a penile/scrotal papular rash and pruritus (plates 25-28, 143, 280).

Montgomery's follicles. Hypertrophied sebaceous glands which appear as lumps scattered throughout the areola surrounding the nipple. A reliable early clinical sign of pregnancy, especially in a primigravida.

Morula. The mulberry-like mass of cells formed by repeated divisions of the fertilized ovum.

Mullerian ducts. Arise in the embryo as invaginations of the surface mesothelium of the intermediate cell mass on the dorsal body wall lateral to both the developing gonad and mesonephric system. They swing medially to unite in the midline, the upper unfused parts giving origin to the Fallopian tubes, the lower fused parts becoming the uterus and upper vagina (plates 34, 60).

Multigravida. A woman who is pregnant for the second or subsequent time.

Myomectomy. Surgical removal of fibromyomas from the uterus in an attempt to preserve a functioning organ (plates 326, 327).

Nabothian follicles. Retention cysts on the cervix; they contain mucus which is secreted by columnar epithelial cells which have become imprisoned by the overgrowth of metaplastic squamous epithelium (plates 40, 41, 89).

Natural birth control. Based on abstinence from coitus during the fertile phase of the menstrual cycle. See also Billings' method.

Neoplasm. A progressive growth. Neoplasm is often used synonymously with the word tumour which, however, means a swelling or enlargement.

Neurectomy. Presacral neurectomy (excision of the presacral nerve plexus) was occasionally performed for severe dysmenorrhoea, especially when associated with endometriosis, before conservative therapy with progestogens became available.

Neurogenic bladder. Urinary retention with overflow incontinence as a result of damage to the nerve supply of the bladder by surgery (radical hysterectomy), disease (paraplegia, diabetes, cerebrovascular disease, multiple sclerosis) or senility.

Oligospermia. Deficiency in the number of spermatozoa in semen. The usual definition is less than 20 million per ml (normal value 40 million/ml). Beware of labelling a male as oligospermic since many women with infertility conceive when the husband's sperm count is less than 20 million/ml!

Oophorectomy. Surgical removal of one or both ovaries.

Oophoritis. Inflammation of the ovary. Usually bilateral and associated with salpingitis. Acute salpingo-oophoritis can result in a tuboovarian abscess and/or chronic pelvic inflammatory disease (plates 136-139, 163).

Oophoron means ovary.

Operculum. The plug of mucus that occludes the cervical canal during pregnancy.

Orrhaphy means to repair, e.g., colporrhaphy, herniorrhaphy.

Otomy means to cut open, e.g., colpotomy, cystotomy, hysterotomy.

Ovarian agenesis. Total failure of germ cells to appear in the genital ridge area. The individual is genetically female and will be tall and eunuchoid in appearance without secondary sex characteristics.

Ovarian cystectomy. Removal of a cyst with conservation of ovarian tissue and function (production of ova and hormones) (plate 344).

Ovarian pregnancy. Ectopic gestation implanted in the ovarian stroma. To confirm the diagnosis, the Fallopian tube must be intact, the pregnancy must be attached to the uterus by the ovarian ligament and microscopically, ovarian tissue must surround the pregnancy sac (plate 115).

Ovulation. Extrusion of the ripened ovum from the Graafian follicle in the ovary into the peritoneal cavity (and then into the tube). Clinical signs that ovulation has occurred are changes in the quality of cervical mucus (loss of spinnbarkeit), vaginal spotting and lower abdominal pain (mittelschmertz). Many women experience none of these signs.

Papanicolaou smear. Cervical smear to collect exfoliated cells for microscopic examination to detect the presence of cancer. Cervical, endometrial, vaginal, tubal and even ovarian malignancies can be detected in this way. The routine 'Pap' smear has decreased the incidence of invasive cervical carcinoma by allowing recognition and treatment of its intraepithelial precursors (plates 259, 260, 262, 265-280, 313, 338).

Paraoophoron. Vestigial remnants of the mesonephric tubules that enter the mesonephric duct (Gartner's duct). These tubules are seen at operation as cords running between the layers of the mesosalpinx.

Pediculosis pubis. Infection of the pubic hair by the crab louse, Phthirus pubis. Its eggs are visible as white 'nits' attached to the base of the hairs.

Perineal body. The wedge of tissue between the vagina and anal canal, the extent of which is best appreciated by palpation between one finger in the vagina and the other in the rectum at the lower level of the rectovaginal septum.

Perineorrhaphy. Repair of a rectocele and/or deficient perineum by suturing the levatores ani muscles together anterior to the rectum and anal canal, followed by repair of torn perineal muscles. Vertical closure of the transverse incision at the introitus narrows the vagina and restores the perineal body (plates 390-392, 410-416).

Period of gestation. The number of completed weeks from the first day of the last menstrual period to the date in question.

Pessary test. A trial of pessary in a patient with a retroverted uterus to see if dyspareunia is relieved by anteverting the uterus. If it is, surgical anteversion of the uterus (ventrosuspension) is indicated.

Pfannenstiel incision. Transverse abdominal incision in the skin crease above the mons pubis, dividing skin, subcutaneous tissues and rectus sheath transversely, with separation of the rectus abdominis muscles and vertical incision of the peritoneum (plates 42, 50).

Placenta. The organ of communication (nutrition and products of metabolism) between the fetus and the mother. Forms from the chorion frondosum with a maternal decidual contribution (plate 10).

Placenta accreta. Absence of decidua basalis, with chorionic villi attached to uterine muscle. In placenta increta the villi are in the muscle wall; in placenta percreta the villi are through the muscle wall (a variety of uterine rupture) (plate 117).

Polycystic ovaries. See Stein-Leventhal syndrome.

Polyp. A pedunculated mass of tissue usually covered by columnar epithelium. Endometrial, endocervical and cervical polyps commonly occur in women aged 35-55 years. Although usually benign, they can be carcinomatous or sarcomatous. Fibromyomatous, adenomyomatous and placental polyps also occur (plates 41, 84-87, 165, 184, 246-258, 330, 331, 333, 341, 348).

Postcoital test. See Huhner's test.

Postmenopausal bleeding. Haemorrhage from the genital tract 6 months or more after the menopause. Dilatation and curettage should always be performed to exclude carcinoma of the body of the uterus or cervix since genital tract cancer is the cause of the symptom in approximately 20% of patients (plates 20, 92-94, 307-312, 315-318).

Pouch of Douglas. The rectovaginal (rectouterine) pouch of peritoneum which can be entered by an incision in the upper third of the posterior vaginal wall. An enterocele is a herniation of this pouch into the vagina. There is considerable variation in the width and depth of the pouch as seen at abdominal hysterectomy in women without uterovaginal prolapse (plates 49, 177, 179).

Premenstrual syndrome. In the 5-10 days before the menses, the patient suffers from nausea, sore breasts, emotional instability and a bloated feeling. Probably the cause is oestrogen-induced fluid shift or retention. Treatment with progestins (last 10 days of cycle, or an oral contraceptive pill) is often effective.

Primigravida. A woman who is pregnant (gravid) for the first time.

Procidentia means prolapse but the word is often used to refer to extensive prolapse (i.e. third degree) with large associated cystocele and/or enterocele (plates 168-172, 393).

Prolapse. Means down out of place and in gynaecology can happen to the uterus, bladder, rectum, pouch of Douglas, ovaries and urethra. The following degrees of uterine prolapse are recognized.
  (a) *First degree.* The uterus descends beyond the normal range of mobility (2 cm) but the cervix does not reach the level of the introitus on straining (plate 3).
  (b) *Second degree.* The cervix appears outside the introitus at least when the patient strains downwards or the cervix is pulled upon gently with a tenaculum (plate 387).
  (c) *Third degree.* The uterus descends so far that the top of the fundus lies below the level of the introitus. The vagina is turned inside out. There is often an associated cystocele, rectocele and enterocele except in the nulliparous patient in whom the uterus descends like an intussusception without prolapse of the bladder or rectum (plates 173, 174, 180-185).

Proliferative phase of menstrual cycle. The interval after menstruation and up to ovulation during which growth of the endometrium is stimulated by oestrogen from the developing Graafian follicle (plates 11, 13, 21).

Prostaglandins. A group of fatty acid compounds found in semen, decidua and many body tissues. They have a role in normal physiological processes involving both smooth muscle contraction and relaxation. They are used as oxytocic agents in induction of abortion or labour and can be administered by many routes (intravenous infusion, vaginal gel, intraamniotic or extraamniotic injection).

Pruritus vulvae. Itching of the external genitalia usually due to trichomonal or monilial vulvovaginitis.

Also occurs with chronic vulval dystrophies or as part of a generalized skin disease (plates 25, 26, 142, 143, 218-220).

Pseudocyesis. A phantom pregnancy — the patient thinks she is pregnant but she is not. A royal illness (Queen Mary) seen typically in the premenopausal nullipara anxious for a child.

Pseudomyxoma peritonei. An uncommon condition where the abdominal cavity is full of jelly (mucin) arising from rupture of a mucinous cystadenoma of the ovary or from a mucocele of the appendix. Although the ovarian tumour is usually benign, the mucin continues to form after its removal due to seeding of mucin-secreting cells throughout the peritoneal cavity. Death occurs due to bowel obstruction or associated ovarian carcinoma.

Puberty. The time during which a girl becomes a woman capable of reproduction. Usually occurs between 11-16 years of age. The age of onset is related to social, racial and environmental factors. The essential features are the appearance of secondary sex characteristics, cyclical hormone production and the onset of menstruation. Ovulation and true sexual maturity is delayed for 1-2 years after the menarche.
  (a) *Delayed puberty.* Non-appearance of secondary sex characteristics and the menarche by the age of 18.
  (b) *Precocious puberty.* Onset of menstruation and secondary sex characteristics before the age of 8. The cause is premature gonadotrophin secretion from the pituitary gland. Endogeneous oestrogen production by an ovarian or adrenal tumour causes *precocious pseudopuberty.*

Pyometra. A collection of pus in the uterine cavity. Occurs when free drainage of the uterine cavity is prevented by cervical stenosis due to carcinoma of the cervix or endometrium, cervical electrocautery, cone biopsy or amputation, postmenopausal atrophy or irradiation therapy (plates 144, 145, 166, 310-312).

Pyosalpinx. Collection of pus in the Fallopian tube which is distended and has occluded infundibular (fimbrial) and isthmic ends due to acute or chronic salpingitis (gonococcal, postabortal, puerperal). There can be an associated tuboovarian abscess and dense adhesions to pelvic viscera (plates 136, 138, 161-163).

Rectocele. Herniation of the rectum into the vagina as a result of damage to levatores ani muscles and rectal fascia during childbirth. Usually associated with a cystocele and uterine prolapse. If severe, the patient may have to push the prolapsus upwards and backwards in order to defaecate (plates 178, 410).

Rectovaginal fistula. An opening between rectum and vagina whch can cause incontinence of faeces and genital tract infection. Usual causes are breakdown of an episiotomy, incomplete repair of a third degree tear after delivery, posterior colporrhaphy, cervical carcinoma, irradiation therapy (plates 196, 197).

Red degeneration. A common complication of large fibromyomas in pregnancy. The cause of pain is ischaemic necrosis — the fibroid has had a 'coronary occlusion' (plates 326, 332).

Retroversion of the uterus. The uterine fundus lies in the rectovaginal pouch of Douglas instead of anteriorly on the bladder. It is a normal finding in 20% of women. If the uterus is fixed and the patient has secondary dysmenorrhoea and dyspareunia, then the condition is pathological and likely to be due to endometriosis or chronic pelvic inflammatory disease.

Rhagia means to flow in a torrent, e.g., menorrhagia — torrential menses!

Rhesus factor. An antigen attached to red blood cells capable of causing production of antibodies when introduced into the circulation of a person lacking this factor (an Rh-negative person).

Rhoea means to flow: hence dysmenorrhoea — pain with the menstrual flow.

Round ligament. A fibromuscular cord, embryologically continuous with the ovarian ligament (gubernaculum), but attached to the cornu of the uterus, the fusion resulting from the Mullerian duct crossing medial to it to fuse with its fellow to form the uterus. The round ligament runs to the internal ring, down the inguinal canal and inserts into the labium majus (plates 44, 100, 130, 133).

Rubin's test (tubal insufflation). Test of tubal patency in which carbon dioxide gas is insufflated into the uterus via the cervical canal at a rate of 60-90ml/minute for a maximum of 2 minutes. The pressure is measured on a gauge. Normally gas enters the peritoneal cavity at pressures less than 100 mm of mercury. Sustained pressure between 100-200 mm indicates blockage of the Fallopian tubes due to spasm or organic pathology. The passage of the gas through the tubes is audible with a stethoscope on the patient's abdomen. The conscious patient will experience shoulder tip pain when she sits up due to irritation of the diaphragm by the gas.

Salpingectomy. Removal of a Fallopian tube, usually as treatment of a ruptured ectopic pregnancy. The operation can be complete or partial, unilateral or bilateral. It is unusual for the operation to be complete (unless hysterectomy is being performed) since the interstitial portion of the tube is buried in the uterine wall (plates 4, 107, 109-112, 114).

Salpingitis. Infection of the Fallopian tube. Usually bilateral, often gonococcal in origin or due to postabortal or puerperal infection. The patient typically has pyrexia, lower abdominal pain (severe if associated with pelvic peritonitis) and purulent vaginal discharge. Treatment with chemotherapy must be prompt to minimize the risk of tubal damage resulting in tubal occlusion, infertility and chronic pelvic inflammatory disease. The disease is predisposed to by all intrauterine contraceptive devices (plates 32, 136-139, 161, 162).

Salpingolysis. Freeing of adhesions about the

Fallopian tube that are causing kinks or blockages or preventing normal apposition of tubal fimbriae to the ovary. This operation can sometimes be performed at the time of laparoscopic investigation of the infertile patient (plate 43).

Salpingostomy. Surgical procedure to create a new ostium at the distal end of a blocked Fallopian tube. It has a low success rate in the treatment of infertility as fimbrial function is lacking. A more effective approach is to locate the former ostium and dissect the fimbriae free; unless significantly damaged they evert like an opening sea anemone.

Salpinx means tube.

Sarcoma. A malignant neoplasm of connective tissue origin (muscle, fibrous tissue, bone, cartilage) (plates 253-258).

Schiller's test. Application of an iodine solution to the cervix. Failure of epithelial cells to stain brown denotes lack of glycogen which may be abnormal; the pale-staining area represents a site for biopsy. Colposcopy when available has superseded this test in detection of sites for biopsy of an abnormal cervix (plates 302, 304, 421).

Secretory (luteal) phase of the menstrual cycle. The interval between ovulation and the succeeding menstrual period during which oestrogen and progesterone from the corpus luteum stimulate growth of the endometrium and glycogen secretion by the glands (plates 8, 9, 12, 14-18, 22).

Senile vaginitis. Occurs after the menopause due to oestrogen lack, with resultant loss of resistance to bacterial infection; on rare occasions results in fusion (conglutination) of the labia minora in the midline (plate 95). See also atrophic vaginitis (plates 92-95, 144).

Shirodkar operation. Insertion of a ligature around the cervix, usually at the 14th - 16th week of pregnancy to prevent abortion in patients with incompetence of the cervix. A similar operation for insertion of a purse-string stitch was described by McDonald (plate 423).

Sim's or Huhner's test — see Huhner's test.

Spinnbarkeit. Ability of cervical mucus to be drawn into threads. This is maximal a day or so before ovulation due to the oestrogen surge from the Graafian follicle. After ovulation this quality is lost and cervical mucus becomes sticky (tacky). Observation of the quality of cervical mucus is the basis of the Billings' method of birth control (abstinence when fertile).

Stein-Leventhal syndrome. Bilateral polycystic ovaries with a thickened tunica albuginea associated with infertility, obesity, hirsutism and oligomenorrhoea-amenorrhoea (plates 82, 83, 128).

Sterilization. The ultimate in barrier methods of contraception. Formerly regarded as permanent, but recent technology (techniques of sterilization and microsurgical repair) gives a 75-90% chance of reversal, whether performed on the Fallopian tube or the vas deferens. Occlusion of the Fallopian tube is effected by ligation, electrocautery, or application of clips or rings at laparotomy or laparoscopy (plates 431-437).

Stress incontinence of urine. Involuntary passage of spurts of urine from the bladder due to raised intraabdominal pressure caused by coughing, sneezing, laughing or even changing from the sitting to the standing position. Associated with loss of the posterior urethrovesical angle (plates 53-56, 198, 199).

Striae (stretch marks). Are red or purple in colour during the pregnancy in which they first appear; later they become white. They are situated on the lower abdomen, breasts, thighs and buttocks. Striae also occur in Cushing's syndrome probably for the same reason — i.e., not mere stretching, but an increased secretion of hormones from the adrenal cortex.

Suction curettage. Removal of a hydatidiform mole, missed abortion, incomplete abortion, or intact pregnancy of less than 14 weeks' maturity via a hollow glass or plastic cannula (curette) attached to a vacuum pump capable of a suction force of 600 mm of mercury. The conventional curette carries a greater risk of haemorrhage and incomplete withdrawal of the uterine contents.

Syphilis. The most ancient and feared venereal disease. It is caused by the spirochaete, Treponema pallidum. The primary chancre appears about 3 weeks after exposure and this is followed by the generalized rash and condylomata lata of the secondary stage, and finally the gummata (necrosis due to endarteritis) of the tertiary stage (plates 156-159, 210).

Testicular feminization syndrome (androgen insensitivity syndrome). In this condition the individual has a normal male genotype (XY), well developed breasts, blind vagina and undescended testes which produce androgen and oestrogen. The genitalia fail to respond to androgens, due to lack of receptors in the cell, but the breasts respond to oestrogens. Primary amenorrhoea is a common presentation if the condition is overlooked in infancy.

Theca-lutein cysts. Polycystic ovaries (up to 15 cm diameter) due to atretic follicles enlarging as a response to high plasma levels of chorionic gonadotrophic hormone — hydatidiform mole, invasive mole, hyperplacentosis (diabetes mellitus, erythroblastosis, multiple pregnancy, large fetus) (plate 121).

Third degree tear. A perineal laceration passing through the anal sphincter and laying open the anal canal. Usual cause is failure to cut an episiotomy before delivery. Can result in rectovaginal fistula if not properly repaired (plates 196, 197).

Thrush. Infection with Candida albicans; usual sites are the mother's vagina and the baby's mouth (plates 25-28, 143, 280).

Transformation zone. This is a colposcopic entity and is the area of the cervix in which squamous cell carcinomas arise. It lies between the original squamocolumnar junction and the most cranial (upper) limit of columnar epithelium undergoing squamous metaplasia. The squamocolumnar junction can be situated in the endocervical canal, at the external os, or on the ectocervix; in the latter case there is the appearance of an 'erosion'. In the neonate the junction often extends onto the vagina (plates 281-285).

Trichomonal vaginitis. Common infection of the vagina with the protozoa Trichomonas vaginalis. Presenting symptoms are offensive discharge and pruritus vulvae. The vaginal epithelium is oedematous, with a strawberry appearance due to engorged capillary loops and petechial haemorrhages. There is a frothy, greenish-coloured discharge. The disease is sexually transmitted and the male partner often has symptoms (penile rash and pruritus) (plates 29, 30, 140-142, 278, 279).

Trimester. A period of 3 months (13 weeks).

Trophoblast or chorion. The cells which line the blastodermic vesicle and surround the embryonic cell mass. Chorionic processes or villi develop, with outer syncytial and inner cytotrophoblastic layers (plate 10).

Tubal ligation. Sterilization by interruption of the continuity of both Fallopian tubes (plate 431).

Tuboovarian abscess. Acute or chronic infection initially affecting the endosalpinx, resulting in formation of pus with secondary involvement of the ovary. Usually bilateral; unilateral infection is often associated with an intrauterine contraceptive device (plates 136, 138, 161, 162).

Turner's syndrome. A genetic abnormality where the individual has 45 chromosomes instead of 46 (XO karyotype) and is sex chromatin negative, despite being female in appearance. There is gonadal failure (primary amenorrhoea), short stature, webbing of the neck and often coarctation of the aorta.

Ultrasonography. Use of high frequency, short wavelength, sound wave reflections to diagnose pregnancy, twins, hydatidiform mole, malpresentations, position of the placenta, amniotic fluid volume and the size of the fetus (hence an assessment of fetal maturity). Used increasingly in gynaecology to diagnose tubal ectopic pregnancy, ovarian cysts, size of ovarian follicle (ovulation induction programmes), presence of enlarged lymph nodes, renal tumours. Useful as a test of fetal viability to distinguish between threatened, incomplete and missed abortion.

Umbilical cord. The connecting lifeline between the fetus and placenta; it contains two umbilical arteries and one umbilical vein encased in Wharton's jelly (plate 118).

Ureter. The epithelial-lined tube carrying urine from the kidney to the bladder. It is much at risk in gynaecological surgery, especially radical (Wertheim's) hysterectomy. It crosses the pelvic brim anterior to the division of the common iliac artery. The uterine artery crosses it anteriorly as it passes 1 cm lateral to the cervix to enter the bladder (plates 5, 43, 365).

Urethral caruncle. Common, cherry-red, polypoid, often asymptomatic lesion at the posterior lip of the external urinary meatus. It is due to postmenopausal atrophy of the vagina (oestrogen deficiency) causing eversion of the meatus; the exposed transitional epithelium can undergo squamous metaplasia (plates 169, 200).

Urethral prolapse. Uncommon lesion seen in the very young and the very old. The urethra is lax and patulous and straining causes an intussusception of its wall (plates 202, 203).

Urethrocele. Prolapse of the lower half of the anterior vaginal wall and urethra into the vagina. It usually occurs together with a cystocele, both being due to tearing of the pubocervical fascia during childbirth. The patient often has stress incontinence of urine (plate 183).

Urethroscopy. Examination of the urethra with an endoscope that can also serve as a hysteroscope.

Urge incontinence of urine. Inability to withhold the passage of urine following the desire to void. It is due to excitability of the bladder detrusor muscle as a result of infection or weakness of the bladder neck which allows urine to enter the proximal urethra.

Uterine prolapse. Descent of the cervix and uterus into the vagina as a result of failure of its direct and indirect supports (transverse cervical ligaments, levatores ani muscles). Usually accompanied by prolapse of anterior and posterior vaginal walls and their underlying structures (bladder, rectum, pouch of Douglas). See also prolapse (plates 3, 168-193, 387-416).

Uterosacral ligaments. The posterior division of the extraperitoneal strong fascial condensation that corresponds to the transverse cervical ligaments The uterosacral ligaments extend from either side of the cervix to the sacrum, forming the lateral boundaries of the pouch of Douglas as they sweep lateral to the rectum. They carry nerves from the pelvic plexus to the pelvic viscera and form a mass of supporting tissue for the cervix and vagina above the level of fusion with the fascia covering the superior surface of the levatores ani muscles (plates 51, 52, 400, 401).

Vaginal adenosis. Cervical columnar epithelium replaces the squamous epithelium of the upper vagina. This epithelium secretes mucus and therefore the patient may complain of leucorrhoea. The area macroscopically resembles severe vaginitis due to its red appearance; it may be confused with adenocarcinoma.

Vaginal cysts. Cysts of Gartner's duct arise in mesonephric remnants and so are located antero-laterally in the vagina. Inclusion dermoids are the result of buried squamous epithelium and usually occur at the site of an episiotomy. Endometriotic cysts are rare. Bartholin's cysts bulge into the lower vagina (plates 61, 167, 206, 211-216, 240).

Vaginal cytology. Study of desquamated cells in the vagina arising from the vagina, cervix, endometrium

14

and occasionally Fallopian tube and ovary. Used for diagnosis of genital tract neoplasia, vaginal infections and hormonal status (cornification index). See also cytology (plates 21-25, 30, 257, 262, 265-280, 313, 338).

Vaginal discharge. Can be physiological (white, nonirritating and seldom copious, except in pregnancy) or pathological due to infection or ulceration (benign or malignant polyps or tumours) (plates 26, 29, 31, 144, 147).

Vaginal prolapse. Descent of vaginal walls due to weakness of supporting fascia and pelvic floor musculature as a result of parturition and postmenopausal atrophy (lack of oestrogen). Usually accompanied by uterine prolapse. See also cystocele, urethrocele, enterocele, rectocele, uterine prolapse (plates 3, 168-184).

Vaginismus. Involuntary spasm of levatores ani muscles attached to the lower third of the vagina at attempted intercourse or clinical vaginal examination. Spasm of adductor muscles of the thighs also occurs in extreme cases. Aetiology can be primarily anatomical (narrow introitus) or psychological.

Vaginitis. Infection of the vagina. Usually sexually transmitted although the term *venereal disease* should be reserved for gonorrhoea and syphilis, neither of which primarily attack the vagina. Common causes are trichomonas, monilia, herpes simplex and wart virus disease. Bacterial infections are usually secondary to ulceration and necrosis caused by neoplasia, trauma or other infections, except in the absence of ovarian function (prepubertal, postmenopausal) when oestrogen-induced glycogen content of desquamated vaginal cells (Doderlein bacillus — vaginal protective acidity) is lacking. All of the above infections are common and are often subclinical, the organisms being identified in routine Papanicolaou smears performed on asymptomatic patients. About 20% of sexually active women harbour trichomonads and/or candida albicans. Acute infection with the onset of discharge and/or pruritus occurs after the trauma of coitus or change in hormonal status (menstruation, pregnancy, oral contraceptive pill) (plates 23-32, 92-95, 142-144).

Varicocele means a tumour of varicose veins. Often varicosity of the ovarian veins in the infundibulopelvic ligament is seen at hysterectomy performed for menorrhagia and chronic pelvic pain. This suggests a cause and effect relationship; ligation of the veins usually relieves the pain (plate 44). Varicocele of the pampiniform plexus of spermatic veins is one of the few treatable causes of male infertility; ligation should be performed if the patient has oligospermia, especially when there is no other apparent cause of infertility.

Varicose veins. Dilatation of veins in the lower half of the body, especially legs and thighs. Usually occur for first time or get worse in pregnancy.

Vault prolapse. A vault is an arched roof and so properly should refer to the posterior fornix rather than the cervix. However, vault prolapse is often used to describe pure uterine prolapse (nulliparous postmenopausal prolapse — caused by atrophy of ligaments due to oestrogen lack) where the uterus telescopes downwards, turning the vagina inside out, without associated cystocele or rectocele because the vagina has never been overdistended. The term is also used to describe prolapse of the vagina occurring after hysterectomy (usually vaginal) when an enterocele develops due to failure to obliterate the pouch of Douglas and support the upper posterior vaginal wall (plates 176, 177, 179, 394, 399).

Ventrosuspension. Operation whereby the uterus is anteverted by shortening the round ligaments. It is performed as part of the conservative surgical treatment of endometriosis so as to avoid postoperative fixation of the uterus in the retroverted position, where ovaries prolapsed into the pouch of Douglas can be the cause of deep dyspareunia. Formerly, the operation was often performed for dyspareunia and infertility for which no cause other than the retroverted uterus was apparent.

Vesicovaginal fistula. An opening between bladder and vagina causing true incontinence of urine. The usual causes are damage to the bladder during pelvic surgery (hysterectomy, anterior colporrhaphy, Caesarean section), neglected obstructed labour, irradiation for carcinoma of the cervix (plates 194, 195).

Virilization. Development of male secondary sexual characteristics in the female due to excessive production of androgens by the adrenal cortex or ovary. There is amenorrhoea, breast atrophy and progressive hirsutism, deepening of the voice, clitoromegaly, temporal hair recession and increase in muscle bulk (defeminization followed by masculinization).

Vulvectomy.
(a) Simple vulvectomy is the removal of all vulval structures — clitoris, labia majora and minora including skin, superficial fat and connective tissue. Performed for intractible pruritus, chronic vulval dystrophy and intraepithelial neoplasia (plates 218-221, 417-419).
(b) Radical vulvectomy is the removal of labia majora and minora, mons pubis, clitoris and subcutaneous fat to the deep fascia and muscles. Usually combined with bilateral inguinal, femoral, and external iliac lymphadenectomy. It is the treatment of choice for carcinoma of the vulva (plates 224-233).

Vulvitis. Inflammation of the vulva often associated with trichomonal or monilial vaginitis and condylomata acuminata. Vulvitis can be part of a generalized skin disease or due to local irritation aggravated by obesity, hot weather, poor hygiene and nylon underclothing. Diabetes predisposes to the condition and in chronic cases should always be excluded by a glucose tolerance test (plates 31, 146-148, 150, 164, 209).

Warts. See condylomata acuminata.

Wart virus disease. Cytological features of this disease (balloon cells with perinuclear halo) are found in 1% of routine cervical smears. The same papilloma virus probably causes the small cervical warts seen at colposcopy as well as the large genital warts (condylomata acuminata) of vulva and vagina. This infection has an association with cervical neoplasia (plates 146-148, 277, 299, 300).

Wolffian ducts. Mesonephric ducts which develop in the urogenital ridge and persist in the male as the vas deferens and epididymis. In the female they degenerate and become Gartner's ducts; they can be seen in the mesosalpinx, and can be traced downward as they run anterolateral to the uterus, cervix and vagina, reaching the midline near the external urinary meatus. Cystic dilatation can occur in any of these areas (plates 61, 167, 240).

Wound dehiscence. Rupture of a wound. Predisposed to by obesity, wound infection, paralytic ileus, a vertical midline incision, postoperative coughing and faulty surgical technique. It usually occurs 6-10 days after operation. A copious, serosanguineous discharge from the wound indicates that the suture in the peritoneum has parted and bowel lies underneath the skin! (plates 428, 429).

Wound granuloma. A heaped-up area of granulation tissue occurring at sites of sutures in wounds. Commoner after vaginal than abdominal incisions. Can cause serosanguineous vaginal discharge and/or postcoital bleeding. Treatment is chemical cautery (silver nitrate stick) or electrocoagulation diathermy under anaesthesia if the lesion is persistent (plate 427).

16

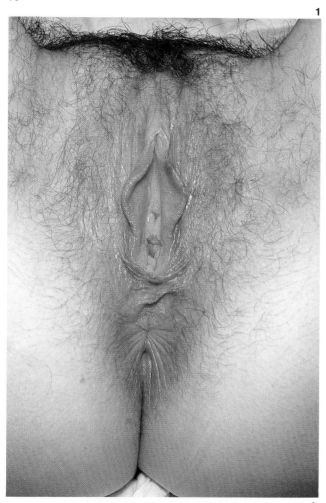

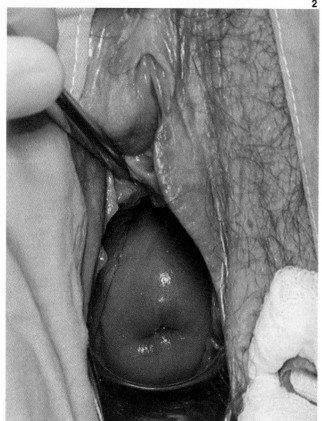

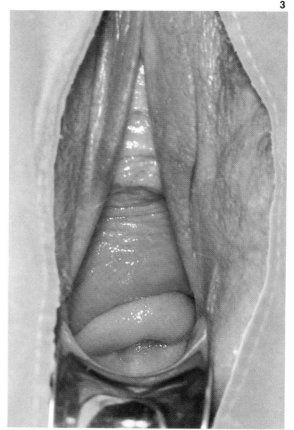

Plate 1 External genitalia in a 34-year-old para 2 with a rather deficient perineal body. The labia minora have been parted to expose the external urinary meatus prior to catheterization. Usually the labia minora are apposed and cover the entrance to the vagina (introitus). Posteriorly they fuse to form the fourchette, seen here as a thin fold of skin. Superiorly the labia minora fuse to form the prepuce of the clitoris.

Plate 2 The same patient as in plate 1, showing a normal cervix exposed by Sims' speculum and vaginal elevator. She had developed heavy, irregular, and painful periods after tubal ligation performed 3 years previously. Normal secretory endometrium was obtained at curettage. At the postoperative visit it was decided to perform an abdominal hysterectomy if the symptoms persisted.

Plate 3 Asymptomatic first degree uterine prolapse and small cystocele in a 47-year-old para 2. Such patients are often referred unnecessarily for Manchester repair or vaginal hysterectomy and repair. This patient had a large, retroverted mobile uterus and presented with a 7-year history of irregular, heavy periods. She had no stress or urge incontinence of urine. Curettage on day 20 of the cycle showed early secretory endometrium. At the postoperative visit, the patient elected to try hormone therapy if menorrhagia persisted.

4

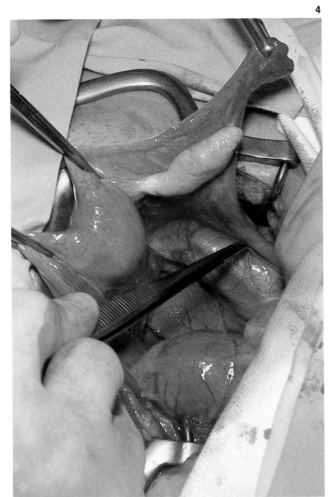

Plate 4 Normal pelvic anatomy in a 32-year-old para 2 having abdominal hysterectomy performed for carcinoma in situ. Abnormal cytology had persisted after cone biopsy of the cervix. The uterus (weight 60g) showed residual carcinoma in situ of the endocervix. The dissecting forceps indicates the infundibulo-pelvic ligament (lateral one-quarter of the broad ligament) as it is ascending towards the pelvic brim; the pampiniform plexus of ovarian veins impart a characteristic bluish colour. Note the attachments of the ovary to the uterus by the ovarian ligament medially and to the posterior aspect of the broad ligament by the mesovarium.

5

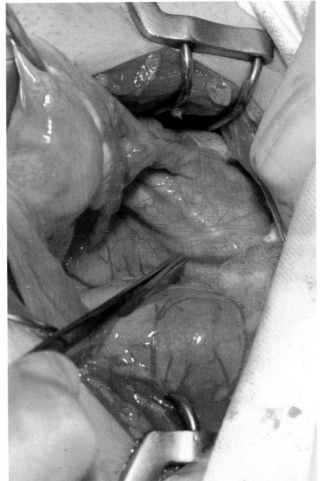

Plate 5 The same patient showing structures on the lateral pelvic wall. The dissecting forceps is resting on the internal iliac artery and is pointing to the ureter which has crossed anterior to the bifurcation of the common iliac artery at the pelvic brim. Then, in ascending order, are the external iliac vein, external iliac artery and infundibulopelvic ligament. These structures are subperitoneal and are loosely connected by investing areolar tissue. The external iliac artery lies at the pelvic brim, but the vein slips below and medial to it and lies on the lateral pelvic wall as it descends to become the femoral vein.

18

6

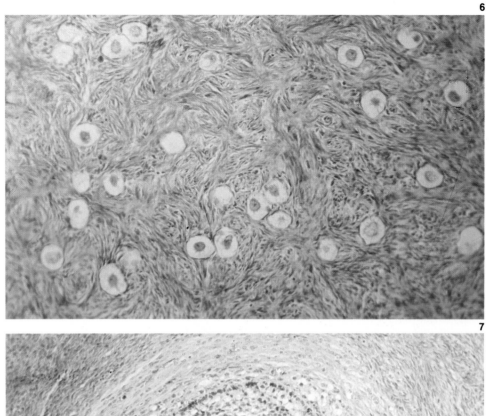

7

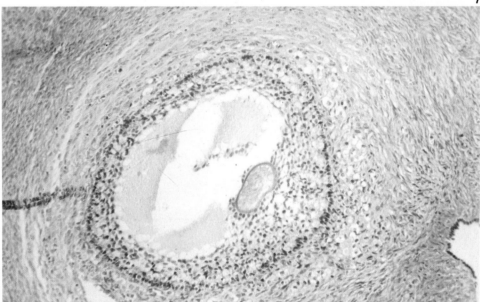

8

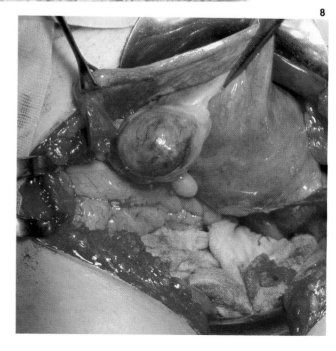

Plate 6 Section of ovary from a 26-year-old patient showing numerous primordial follicles. These have a single layer of follicular cells which proliferate and become stratified as the follicle develops. Note the typical spindle cells of ovarian stroma which, with development of the follicle, will form the theca interna and theca externa. (Magnification × 200).

Plate 7 Developing Graafian follicle showing the ovum with subjacent cumulus oophorus or heap of follicular (granulosa) cells, external to which are the ensheathing rings of theca interna and theca externa, the cells of these layers having differentiated from the ovarian stroma. Theca interna is more cellular than theca externa which merges with the stroma. Oestrogen is secreted by granulosa cells of the developing follicle. After ovulation occurs, the granulosa cells become luteinized and produce progesterone in addition to oestrogen. (Magnification × 40).

Plate 8 Corpus luteum in the left ovary seen at the time of abdominal hysterectomy performed for menorrhagia and dys-menorrhoea in a 43-year-old para 2 who had an intrauterine device in situ. Intramural fibromyomas have enlarged the uterus to the size of a pregnancy of 10 weeks' maturity. Note that a corpus luteum is not a 'yellow body' unless sectioned (plates 9 and 114). This corpus luteum is unusually large and prominent and could be mistaken for a tumour and needless oophorectomy performed. Plate 113 shows the usual appearance of a corpus luteum.

9

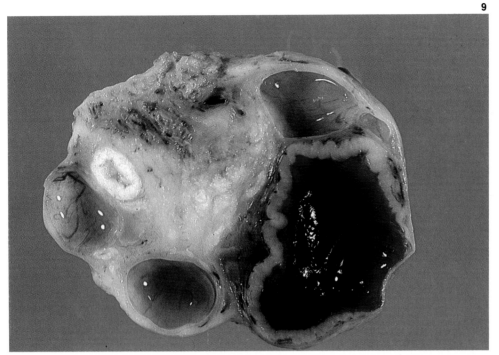

Plate 9 Section of an ovary removed at the time of hysterectomy for fibromyomas from a 40-year-old woman. A haemorrhagic corpus luteum (1 × 1.5cm) with typical yellow crenated wall, several cystic follicles and a corpus albicans are shown.

10

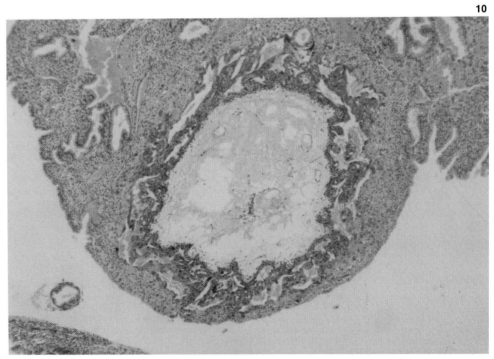

Plate 10 Cross-section of an early embryo soon after embedding into the uterus (8 to 10 days after fertilization) obtained when curettage was performed 3 days premenstrually at the time of cervical diathermy in a 29-year-old para 3 who had gross cervicitis and cervical hypertrophy. The patient was taking the oral contraceptive pill and had a recent history of scanty periods. The embryonic disc is only partly represented in the plane of this section. The yolk sac lies beneath the disc and pink-staining embryonic mesoderm is seen that would have formed the core of eventual chorionic villi. Note that the trophoblast has eroded maternal vessels, forming blood lakes. The endometrium shows glands in the secretory phase and the stroma shows a well-marked decidual reaction. (Magnification × 40).

11

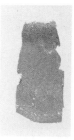

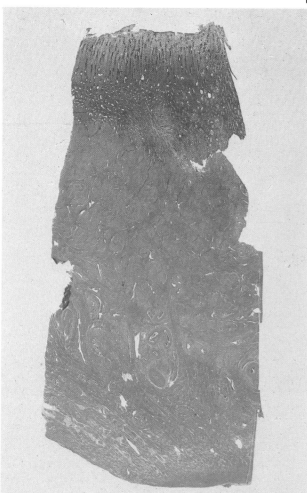

Plate 11 Photograph of mounted section of uterine wall showing endometrium during the proliferative phase (day 12-13) of the menstrual cycle shortly before ovulation. The outer half of the endometrium is the functional zone, the inner being the basal layer that remains after endometrial shedding at menstruation. Note numerous blood vessels in the deeper layers of the myometrium. (Magnification × 5). The inset shows the actual thickness of myometrium and endometrium.

12

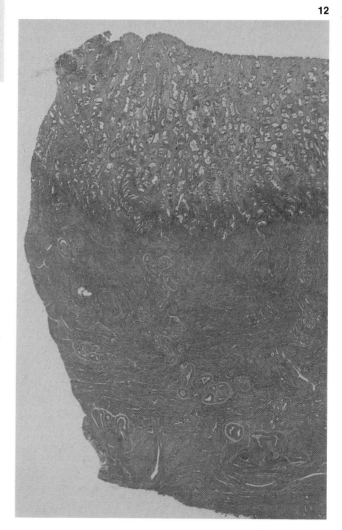

Plate 12 Photograph of mounted section of uterine wall showing thickened endometrium of the mid-secretory phase (day 20-21). The endometrial glands are saw-tooth in shape and contain ecretion, except in the darker staining basal layer that is less responsive to progesterone secreted by the corpus luteum. Note the series of cross-sections of a myometrial artery as it spirals through the myometrium to the basal layer of the endometrium. (Magnification × 9).

13

14

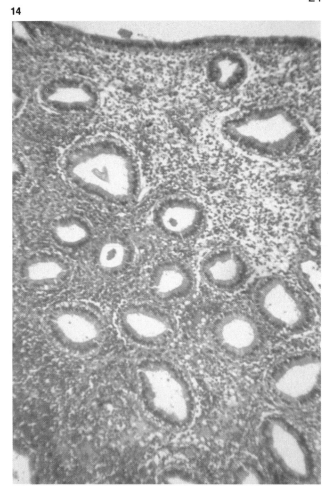

Plate 13 Late proliferative phase. There is stratification of cells in the endometrial gland and numerous mitoses are seen in cells of both gland and stroma; the latter contains blood (bottom right) due to trauma of the curette. (Magnification × 250).

Plate 14 Early secretory phase. The glands are numerous and the nuclei show as a basophilic ring since secretion has collected beneath them. The glands are not yet tortuous and the subnuclear vacuoles are indicative of day 16-17 of the cycle. (Magnification × 120).

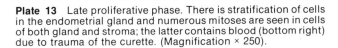

Plate 15 Early secretory phase at higher magnification. Subnuclear vacuoles have displaced the nuclei to the mid-portion of the cells. The surface of the cells lining the lumen of each gland is unbroken since secretion has not yet been extruded. (Magnification × 250).

15

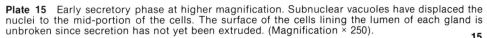

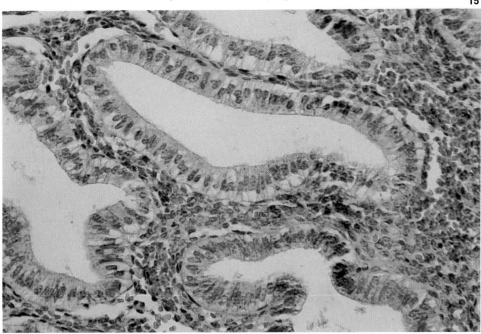

16

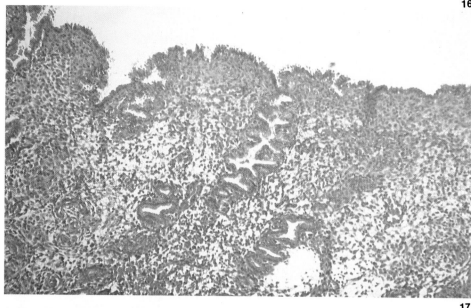

17

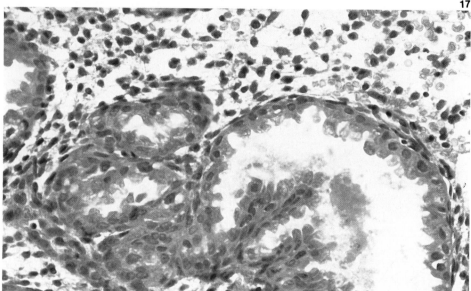

Plate 16 Late secretory phase. The glands are convoluted and show a saw-tooth pattern in longitudinal section. The stroma shows a decidual reaction in the compact superficial zone. (Magnification × 120).

Plate 17 Late secretory phase at higher magnification on day 24-25 of the cycle. The luminal aspect of the glandular cells is irregular due to shedding of secretion into the lumen. The nuclei are again basal in position. (Magnification × 250).

18

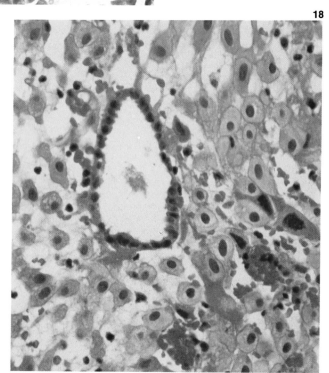

Plate 18 Decidual reaction of the stroma seen in premenstrual endometrium is a response to progesterone from the corpus luteum. The enlargement of the stroma cells is due mainly to accumulation of cytoplasm. The decidual reaction first occurs around vessels and then extends to the surface of the endometrium. The typically 'spent' endometrial gland seen in cross-section has basal nuclei and scant cytoplasm. Premenstrually, the endometrium has a compact superficial layer, a middle spongy layer with tortuous glands, and a basal layer that is inactive since these cells do not respond to progesterone. These 3 layers are more pronounced in the decidua of early pregnancy. (Magnification × 250).

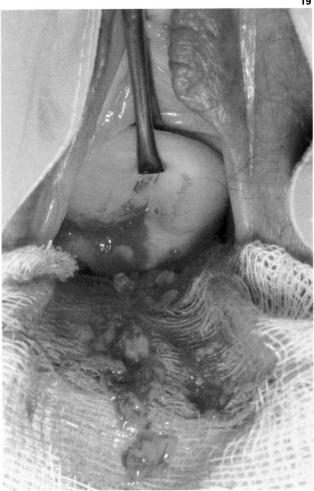

Plate 19 Unusually thick, red (but nonpolypoid) premenstrual curettings from a 43-year-old para 3 who presented with menorrhagia (duration of menses 17 days). Her uterus was bulky and her left ovary was enlarged × 3, probably due to a follicular cyst (anovulation) since histology showed cystic hyperplasia of the endometrium. Traction with the volsellum is causing the apparent prolapse. Menses became more satisfactory after curettage and she decided against hysterectomy. She had hot flushes as do many women during the climacteric when they are still producing sufficient oestrogen to menstruate.

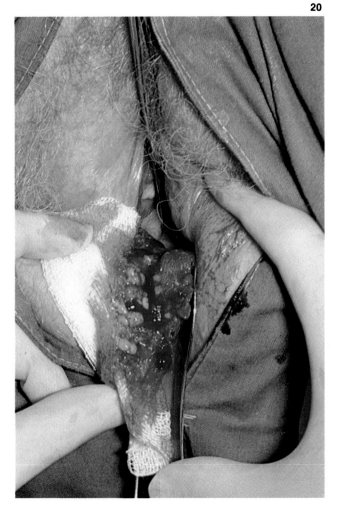

Plate 20 Adenocarcinoma of the endometrium in a 71-year-old para 3 who presented with intermittent vaginal bleeding for 2 months. She had a past history of 2 myocardial infarcts. The Papanicolaou smear was negative as in 40-60% of such carcinomas. The uterus was mobile and bulky. The curettings were typically yellow, profuse and crumbly; often they are even paler and so friable that a semisolid fluid resembling thick pus is obtained. Glucose tolerance testing revealed a diabetic curve as in a high proportion (20%) of patients with this disease, many of whom are elderly. Abdominal hysterectomy and bilateral salpingo-oophorectomy was performed. The uterus contained a fungating, polypoid tumour that had not invaded the myometrium. Four weeks after operation irradiation to the upper vagina with caesium was given to reduce the risk of vault recurrence (from 8% to 1%).

21

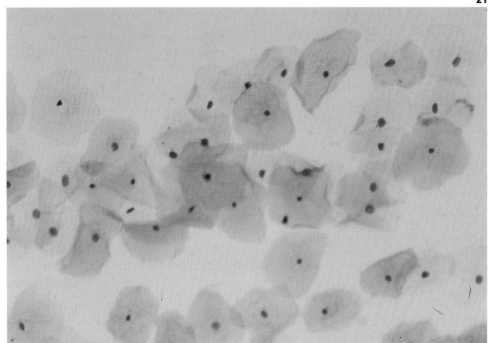

Plate 21 Papanicolaou stain of a vaginal smear taken during the late follicular phase of the menstrual cycle (day 12) showing the oestrogenic pattern. There is a preponderance of superficial mature squames with pyknotic nuclei. Many squames are eosinophilic, keratinized, thin plates. In the absence of inflammation (no polymorphs), the staining pattern of the cells reflects the hormonal status of the patient. (Magnification × 250).

22

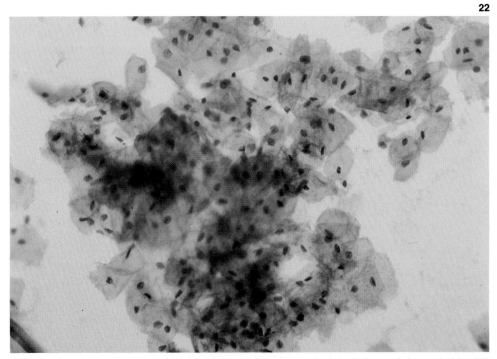

Plate 22 Papanicolaou stain of a vaginal smear taken during the luteal phase of the cycle (day 20) showing the progestogenic effect. There is a preponderance of intermediate-type squames that show typical folding, with the cells curled over each other (navicular or boat-shaped cells). The smear is unusually 'clean' without evidence of inflammation. (Magnification × 250).

23

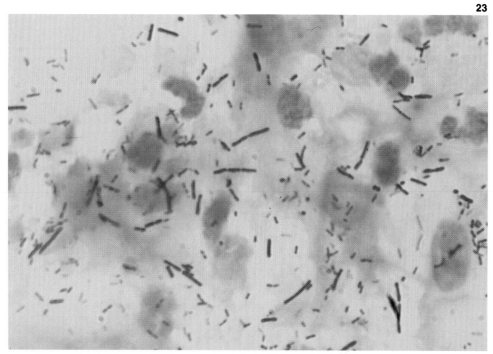

Plate 23 Gram stain of a vaginal smear showing normal flora of Doderlein's bacilli which appear as plump Gram-positive bacilli, often in lines of 2 or 3 forming a chain. These organisms do not incite phagocytosis. The high acidity of the vagina during the reproductive years is due to these bacteria forming lactic acid from glycogen within vaginal squames; the glycogen content is an effect of oestrogen secreted by the ovary. The large eosinophilic cells are squames, the smaller denser ones being polymorphs. (Magnification × 1,000).

24

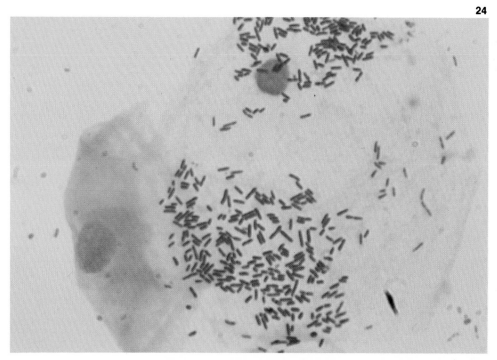

Plate 24 Gram stain of a vaginal smear showing normal vaginal flora. Hundreds of phagocytosed Gram-positive bacilli are shown within 2 polymorphs. These organisms are Corynebacteria (diphtheroids) and are not necessarily indicative of infection. They are smaller than Doderlein's bacilli and have a characteristic 'Chinese letter' or palisade formation. (Magnification × 3,000).

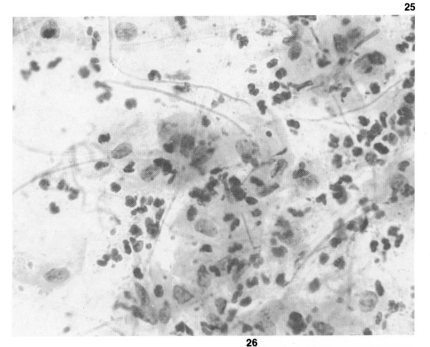

Plate 25 Gram stain of a vaginal smear taken from a patient who complained of a vaginal discharge. Note the contrast to the clean smears shown in plates 21 and 22. The field contains a few basophilic squames but mainly polymorphs. There are a number of pseudohyphae indicating that Candida albicans was the likely cause of the vaginitis. These pseudohyphae are Gram-positive, but with age lose the ability to retain the stain. (Magnification × 1,000). Although most vaginal smears do not show infection (due to pathogens), it is uncommon to get clean smears allowing hormonal assessment, because there is a background of inflammation associated with normal vaginal flora; i.e. there are bacteria and polymorphs but no bacteriological evidence of pathogens or clinical symptoms of infection.

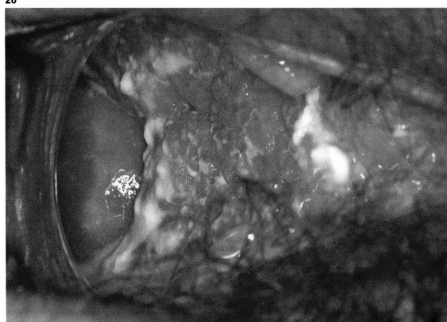

Plate 26 Monilial vaginitis in a 25-year-old para 1 with gestational diabetes at 31 weeks' pregnancy. She complained of discharge and pruritus vulvae. The patient is shown in the left lateral position with a Sims' speculum exposing the cervix (blue due to pregnancy-induced vascularity) and oedematous anterior vaginal wall epithelium with monilial milk-like curds attached. Gentian violet (1% aqueous solution) was applied with immediate relief and Mycostatin pessaries (nystatin 100,000u), 1 at night for 2 weeks, were prescribed.

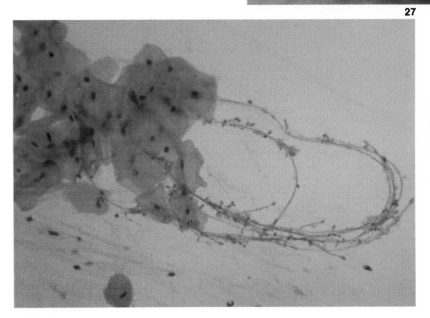

Plate 27 Papanicolaou stain of a vaginal smear from a patient with vaginitis due to Candida albicans. The fungus is shown as branching, broad-looped filaments of pseudohyphae and budding organisms. The group of vaginal epithelial squames show excessive keratinization as is often seen in the presence of monilia. (Magnification × 400).

Plate 28 Candida albicans. Gram stain showing a chain of budding yeasts that would under appropriate culture conditions produce single threads of pseudohyphae. These organisms stain strongly and so appear dark purple in colour. (Magnification × 3,000).

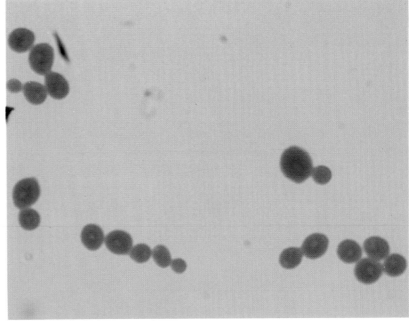

28

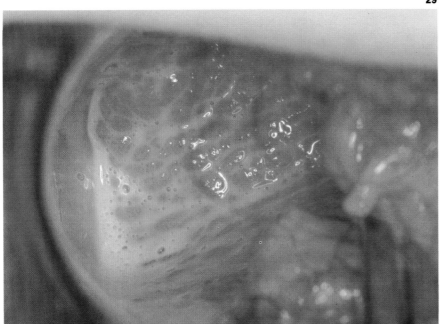

29

Plate 29 Trichomonal vaginitis in a 26-year-old para 2 at 19 weeks' gestation. She complained of irritating vaginal discharge and pruritus vulvae. This close up view, magnification × 2, with the patient in the left lateral position, shows the typical frothy greenish-yellow discharge and the reddened, oedematous 'strawberry-like' vaginal wall Pregnancy-induced vascularity accounts for prominence of the vaginal rugae. The husband was asymptomatic. The infection responded promptly to oral metronidazole, 200 mg 3 times daily for 7 days.

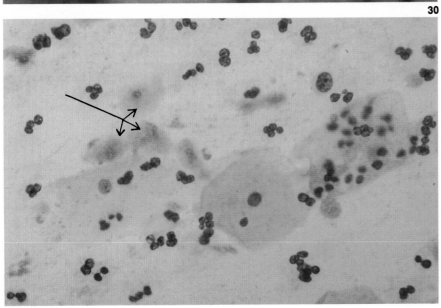

30

Plate 30 Numerous trichomonads are shown in this Papanicolaou-stained cervical smear as pear-shaped grey or bluish bodies 10-30μ in diameter, and thus larger than the polymorphs scattered over the field. This is an unusually severe infestation. The cervical squames are of intermediate type with large nuclei. Note the oval, eccentric nuclei of the trichomonads; their characteristic flagella are not seen in fixed preparations. Trichomonas or any other infection renders hormone evaluation of a vaginal smear impossible, since inflammation produces nuclear changes and alteration in staining qualities of the exfoliated squamous cells. (Magnification × 400).

28

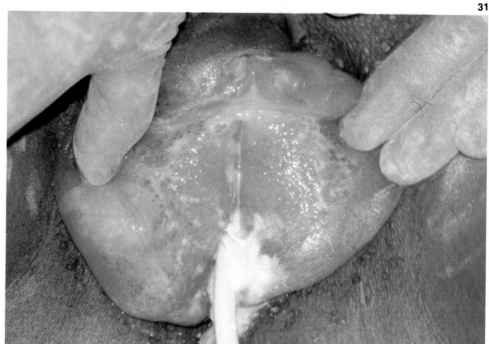

Plate 31 Acute gonococcal vulvovaginitis. This 19-year-old primigravida presented at 26 weeks' gestation with a vaginal discharge, vulval swelling and acute urinary retention (hence the indwelling catheter). There was a copious, thin, yellow vaginal discharge and marked oedema of the labia. Microbiological study identified Gram-negative, intracellular diplococci and there was secondary infection of the excoriated tissues. Spontaneous labour and delivery followed 2 days after commencement of antibiotic therapy.

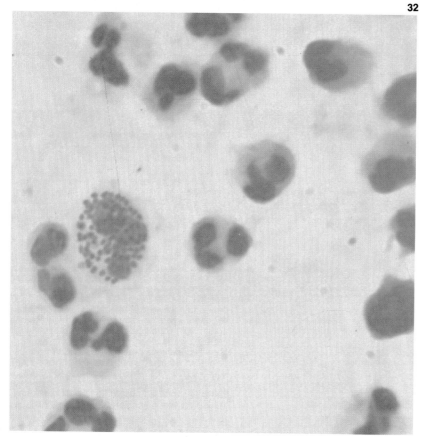

Plate 32 Gonorrhoea. Dozens of pairs of Gram-negative diplococci are shown phago-cytosed within a single polymorph. In most infections only 1 or 2 pairs of diplococci are seen within polymorphs. Even in severe infections such as the one shown here the bacteria are present in only a small proportion of polymorphs, presumably due to the immune competence of the polymorphs concerned. It is difficult to focus on individual members of the pairs in which these bacteria occur so they appear fat in this photomicrograph. (Magnification × 3,000).

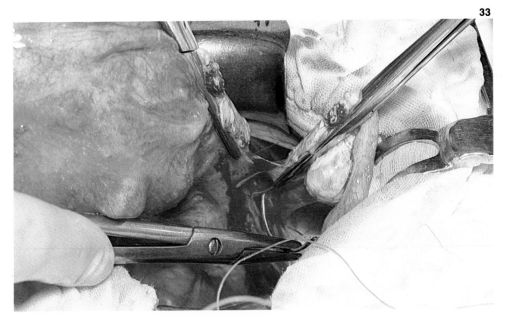

Plate 33 Anatomy of the upper part of the broad ligament as seen during total hysterectomy with conservation of the ovaries. The 2 straight forceps grasp Fallopian tube, round ligament and ovarian ligament, their tips lying above the uterine vessels which are crossing the terminal ureter at a lower level. Note the multiple uterine fibromyomas and the several ovarian veins and artery. The tube pouts where it has been sectioned showing the small diameter that must be handled when tubal reanastomosis is performed in patients who request reversal of sterilization.

Plate 34 Uterus didelphys or double uterus due to failure of fusion of the Mullerian ducts. The patient was a 40-year-old para 4 who came to hysterectomy because of menorrhagia and severe secondary dysmenorrhoea. She also had a double vagina, but the septum was displaced to the left by coitus and did not cause dyspareunia — hence the preoperative swabbing with Bonney's blue has coloured the cervix only on this side. All her pregnancies were in the right-sided uterus and when tuboovarian infection occurred it also was confined to this side and was the reason for salpingo-oophorectomy. (Courtesy of Dr Kevin Barham).

34

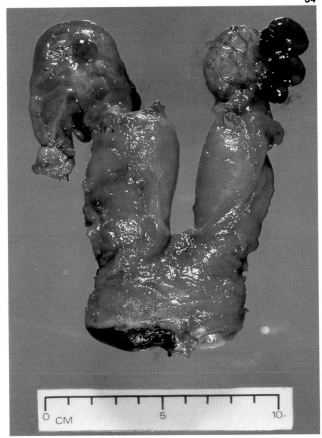

Plate 35 Midline vaginal septum in a 23-year-old woman who presented with primary infertility. Hysterosalpingography showed patent tubes and a normal-shaped uterine cavity. The uterus was anteverted and regular. This illustrates that a septate vagina is not always associated with a uterine abnormality. The husband's seminal analysis was normal (volume 4.5 ml, motility 75%, count 200 million per ml). The septum connected the middle of the anterior to the posterior vaginal wall, was 1 cm thick and extended 4 cm up the vagina. The patient denied dyspareunia although the septum shows no evidence of lateral displacement by coitus. Note normal rugae of vagina. The patient subsequently had 4 normal confinements of surviving infants.

35

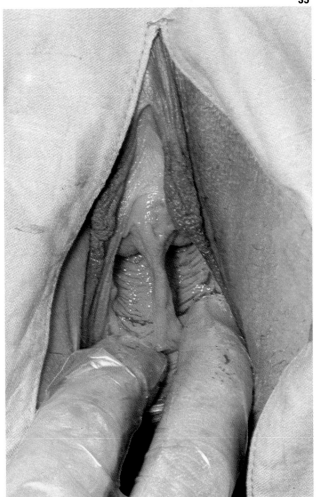

36

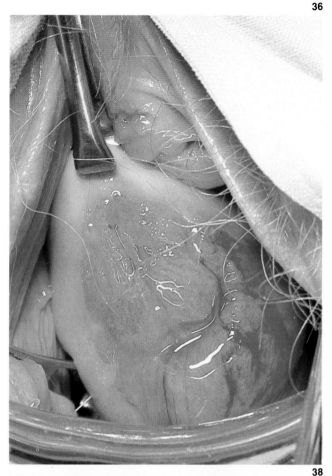

37

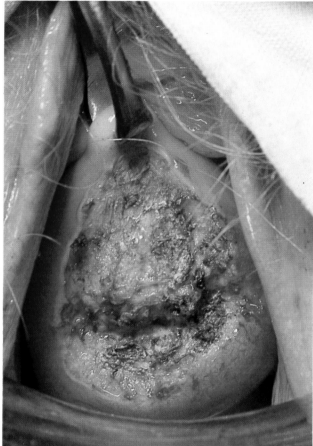

38

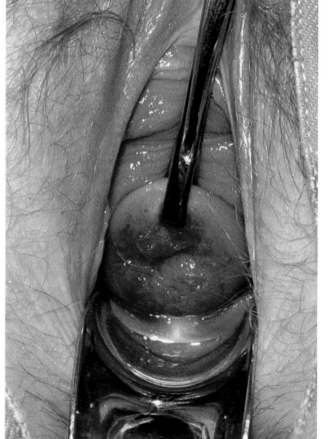

Plate 36 Cervical ectropion in a 31-year-old para 2 who presented with a history of postcoital and spontaneous intermenstrual bleeding. She also had a clear, nonirritating vaginal discharge of the mucus seen glistening in the endocervical canal. Cervical cytology was normal.

Plate 37 Appearance of the cervix after extensive electrocautery to the delicate (hence bleeding with trauma) exposed endocervical columnar epithelium. A uterine dilator was passed to ensure patency of the canal and to prevent cervical stenosis. It is also wise to pass a uterine sound at the postoperative visit to exclude this complication. The cervix appeared normal 8 weeks later. Once healing is complete (by squamous metaplasia), the ectropion does not recur and the destruction of the endocervical glands by electrocautery means that retention cysts (plate 40) will not develop.

Plate 38 Another example of columnar epithelium on the ectocervix (ectopy). These common lesions vary enormously in size and colour, largely due to the presence of chronic inflammation and beginning of healing by squamous metaplasia. The patient was an asymptomatic, 25-year-old, para 2 widow with regular menses, whose routine cervical smear was indicative of dysplasia. Cervical biopsy and electrocautery were performed. The biopsy revealed polypoid columnar epithelium. Follow-up cytology was normal. Note the macroscopic similarity to the cervical lesion shown in plate 318. To distinguish benign from malignant lesions, cytology, colposcopy and biopsy are necessary. A visible lesion on the cervix requires more than cytology to exclude malignancy.

39

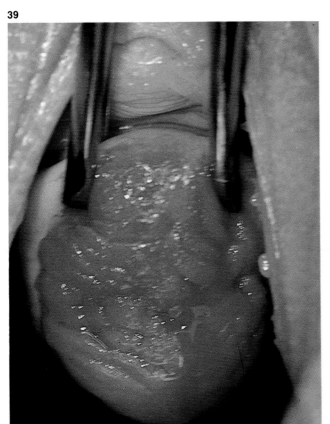

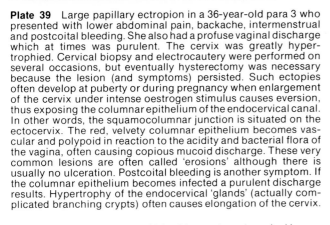

Plate 39 Large papillary ectropion in a 36-year-old para 3 who presented with lower abdominal pain, backache, intermenstrual and postcoital bleeding. She also had a profuse vaginal discharge which at times was purulent. The cervix was greatly hypertrophied. Cervical biopsy and electrocautery were performed on several occasions, but eventually hysterectomy was necessary because the lesion (and symptoms) persisted. Such ectopies often develop at puberty or during pregnancy when enlargement of the cervix under intense oestrogen stimulus causes eversion, thus exposing the columnar epithelium of the endocervical canal. In other words, the squamocolumnar junction is situated on the ectocervix. The red, velvety columnar epithelium becomes vascular and polypoid in reaction to the acidity and bacterial flora of the vagina, often causing copious mucoid discharge. These very common lesions are often called 'erosions' although there is usually no ulceration. Postcoital bleeding is another symptom. If the columnar epithelium becomes infected a purulent discharge results. Hypertrophy of the endocervical 'glands' (actually complicated branching crypts) often causes elongation of the cervix.

Plate 40 Large, numerous Nabothian cysts and cervical hypertrophy in a 42-year-old para 2 who presented with menorrhagia and dysmenorrhoea of 6 months' duration. Treatment consisted of dilatation and curettage followed by cervical biopsy and cauterization during which thick clear mucus escaped from the retention cysts (mucus secreting columnar cells covered by squamous epithelium). This appearance is the end result of spontaneous 'healing' of an ectopy by squamous metaplasia. The squamous epithelium obstructs the crypts of the endocervical glands and the Nabothian retention cysts result. These cysts are very common, often asymptomatic, and usually smaller and less numerous than in this patient.

Plate 41 Large polypoid Nabothian cyst in a 40-year-old para 2. This lesion was seen at routine examination for cervical cytology. Treatment was excisional biopsy and cautery.

40

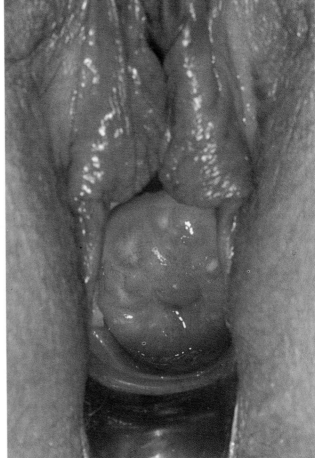

41

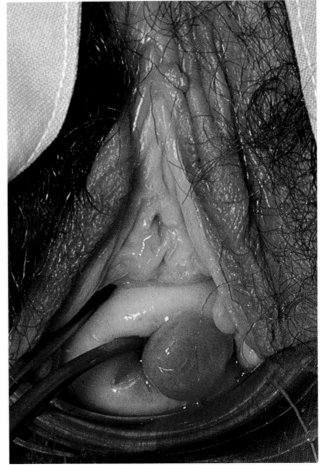

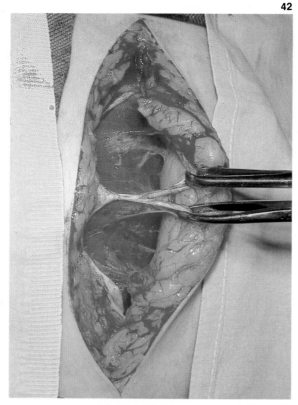

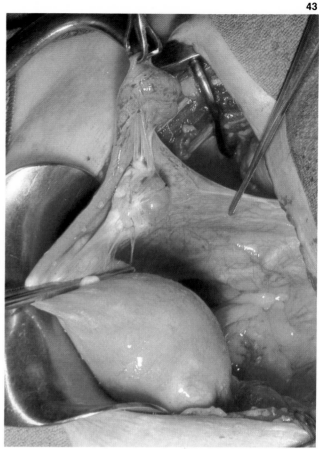

Plate 42 Total abdominal hysterectomy and bilateral salpingo-oophorectomy. The views are from the left hand side of the patient where the operator is usually situated. The patient was a 48-year-old para 2 who presented with severe anaemia (haemoglobin value 5.9 g/dl before pre-operative blood transfusion) due to menorrhagia. She had a bulky, mobile uterus and profuse curettings typical of cystic glandular hyperplasia. Pfannenstiel incision is shown with skin, subcutaneous fat and aponeuroses of oblique muscles and rectus sheath incised transversely. Rectus sheath (held by tissue forceps) is dissected off the linea alba and rectus abdominis muscles which are then separated and the peritoneum is incised vertically.

Plate 43 Uterus held anteriorly by a long, straight clamp applied laterally to grasp the right round ligament (obscured anteriorly), Fallopian tube and ovarian ligament. Adhesions from ovary to uterus and mesosalpinx, and bulbous end of Fallopian tube are evidence of previous inflammatory disease. The dissecting forceps indicates the infundibulopelvic ligament stretching to the pelvic brim. Just below the tip of the forceps is one of the ovarian veins running up to the inferior vena cava; below and diverging from it is the ureter which lies on the lateral pelvic wall. It exhibits a characteristic pallor and is tortuous with peristaltic wave.

Plate 44 Front of the broad ligament. A single ligature has been placed on the left round ligament which is left long and a double ligature on the left infundibulopelvic ligament (large blood vessels merit double ligation). The next step is division of the broad ligament between these ligatures and the medial straight clamp. The ovary and tube were then excised as already performed on the right side to facilitate the demonstration. Note that the ovary is hidden in this anterior view, for it lies behind the posterior leaf of the broad ligament peritoneum, attached by mesovarium and ovarian ligament.

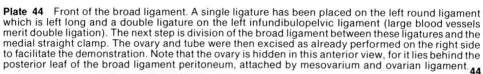

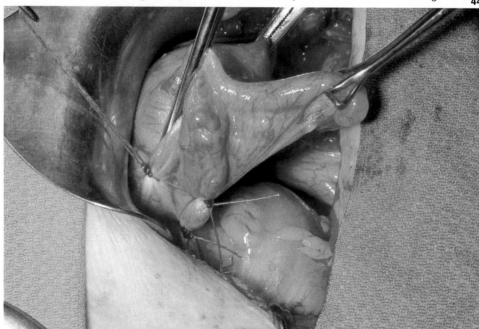

45

Plate 45 With the ligature on the round ligament held laterally, the uterovesical fold of the peritoneum is incised, exposing the loose areolar tissue between the uterus and bladder. Above this fold the peritoneum is firmly adherent to the uterus. The uterus is held upwards with the 2 straight clamps and the bladder is then pushed off the cervix with a gauze swab held in sponge-holding forceps.

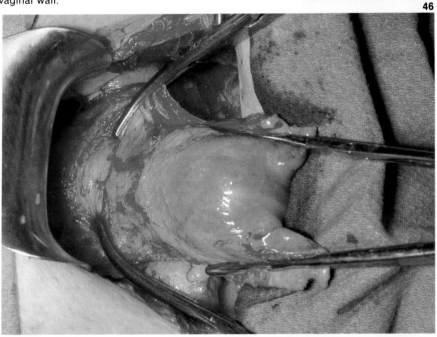

Plate 46 The uterus is drawn upwards and with the bladder already pushed off the cervix, the uterine vessels are clamped lateral to the cervix with curved Kneale's forceps which has vertical grooves on its jaws to minimize risk of a pedicle slipping through. These pedicles are cut and ligated and the bladder is pushed down further to expose the longitudinal muscle fibres of the anterior vaginal wall.

46

47

Plate 47 The curved clamps have now been applied on each side to the lateral aspect of the vaginal vault at the lower level of the cervix, grasping the transverse cervical (cardinal) ligaments. Note that these clamps are applied medial to the ligatures on the uterine vessels which cross anterior to the ureters; the latter are displaced downwards and laterally to safety beyond the reach of the clamp on the lateral angle of vagina.

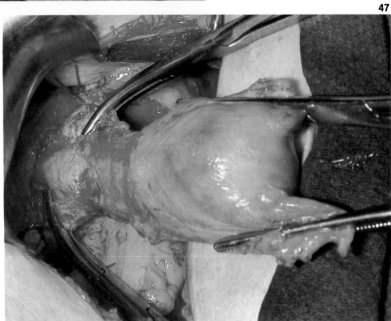

34

48

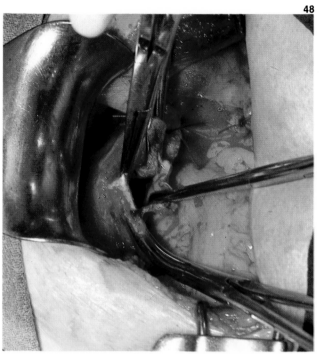

Plate 48 The uterus has been removed by cutting across the vaginal vault between the clamps holding the lateral angles. Two straight Kocher's forceps hold the vaginal vault open, demonstrating the vaginal epithelium coloured by preoperative swabbing with Bonney's blue to allow its ready identification when incised.

Plate 49 The vagina and lateral angles of the vault have been sutured and covered by pelvic peritoneum as the anterior and posterior surfaces of the broad ligament were drawn together by a continuous suture passing from right to left across the pelvis. The sigmoid colon is seen passing over the pelvic brim. The site of the rectosigmoid junction is in the lower part of the picture. The rectum is apposed to the middle third of the posterior vaginal wall after contributing to the posterior wall of the rectovaginal pouch of Douglas shown here.

Plate 50 Pfannenstiel incision with skin closure completed. This incision has cosmetic advantage (scar hidden by Bikini bathers), less postoperative pain (and hence better postoperative deep breathing and coughing), and a lesser incidence of wound dehiscence and incisional hernia in comparison with vertical incisions. Disadvantages are a greater incidence of wound haematoma (bleeding from vessels damaged during reflection of rectus sheath off rectus abdominis muscles) and inadequate exposure when there is a large tumour (uterus or ovary) extending above the level of the umbilicus.

49

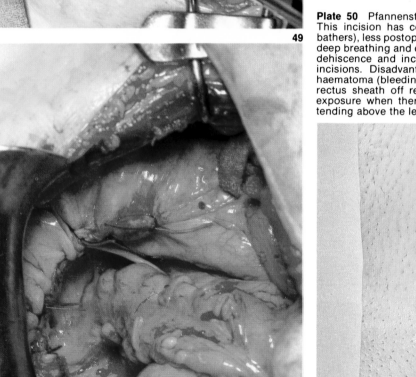

50

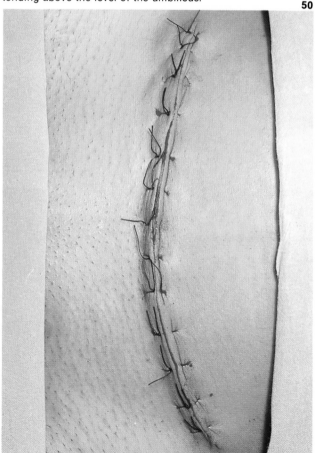

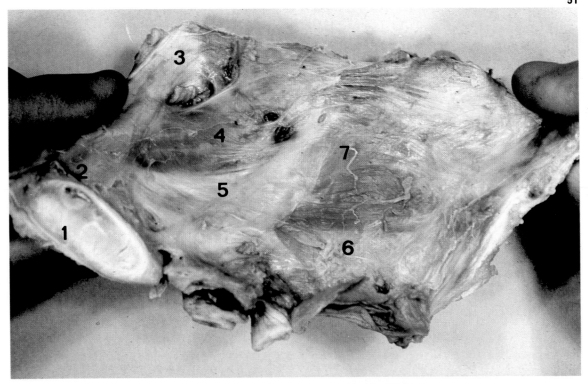

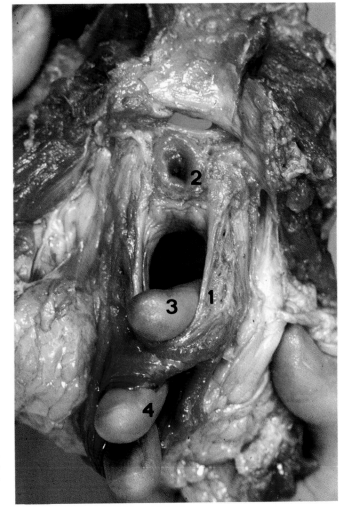

Plate 51 Pelvic view of right hemipelvis showing, from left to right, pubic symphysis (1), superior pubic ramus (2), obturator vessels (3), obturator internus muscle (4) covered by obturator fascia, thickened to form the white line of origin of levator ani (5), and between ischial spine and sacrum the coccygeus (6), and piriformis muscles (7) forming the posterolateral wall of the pelvis. The levator ani muscle arises anteriorly, on each side, from the inner surface of the pubic bone, posteriorly from the base of the ischial spine and between these 2 bony points it arises from the white line of thickened obturator internus fascia. The muscle sweeps downwards and backwards, fusing with its fellow of the opposite side, the medial margins forming the levator hiatus; the puborectalis sling assists the internal sphincters of the rectum and bladder and help to maintain vaginal tone. The levators complete the pelvic diaphragm posteriorly by inserting into the anococcygeal raphe.

Plate 52 View from above of a section through the lower pelvis. Gloved fingers in vagina and rectum illustrate the thick medial aspect of the levatores ani muscles (1) (puborectalis) as they fuse to form the levator hiatus, through which urethra (2), vagina (3), and rectum (4) pass from the pelvis to the perineum. The main bulk of the muscle then sweeps downwards and posteriorly to fuse and insert into the medial anococcygeal raphe between coccyx and anal canal. Note the dense adhesion of the levator fascia to the rectum and vagina as they pass through the hiatus. The cervix and upper vagina are suspended in the pelvic cavity by the ligamentous pelvic cellular tissue (pubocervical, lateral cervical and utero-sacral ligaments), whereas the lower vagina is firmly supported at the junction of its middle and lower thirds by fusion with the margins of the levatores ani muscles. The levatores ani thus provide direct muscular support to the vagina, and indirect support to the uterus, since the cervix inserts into and is fused with the upper, anterior vaginal wall.

36

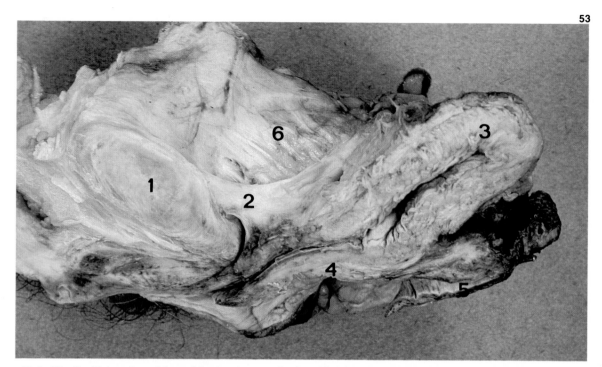

Plate 53 Sagittal section of the pelvis showing symphysis pubis (1), pubourethral ligament (2), bladder (3), urethra (4) and vagina (5) posteriorly. Note the triangular shape of the pubourethral ligament with the apex attached to the pubic bone and the wide basal attachment embedded in the upper paraurethral tissues. The medial borders of these ligaments outline a space that transmits the dorsal vein of the clitoris. The fascia overlying the levator ani muscle is shown lateral to the pubourethral ligament (6).

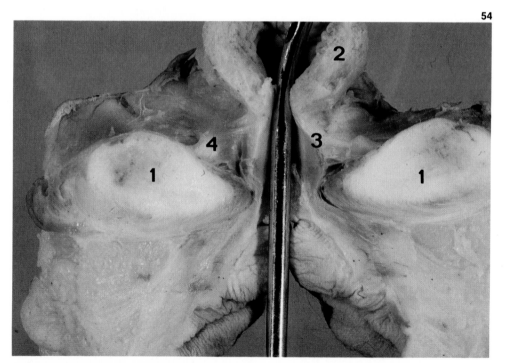

Plate 54 Autopsy view of the pelvis in a 12-year-old girl. An incision has passed through the symphysis pubis (1) into bladder and the halves have been separated. A metal catheter lies in bladder (2) and urethra (3). The pubourethral ligament (4) is shown as a medial condensation of the fascia overlying the levator ani muscle. It passes from the posterior aspect of the pubic symphysis to fuse with the urethra at the junction of its upper and middle thirds, below the level of the posterior urethrovesical angle which nonetheless is maintained by this important ligamentous support of the urethra.

55

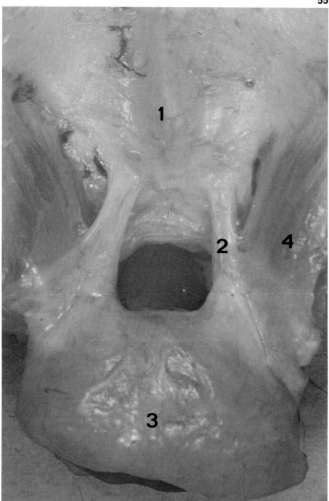

Plate 55 View from above of the posterior surface of the pubic symphysis (1), in an Occidental female, showing the origins of unusually well developed pubourethral ligaments (2) and their attachment to upper paraurethral tissues, with bladder (3) above. The lateral margins of the ligaments have a free edge initially, but are then continuous with the thinner fascia overlying the levatores ani muscles (4), whose fibres are running in a different direction as they pass medially to form the levator hiatus. In the living patient, the urethra is held firmly against the subpubic arch by the suspensory mechanism and the retropubic space shown here is more apparent than real.

Plate 56 View from above of pubic symphysis and levatores ani muscles in a Chinese female. A plastic catheter outlines the urethra (1). Genital prolapse and stress incontinence of urine are exceedingly uncommon in Chinese women who have poorly developed posterior pubourethral ligaments as shown in the picture. However, hard work, perhaps different diet with absence of obesity, and the squatting posture adopted for resting has resulted in muscular excellence of the levatores ani. The levatores ani fascia forms a dense plate (2) that attaches to the paraurethral tissues at the junction of upper and middle thirds of the urethra. This maintains urinary continence by acting as a trampoline elevating the bladder neck area during coughing or straining. (Zacharin, R.F. Aust. N.Z. J. Obstet. Gynaec. 17:1, 1977).

56

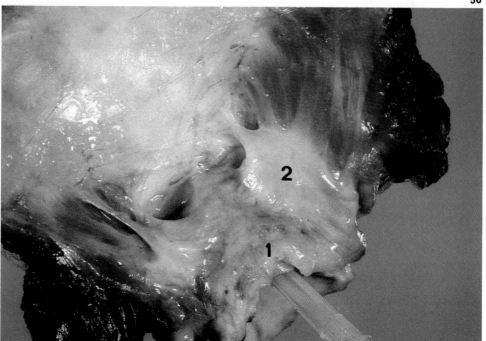

38

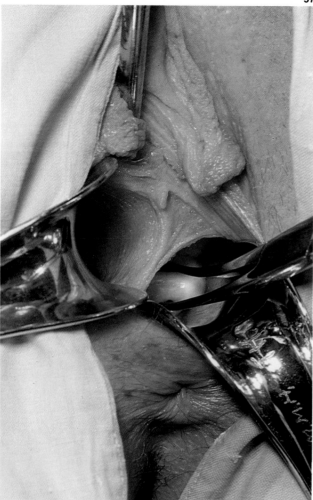

Plate 57 Midline vaginal septum (double vagina) in a 21-year-old woman who presented with recurrent cystitis and dyspareunia 3 months after marriage. The septum was clamped, divided and ligated in steps. The septum stopped 1 cm below a single normal cervix. The uterus was regular, small and mobile. Intravenous pyelography demonstrated a right-sided double collecting system. There is no need to excise such vaginal septa completely, since the divided flaps seem to take up into the vaginal wall with coital dilatation. Sometimes the septum is displaced laterally by coitus and causes no problem until obstruction occurs in the second stage of labour.

Plate 58 Imperforate hymen in a 15-year-old girl admitted to hospital with sudden onset of right iliac fossa pain and a palpable mass arising to the level of the umbilicus. There had been no previous episodes of pain. Examination of the vulva confirmed the diagnosis of haematocolpos suggested by rectal examination. The bulging hymen is shown. Presentation of the patient is sometimes due to acute retention of urine as the bulging haematocolpos occludes the urethra.

Plate 59 Incision of the occluding membrane by the scalpel released a copious volume of typical chocolate-coloured, fluid, old blood. The membrane was excised and chemotherapy given to reduce the risk of infection. Histology showed squamous epithelium on both surfaces of the membrane. Usually cryptomenorrhoea is due to a transverse vaginal septum above the level of the hymen. Such membranes sometimes have columnar epithelium on the superior surface and squamous epithelium on the inferior surface.

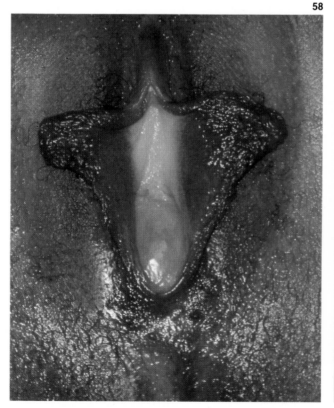

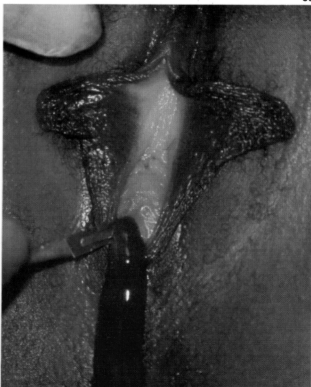

60

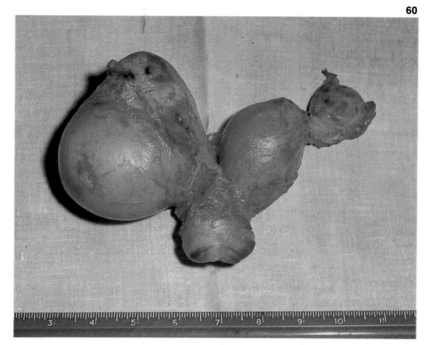

Plate 60 Uterus didelphys (complete duplication of uterus and cervix) associated with fibromyomas, menorrhagia and dysmenorrhoea in a 42-year-old para 3. The specimen shows 2 uterine bodies, 2 cervices (coloured blue by preoperative swabbing) and attached left ovary. A double vagina (plates 34, 35 and 57) often co-exists with this malformation, but was not present in this patient.

Plate 61 Bilateral cysts of Gartner's ducts in a 29-year-old para 1 who had for 2 weeks noted lumps in her vagina which disappeared when she lay down. There was no dyspareunia. The cysts, 2 to 3 cm in diameter, were lateral to the cervix (2 on the right side, 1 on the left, but only 2 are visible here). These cysts were typically anterolateral to cervix and are displaced posteriorly by the cervix being held forwards by the volsellum for photography. Note the exposed endocervical epithelium (ectropion) and pink rugae of a healthy oestrogenized vagina in a young woman. The cysts were excised and the defects in the vagina oversewn. The cysts contained thick clear mucus and histology showed a lining of columnar epithelium.

61

Plate 62 Congenital absence of the vagina in a 32-year-old Italian woman who presented 4 years after marriage with primary amenorrhoea and because she thought intercourse 'should be a lot easier'! She had normal breast development and external genitalia. Laparoscopy revealed normal ovaries and absence of uterus and tubes. A transverse incision was made at the top of the 4 cm deep perineal pouch; bladder and rectum were separated until peritoneum was reached. The cavity was packed for 48 hours, then dilators were used for 4 weeks, then coitus was resumed. The vagina epithelialized without grafting. Chromosome analysis showed a normal female karyotype.

62

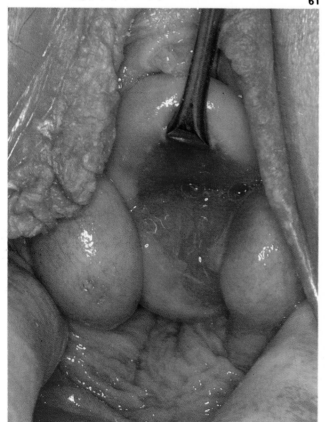

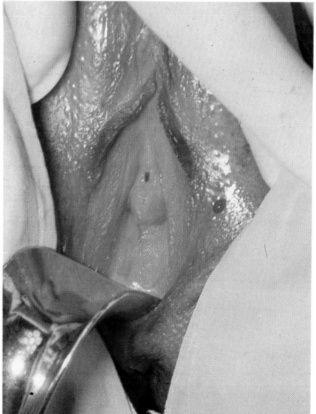

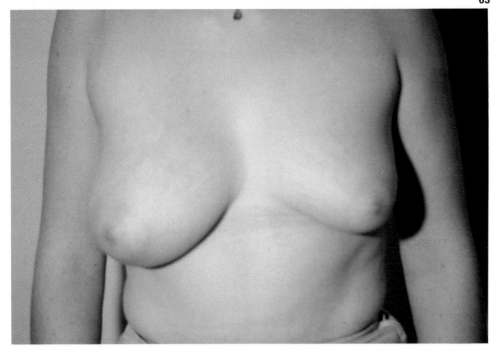

Plate 63 Unilateral hypoplasia of the left breast in a 19-year-old woman who was not sufficiently concerned by the asymmetry to request surgical correction, although referred for consideration of surgery by her family physician. Asymmetry merits surgery when it is psychologically unacceptable or physically unmanageable. The aesthetic standards relevant are those of the patient, not the surgeon.

Plate 64 This 20-year-old woman presented with symmetrical hypertrophy of the breasts and requested bilateral reduction mammoplasty. The line drawn on the breast indicates preoperative planning that must be done with the patient standing. Females view their breasts from above, and from the mirror. The surgeon must remember it is the patient who must be satisfied with the final result!

Plate 65 Same patient shown in plate 64 after reduction mammoplasty. Cosmetic breast surgery is about as commonly performed as cosmetic surgery on the nose. The indications in one series of over 900 patients were post-radical mastectomy (5%), asymmetry (10%), reduction mammoplasty (30%) and augmentation mammoplasty (55%). (Courtesy of Dr John Hueston).

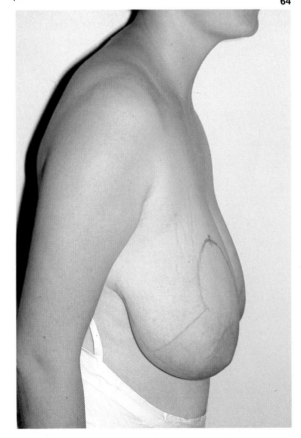

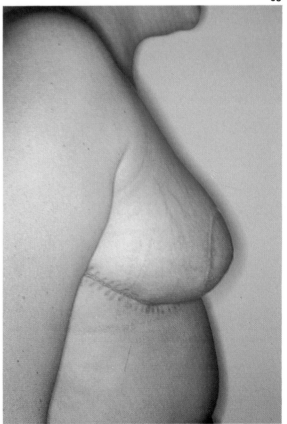

67

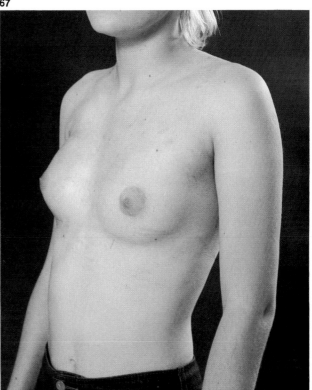

66

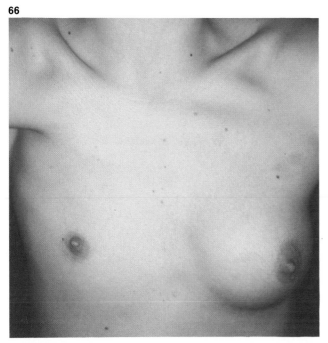

Plate 66 Unilateral complete absence of breast tissue in a 17-year-old woman. Pubertal breast development occurs an average of 2 years before the first menstruation (range 6 months to 6 years). Plastic surgery for breast asymmetry is usually performed in the late teens, when the appearance in beachwear and party dress becomes of paramount importance.

Plate 67 Same patient shown in plate 66 after augmentation mammoplasty of the right breast with a 225 cc silastic prosthesis. Introduction of the silastic Cronin prosthesis has rendered free fat grafting obsolete except after extremely radical mastectomy. Asepsis is especially important when a foreign material is introduced into the body, and prophylactic broad spectrum chemotherapy is the rule. Note that the prosthesis has resulted in expansion of the areola and accentuation of the nipple.

Plate 68 Congenital absence of the left breast associated with absence of pectoralis major muscle. There is also a degree of postlactational ptosis of the right breast due to excessive involution, although poor support of the breasts during pregnancy and lactation is often the cause. Postlactational involution is unpredictable, but sometimes progressively, with successive pregnancies, results in small flabby breasts in previously well endowed women. Many women refuse to breast feed because they are fearful of becoming flat-chested. Absence of the breast is often associated with other connective tissue deficiencies involving underlying ribs and intercostal muscles as well as pectoralis major. This patient was treated by prosthetic augmentation of the aplastic side.

68

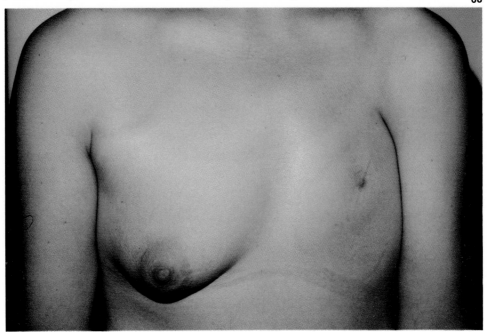

42

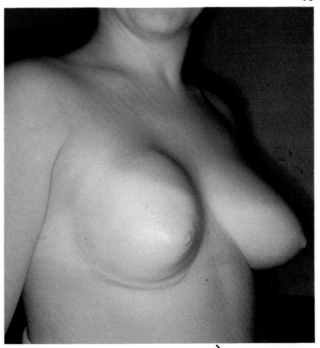

Plate 69 Breast asymmetry in the only daughter of a wealthy family, resulting in pathological antisocial behaviour. Note that the nipple is smaller and higher on the hypoplastic side.

Plate 70 Same patient shown in plate 69 after augmentation of the right breast by insertion of a silastic prosthesis. Her psyche and social behaviour were restored to normal. The deficiency of contour at the right upper margin of the prosthesis might have been avoided by placement of this portion behind the pectoralis major. (Courtesy of Dr John Hueston).

Plate 71 Postlactational involution of asymmetrical breasts, the right being only 25% of the volume of the left. The wishes of the patient often surprise the surgeon. Lack of preoperative communication rather than lack of postoperative contour causes patient dissatisfaction. Some patients with breasts of such proportions elect to have both augmentation of the smaller breast and reduction in the volume of the large breast. Others with breast asymmetry have such an aversion of artificiality that they elect to have reduction mammoplasty of the normal breast to match the volume of the hypoplastic one.

71

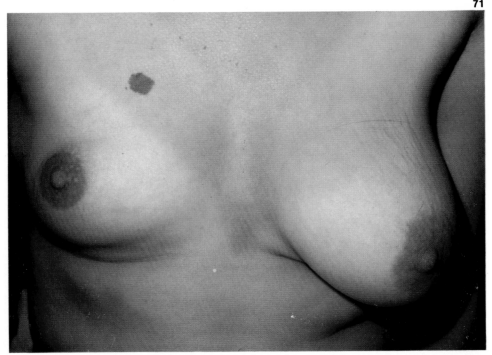

72

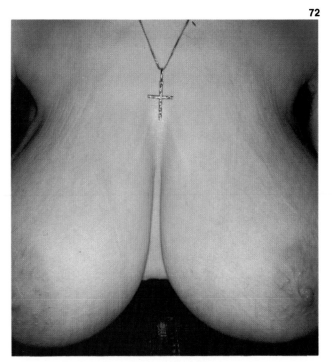

73

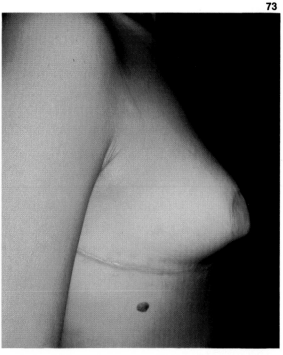

Plate 72 Huge, symmetrical, pendulous breasts showing post-lactational involution. This patient's breasts hypertrophied during pregnancy, but did not enlarge significantly during lactation. Lactational hypertrophy is a common occurrence. Often the sudden change in dimensions of the breasts alarms and embarrasses the patient and her husband. Suppression of lactation is sometimes requested on account of this.

Plate 73 Same patient shown in plate 72 after bilateral reduction mammoplasty. Preoperative planning must consider how much shall remain, rather than how much shall be removed. The volume which remains must be as equal as possible on both sides.

Plate 74 Pregnancy-induced gigantomastia (diffuse hypertrophy) in a 27-year-old multigravida at 28 weeks' gestation. This condition is exceedingly uncommon (1 in 30,000 pregnancies). The breasts had not enlarged excessively in the previous pregnancy. Bromocryptine was administered during pregnancy without demonstrable effect on dimensions of the breasts. Reduction mammoplasty was performed 6 months after delivery. (Courtesy of Professor Roger Pepperell).

74

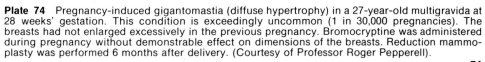
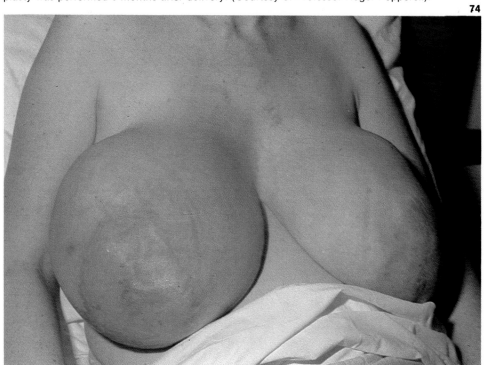

44

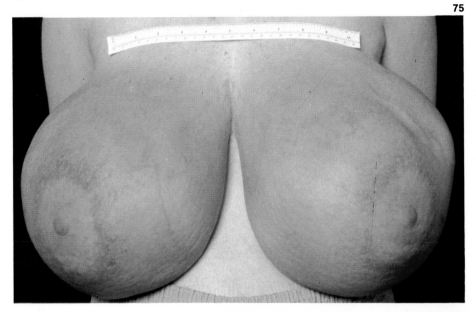

Plate 75 Pregnancy-induced gigan-tomastia in a 24-year-old primigravida. Previously, when taking the contra-ceptive pill, her breasts had enlarged from brassiere size 32A to 36B. They returned to size 32A when the pill was discontinued. This condition can also occur at puberty. During pregnancy the breasts hypertrophied to size 46DD by 20 weeks' gestation. At this time the right breast weighed 4.3 kg and the left 4.7 kg when assessed by displace-ment into buckets of water. Thereafter, breast size remained unchanged. Pro-posed management was suppression of lactation with bromocryptine and reduction mammoplasty according to the degree of postpartum involution. (Courtesy of Professor Roger Peppe-rell).

Plate 76 Bilateral accessory axillary breasts in a 38-year-old lactating multi-gravida photographed 5 days after de-livery. The ectopic breast tissue had enlarged to a lesser extent during pre-vious lactations. The axillary breasts were tender and engorged but non-functional since they lacked nipples. Excision was planned as the lumps were tender and an embarrassment to the patient. Accessory breasts are less common than accessory nipples and are usually located in the axilla.

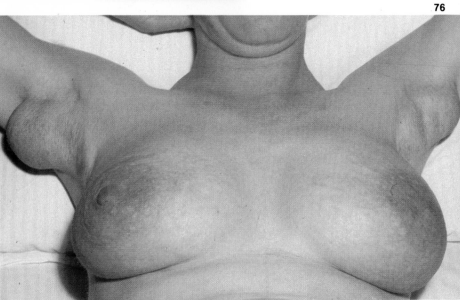

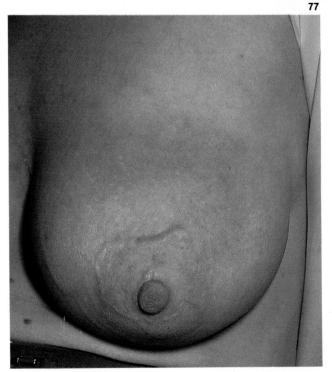

Plate 77 Acute infection of the upper lateral quadrant of the left breast 15 weeks after delivery. Usually serious breast infection occurs about 6 weeks after the onset of lactation, although cracking of the nipples can result in infection 3-6 days after delivery, during the time of breast engorgement. The baby ac-quires Staphylococci from the hospital environment and trans-mits them from his nasopharynx via a cracked nipple during feeding. Note enlarged veins typical of lactation. A tender mass was palpable beneath the reddened skin due to retention of milk within the affected segment. Erythromycin caused complete resolution. Incision and drainage is always required once pus collects and forms an abscess. Pus can point superficially, extend laterally causing breast destruction, or extend to the fascia overlying pectoralis major causing the breast to protrude from the chest wall. Breast abscess is a painful, serious illness that can be averted by prompt treatment at the first sign of infection.

Plate 78 Normal mammograph. This lateral projection mam-mograph shows the architecture of the normal breast. The nipple is shown and the skin covering the breast is of uniform thickness. The trabeculated appearance is due to connective tissue stroma between the segments of breast tissue. The blood vessels are also outlined, their calibre narrowing as the periphery is approached. There is no area of increased density suggestive of a mass. Carcinoma of the breast is the commonest malignancy affecting women; 7% develop it and 4% die from it. Prognosis depends upon early diagnosis, regular self-examination and special sur-veillance (mammography, ultrasonography) in high risk patients (positive family history, chronic mastitis). All women should have regular gynaecological assessment (1-2 years) including cervical cytology and palpation of the breasts. *(See next page)*.

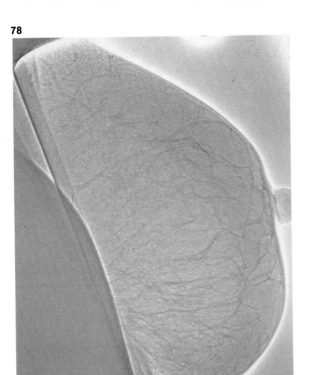

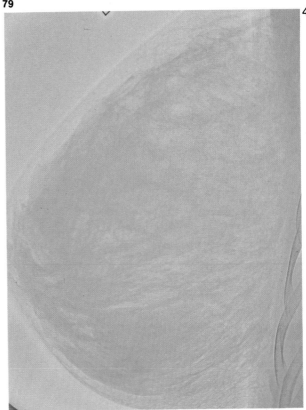

Plate 79 Lateral mammograph in a 24-year-old woman who presented to a plastic surgeon for reduction mammoplasty. Palpation revealed diffuse ropiness in both breasts, and a discrete mass in the lower part of the left breast suggestive of a fibroadenoma. Mammography was performed to exclude other pathology. It shows increased density of the breast, as in dysplasia, with a well defined area of increased density in the lower quadrant, suggestive of a cyst or fibroadenoma. Needle biopsy or ultrasonography can be employed in such patients to distinguish between cystic and solid swellings.

Plate 80 Superior view mammograph in a 69-year-old nullipara, with a strong family history of breast cancer, who years ago first noticed a lump in the right breast following an injury to it! There was a palpable mass 1-2 cm in diameter, not obviously malignant. This picture shows a poorly defined mass with spiculated border (crab-like), an appearance associated with a 95% risk of malignancy. The rest of the breast shows normal stromal pattern, vascularity and benign calcification.

Plate 81 Lateral mammograph in a 52-year-old woman who had noted a lump in the breast for 2 weeks. The nipple is retracted and continuous with a large mass beneath it. Although the mass has well defined borders, malignancy was suggested by the nipple retraction and thickening of the overlying skin. Biopsy and frozen section revealed invasive carcinoma. A Patey mastectomy was performed. The axillary lymph nodes were not involved. The patient remained well but developed carcinoma of the thyroid 2 years later.

80

81

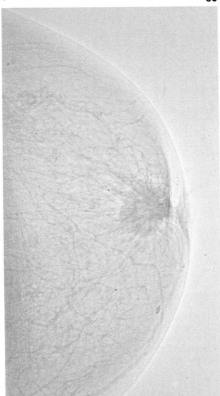

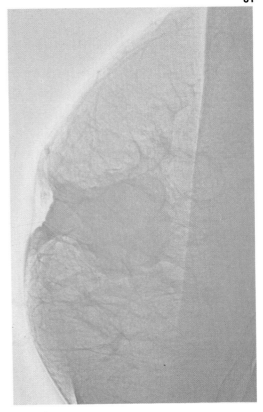

82

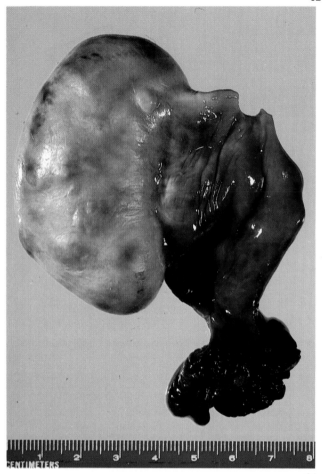

83

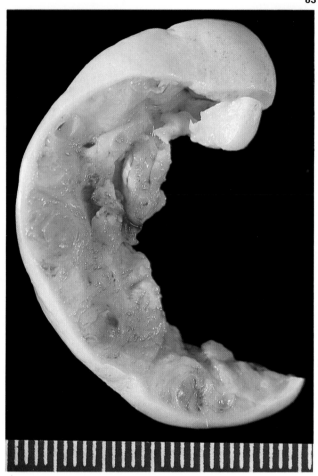

84

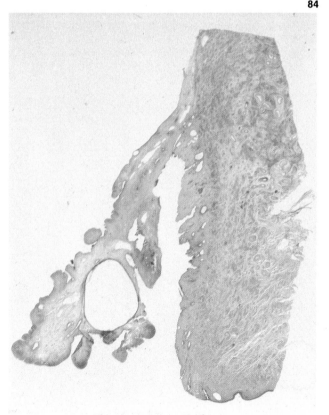

Plate 82 Gangrenous polycystic right ovary and Fallopian tube removed from a 20-year-old single girl with menstrual irregularity who presented with a 12-hour history of pain in the right iliac fossa. Laparotomy was performed immediately, but torsion of the enlarged ovary and tube had resulted in ischaemic infarction.

Plate 83 Wedge biopsy taken from the polycystic left ovary of the same patient described in the legend of plate 82. The thickened tunica albuginea prevents ovulation, and results in the multiple follicular cysts characteristic of the Stein-Leventhal syndrome. The wedge allows exclusion of tumour (cystic teratoma), histological diagnosis, and restores ovulatory menstruation in 50-80% of patients. In this condition the ovaries are unduly mobile and subject to torsion.

Plate 84 Benign endometrial polyp arising near the isthmus. Note the fibrotic uterine wall as seen in postmenopausal patients. The polyp contains a cystically dilated gland and inflammation has resulted in squamous metaplasia. The squamocolumnar junction at the external os is seen at the bottom of the section. Note the inactivity of the endocervical glands. (Magnification of mounted section × 2).

85

86

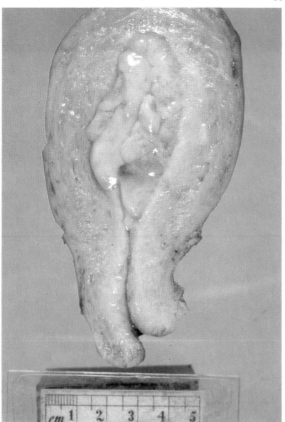

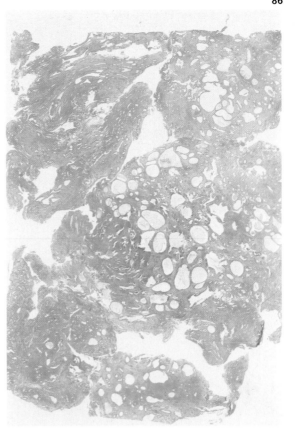

Plate 85 Cystic hyperplasia of the endometrium and hypertrophy of the myometrium in a 41-year-old para 6 with hypertension. She had suffered from menorrhagia for 6 years and had received 3 blood transfusions in the previous 2 years. Her haemoglobin value was 9.8 g/dl. At hysterectomy, her ovaries appeared normal and were conserved.

Plate 86 Cystic glandular hyperplasia in curettings from a 63-year-old woman with a history of postmenopausal bleeding for 18 months. The curettings are typically bulky with polypoid formation. Note that there is *stromal* as well as glandular hyperplasia. The section shows cystic glands (Swiss cheese pattern) and higher magnification in other areas showed adenomatous hyperplasia and atypical hyperplasia, but no carcinoma. These findings warrant hysterectomy. (Magnification of mounted section × 3).

Plate 87 Polypoid endometrium and thickened myometrium in a uterus (9 × 4 × 3 cm) removed from a 45-year-old woman because of menorrhagia. Histology showed a thickened secretory endometrium, the pattern corresponding to day 21 of a 28-day cycle. In spite of the extremely polypoid nature of the surface, the glands were arranged perpendicular to the wall of the uterus. The ovary contained follicular cysts and a corpus luteum. This unusual specimen illustrates that polypoid endometrium is not always associated with anovulation and cystic glandular hyperplasia (plates 85 and 348).

87

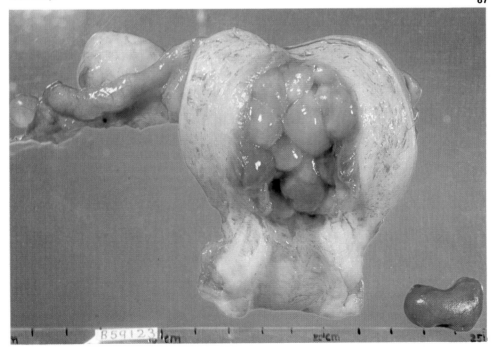

88

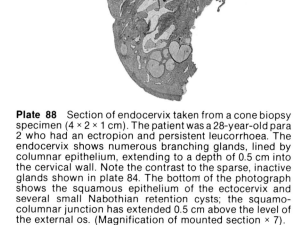

89

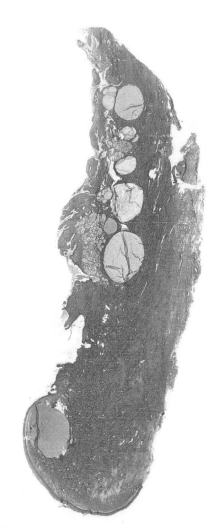

Plate 88 Section of endocervix taken from a cone biopsy specimen (4 × 2 × 1 cm). The patient was a 28-year-old para 2 who had an ectropion and persistent leucorrhoea. The endocervix shows numerous branching glands, lined by columnar epithelium, extending to a depth of 0.5 cm into the cervical wall. Note the contrast to the sparse, inactive glands shown in plate 84. The bottom of the photograph shows the squamous epithelium of the ectocervix and several small Nabothian retention cysts; the squamo-columnar junction has extended 0.5 cm above the level of the external os. (Magnification of mounted section × 7).

Plate 89 Section of endocervix showing Nabothian cysts (plates 40 and 41). The patient was a 51-year-old para 3 with menorrhagia and dysmenorrhoea. Hysterectomy was performed because bleeding had persisted for 6 months in spite of curettage. The uterus weighed 175 g and showed adenomyosis with glands and stroma extending deep into the myometrium (hence the dysmenorrhoea). The endometrium was 0.5 cm thick and showed cystic glandular hyperplasia. The endocervical canal shown here was 3.5 cm long with orderly, stratified squamous epithelium extending over the cervix above dilated endocervical glands. When this condition is treated by electrocoagulation the probe must extend deep into the cervix to reach the dilated glands. (Magnification of mounted section × 5).

90

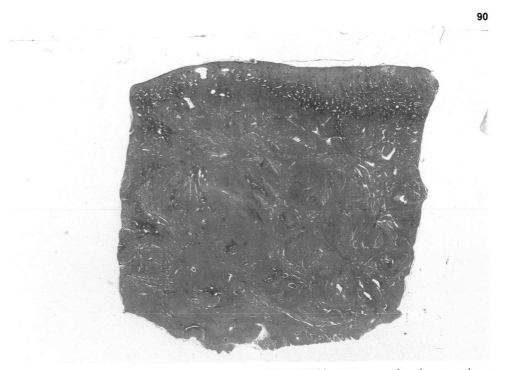

Plate 90 Adenomyosis. The patient was a 40-year-old para 1 with severe secondary dysmenorrhoea and a bulky, tender uterus. Hysterectomy was difficult due to dense adhesions caused by pelvic endometriosis, which often coexists with adenomyosis. This section of uterine wall shows early secretory endometrium, 0.3 cm thick, and extensive adenomyosis, seen as islands of endometrial glands and stroma extending throughout the 2.5 cm thickness of the myometrium. It is easy to appreciate that swelling of these islands of ectopic endometrium causes severe uterine pain during menstruation. Often dark blood wells from these islands when the uterine wall is sectioned after hysterectomy. (Magnification of mounted section × 5).

91

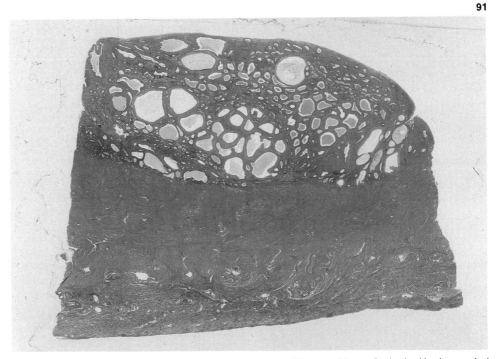

Plate 91 Cystic glandular hyperplasia. The patient was a 55-year-old para 3 who had had no period for 11 years. She presented with abdominal distension and vaginal spotting for 2 months. She had a large (1,250 g) multilocular mucinous cystadenoma of the right ovary. Hysterectomy and bilateral salpingo-oophorectomy was performed. Such tumours sometimes produce oestrogen which could account for the cystic hyperplasia of the endometrium shown here. The myometrium was 1 cm thick. (Magnification of mounted section × 5).

50

92

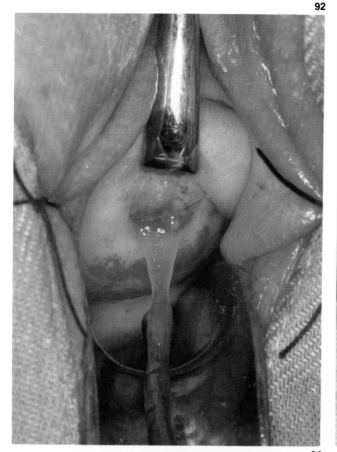

93

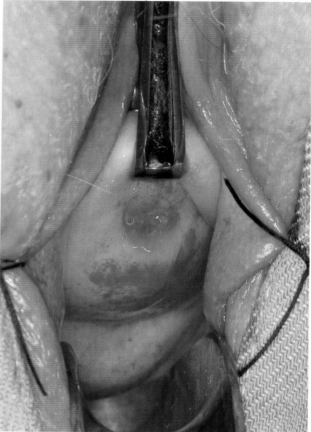

94

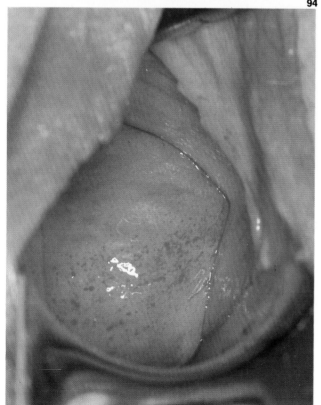

Plate 92 This 78-year-old para 2 presented with a history of vaginal spotting and vulval lump. However mild, postmenopausal bleeding always merits curettage, because 1 in 5 patients with this symptom have endometrial or cervical carcinoma. The lump she had noticed was a cystocele and grade 1 uterine prolapse, the cervix descending almost to the introitus.

Plate 93 Same patient shown in plate 92 with Sims' speculum partly withdrawn to display a small rectocele and area of senile vaginitis on the posterior lip of the cervix that was the likely source of the bleeding. Note the thick tenacious mucus seen when the uterine sound was withdrawn. Curettage obtained mucus alone and no endometrial tissue, which is the commonest result when postmenopausal bleeding is investigated. In such patients, always consider the possibility of the blood having issued from nearby orifices (tumour of bowel or bladder).

Plate 94 Senile vaginitis seen as multiple petechial haemorrhages in thin, shiny, postmenopausal vaginal epithelium, bulged forward by a rectocele in a 62-year-old para 2 who presented with a second degree uterine prolapse. She had not had any vaginal bleeding. When senile vaginitis is symptomatic (discharge, dysuria, dyspareunia, pruritus vulvae, bleeding) local treatment (other than curettage to exclude cancer) is oestrogen cream (0.01% dienoestrol) inserted with a finger (mechanical applicators cause trauma in an aged female with narrowed, dry introitus) once daily. Antibiotic cream (sulphonamide — Sultrin) is also effective, but less physiological in its action.

95

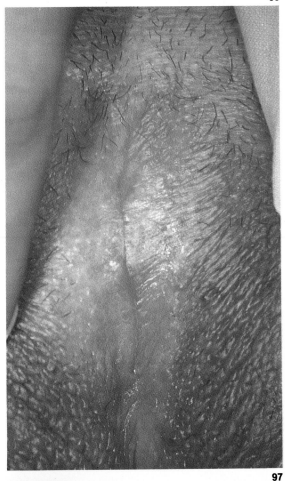

96

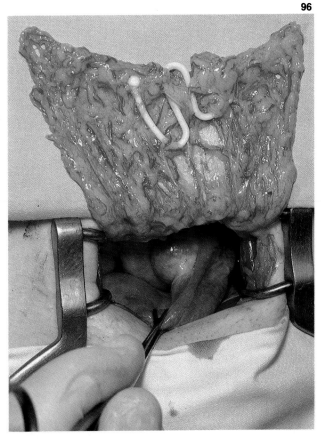

97

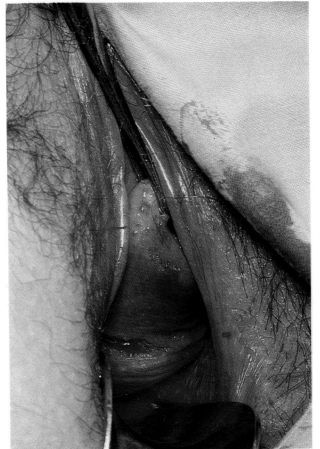

Plate 95 Fusion of labia minora in a 64-year-old nullipara who presented with a 9-month history of dysuria. She thought there was a 'blockage' in her urinary tract. This condition also occurs in young girls. Treatment with oestrogen cream locally is as effective as surgical separation and is less painful.

Plate 96 Lippes loop embedded in omentum. It was inserted at the 6-week postnatal visit in a 32-year-old para 2 who returned 2 years later with 8 weeks' amenorrhoea. Following suction curettage, the loop was removed at laparotomy. Devices lying free in the peritoneal cavity can be removed via the laparoscope. In a series of 620 patients with missing Lippes loop threads, there were 44 with unrecognized expulsion, 41 in the peritoneal cavity, 242 free in the uterus with drawn up threads (coital suction) and 293 embedded in the uterine wall. (Gunaratne, M. Aust. N.Z.J. Obstet. Gynaec. 18: 268, 1978). If a loop does not pull out readily, it should be presumed to be embedded in the uterine wall and it is safest to perform laparotomy and incise the uterine wall to remove it (required in 123 patients in above series).

Plate 97 Coital laceration of the vagina in a single, 28-year-old woman. She was not virginal, but experienced severe deep pain during savage intercourse with a casual acquaintance during a visit by ship to Melbourne. She presented 2 days later because of the sudden onset of heavy vaginal bleeding. The 6 cm tear in the posterior fornix behind the cervix (held forwards with volsellum), more to the right than the left, is shown. There was another tear, 3 cm long, halfway up the left vaginal wall. Interrupted sutures were inserted. There was no bruising or evidence of trauma at the vulva. Such lacerations are often not due to direct injury (genital disproportion), but to levatores ani spasm causing tearing of the unsupported upper vaginal wall. In a series of 15 cases of coital laceration the tears were single in 10, multiple in 5, and were situated in posterior fornix (10), perineum (2), lateral wall (1), hymen (1), and fourchette (1). (Courtesy of Dr Gerald Manly).

98

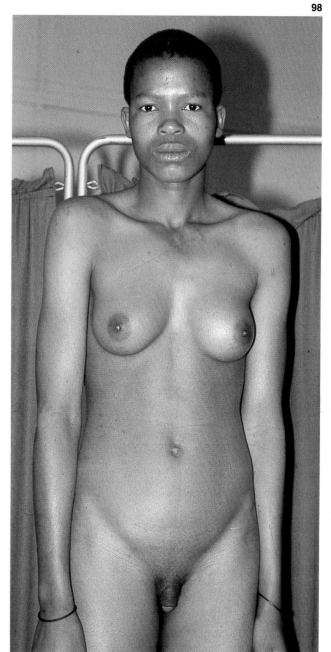

Plate 98 True hermaphrodite. This 20-year-old patient was raised as a male from birth, and presented to hospital 5 years after commencement of breast enlargement and regular menstruation. The 179 cm tall patient had well developed breasts, phallus of normal dimensions but with pronounced bowing (chordee), no palpable gonads in the labioscrotal folds, and what appeared to be a perineal hypospadias.

99

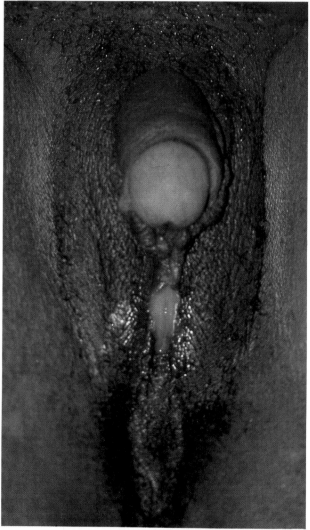

Plate 99 At examination under anaesthesia, a uterus was felt on rectal examination. There was only 1 opening on the perineum. This was a urogenital sinus with the external urinary meatus opening into its anterior wall. Endoscopy through the urogenital sinus revealed a narrow vagina and cervix. Chromosome culture of blood revealed a normal female karyotype, 46 XX. Gonadotrophin levels were low and urinary 17- oxogenic steroids were in the normal range. This view shows the bowed phallus and apparent hypospadias.

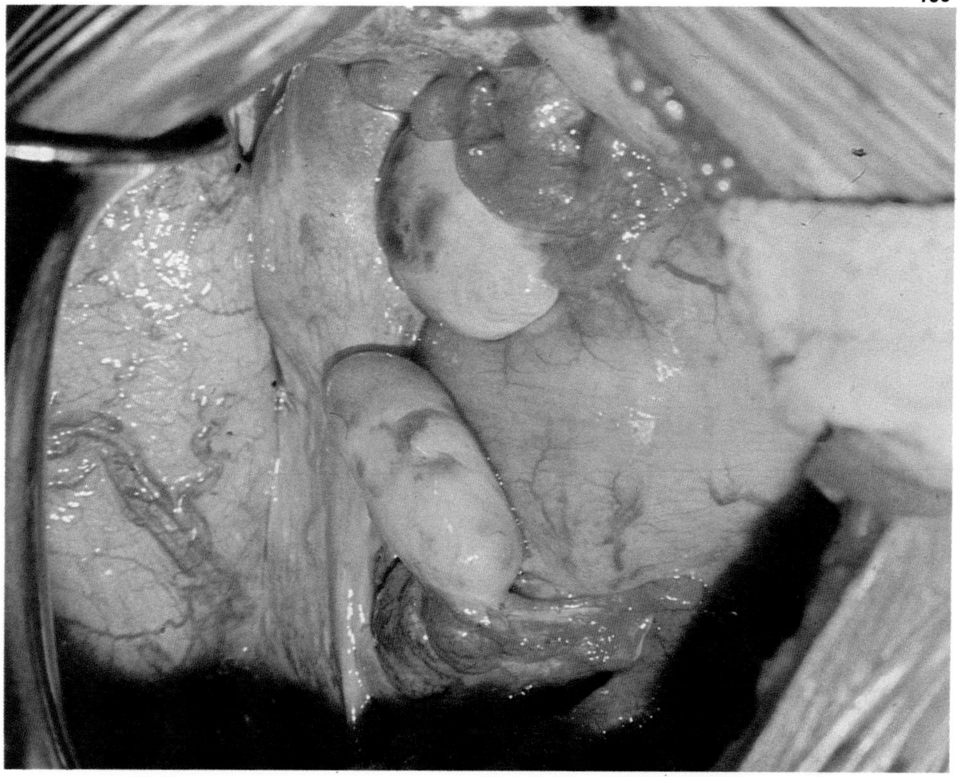

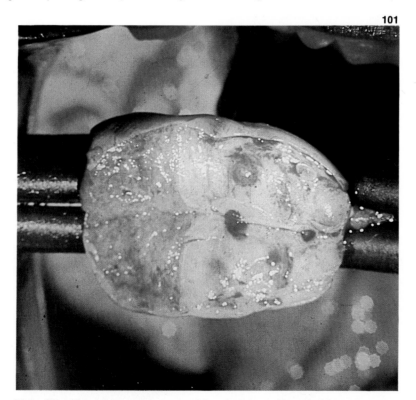

Plate 100 View of this patient at laparotomy showing normal female pelvic anatomy. From left to right the photograph shows veins coursing in the peritoneum covering the bladder, uterus with the left round ligament passing laterally into the inguinal canal, large ovaries and normal Fallopian tubes.

101

Plate 101 The right ovary was normal, but the left, as shown in this section, was an ovotestis. Histology of this gonad showed primordial follicles in the ovarian segment, and seminiferous tubules in the testicular segment. Surgical correction to the sex of rearing was performed and entailed total hysterectomy and bilateral gonadectomy (it was not possible to retain an adequate vascular supply to the testicular portion of the left gonad following removal of the ovarian tissue). Bilateral mastectomies were performed through subareolar incisions and silastic testicular prostheses were placed in the labioscrotal folds. Correction of the 'hypospadias' also necessitated vaginectomy.

54

102

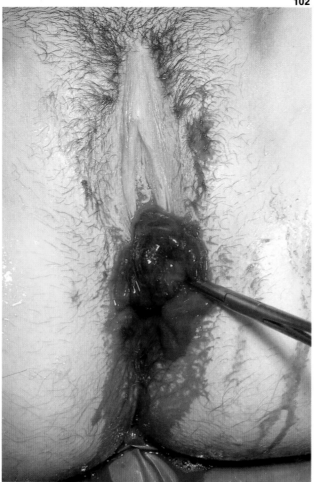

Plate 102 Incomplete abortion in a 21-year-old primigravida who presented with heavy vaginal bleeding and lower abdominal pain after 10 weeks' amenorrhoea. The cervix was 2 cm dilated so the patient was taken to theatre for curettage. This photograph illustrates the common finding in such patients of a dilated vagina filled with blood clot.

Plate 103 After administration of ergometrine (ergonovine), 0.5 mg by intravenous injection, the uterus contracted and placental tissue was seen protruding through the cervix.

Plate 104 The anterior lip of cervix is held with a volsellum, and sponge-holding forceps grasp and remove the placental tissue; preliminary cervical dilatation is usually unnecessary once spontaneous abortion has begun. These steps can be performed in the conscious patient in the left lateral or dorsal position as emergency treatment to halt haemorrhage and treat shock due to placental tissue jammed in the cervix. Resuscitation with intravenous fluid or blood is performed if the patient is shocked, but was not required in this case.

103

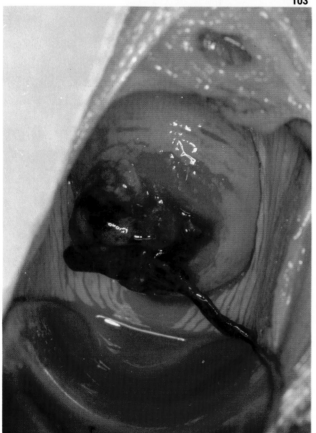

104

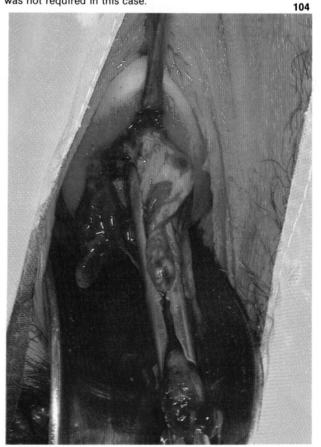

105

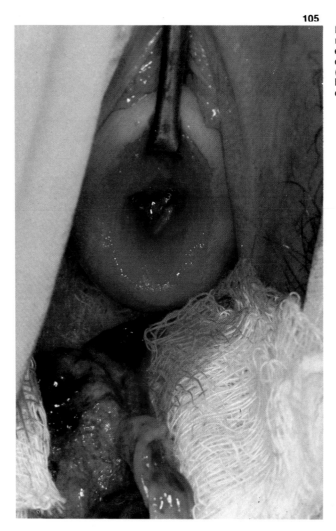

Plate 105 Curettage has been performed to ensure complete removal of placental fragments. Note the dilated external os and extension of endocervical columnar epithelium onto the ecto-cervix as is commonly seen in pregnancy. There was no embryo (blighted ovum) as is usual (70%) in first trimester abortions. Microscopy confirmed the presence of placental villi and absence of abnormal trophoblastic proliferation.

106

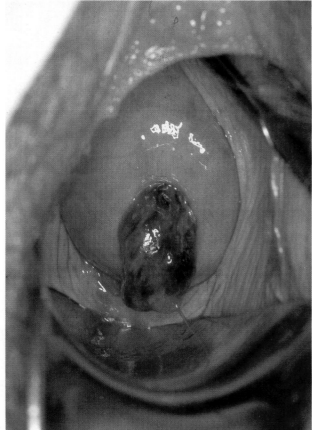

Plate 106 Haemorrhagic decidua and secretory endometrium protruding through the cervix and simulating an incomplete abortion. The patient was a 27-year-old para 1 who presented with 5 days' bleeding (similar to menses) after 12 weeks' amenor-rhoea. The uterus was the size of a pregnancy of 10 weeks' maturity. The diagnosis of incomplete abortion was refuted by histological absence of placental villi or fetal parts. Extrauterine pregnancy could account for the amenorrhoea, uterine enlarge-ment and extensive decidua formation. The message is that histology is required to diagnose early placental tissue. Another possibility is that the patient passed placental tissue unobserved (or resorbed it) and that the thickened endometrium seen here was the result of an intrauterine pregnancy.

56

107

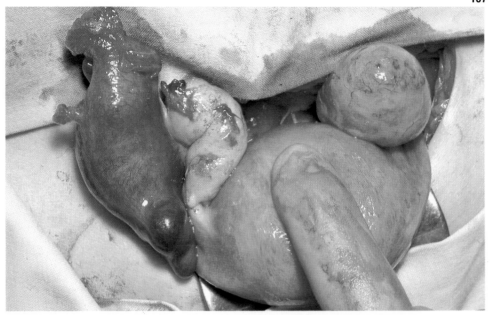

Plate 107 Unruptured right tubal pregnancy. The patient presented with a 3-hour history of abdominal pain, 10 weeks' amenorrhoea and vaginal bleeding for 9 days. The left ovary was larger than the right and contained the corpus luteum. Transperitoneal migration of a fertilized ovum to the contralateral tube seems to have occurred. Right partial salpingectomy was performed. Note uterine enlargement, due to increased vascularity and decidual formation, almost commensurate with an intrauterine pregnancy of the same maturity.

108

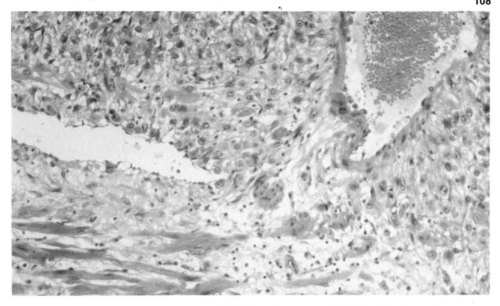

Plate 108 Section of tubal wall showing invasion by a mass of trophoblastic tissue from a 36-year-old patient who developed an acute haemoperitoneum due to rupture of this tubal pregnancy (her second ectopic). Note muscle fibres lower left. These histological features can easily be mistaken for choriocarcinoma, but the typical haemorrhagic necrosis is lacking.

109

Plate 109 Longitudinal section of unruptured tubal pregnancy showing clotted blood and embryo 12 mm in length. The patient was a 36-year-old para 8 with a Lippes loop in situ who presented with irregular vaginal bleeding and abdominal pain for 3 weeks. The uterus was bulky and moving the cervix caused severe pain. Laparotomy was performed the next day when there was no response to antibiotics, the initial diagnosis having been salpingitis, although there was no history of purulent vaginal discharge. There was a 60 ml haemoperitoneum and clotted blood extruded from the fimbrial end of the intact expanded Fallopian tube.

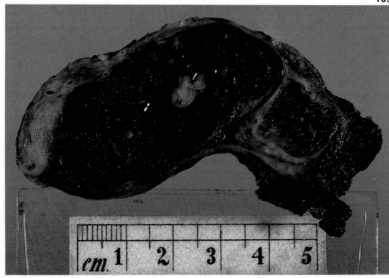

110

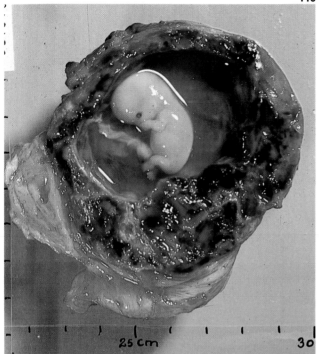

25 cm   30

Plate 110 Ruptured tubal pregnancy and left ovary from a 29-year-old patient with a past history of tuberculous peritonitis and primary infertility. Fetal size corresponded to 8 weeks' maturity but the duration of amenorrhoea was 12 weeks before the onset of acute abdominal pain and shock. Occasionally, peritubal haematoma formation involves the ovary which is thus difficult to conserve.

111

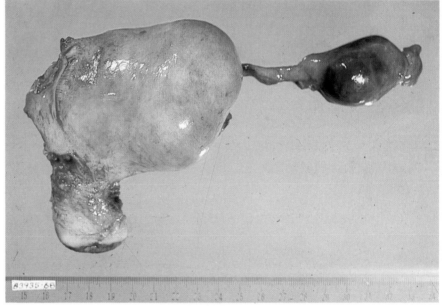

Plate 111 Uterus and left Fallopian tube removed from a 42-year-old patient known to have calcified fibromyomas for 7 years. Operation was performed because of abdominal pain. The outer one-third of the tube contains an ectopic pregnancy which has ruptured into the mesosalpinx; there was no blood in the peritoneal cavity.

112

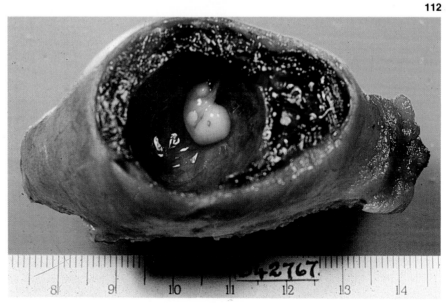

Plate 112 Section of Fallopian tube showing a 6-week-old fetus and intramural haemorrhage. The patient was aged 35 years and previous investigation for infertility had shown blocked tubes. She presented with vaginal bleeding and lower abdominal pain. A small, tender mass was palpable bimanually and at laparotomy there was 500 ml of blood in the peritoneal cavity.

58

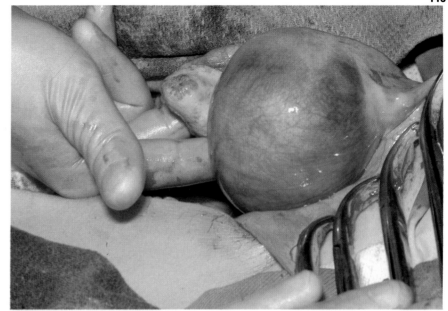

Plate 113 The left ovary shows the puckered surface of a corpus luteum. The patient was aged 23 years and 6 weeks' pregnant. Clamps display the pedicle where a 4,980 g mucinous cystadenoma of the right ovary had been removed. The patient married and was delivered of a normal infant at term.

114

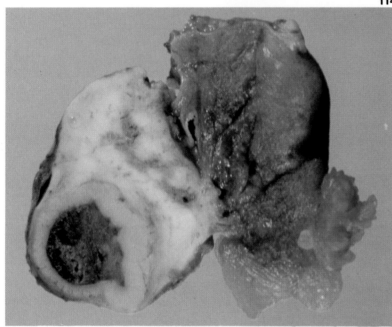

Plate 114 Tubal pregnancy. The patient was aged 35 years and had a history of 2 weeks' lower abdominal pain. At operation there was a haemoperitoneum and the right tube and ovary were matted together within an old blood clot and were removed. Section shows a large corpus luteum (2.5 cm diameter) with typical crenated yellow walls and central blood clot. The ectopic pregnancy lies within the attached distal end of the swollen Fallopian tube.

115

Plate 115 Ovarian pregnancy from a 33-year-old para 2 who presented with lower abdominal and shoulder-tip pain, suggestive of haemoperitoneum (diaphragmatic irritation). She had 6 weeks' amenorrhoea and no vaginal bleeding. There was a fullness in the posterior fornix and extreme pain on rocking the cervix. At operation, the left ovary and both tubes were normal and the haemorrhagic right ovary was removed (although it could have been conserved). The section shows a large recent corpus luteum and haemorrhagic implantation site that contained chorionic villi.

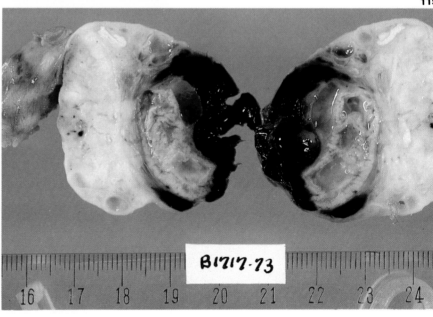

116

Plate 116 Cervical ectopic pregnancy. The patient was a 29-year-old para 1 with a past history of a tubal ectopic pregnancy and a spontaneous abortion. Two months of intermittent vaginal bleeding, followed by recent onset of colicky, lower abdominal pain and identification of placental tissue in the external os, led to the diagnosis of incomplete abortion. At curettage, cervical pregnancy was suspected when placental tissue was noted to be attached to the cervix. After packing of the cervix twice, bleeding ceased. Six weeks later the patient presented with heavy vaginal bleeding for which total abdominal hysterectomy was eventually required. This operative specimen confirmed the diagnosis of cervical pregnancy, which unexpectedly, and uniquely, was a choriocarcinoma! Subsequent chest radiography and tests for urinary chorionic gonadotrophic hormone were negative.

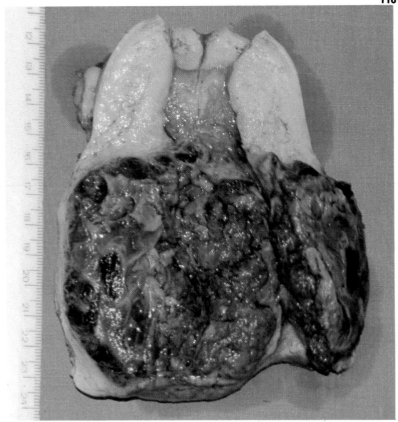

117

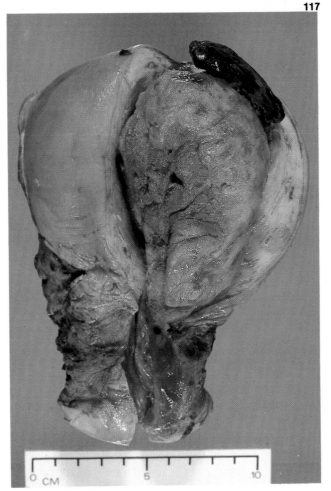

Plate 117 Infected, oedematous placental polyp which was morbidly adherent (accreta). The patient was a 22-year-old para 1 (plus 2 previous terminations) who bled continuously for 18 days after a normal delivery. Local and general signs of sepsis persisted in spite of chemotherapy, curettage and blood transfusion (8,000 ml). Hysterectomy was performed as a life-saving procedure. The presence of the placental tissue as well as the infection was responsible for subinvolution of the uterus (560 g).

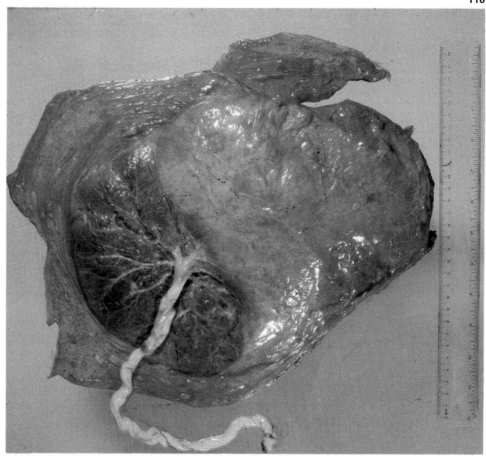

Plate 118 Hydatidiform mole (1 in 700 pregnancies in Australia, more common in other Asian countries and less common in Europe and North America) is associated with a fetus in 6% of cases. In this case the infant survived and was a normal male. The mother was a multigravida. Signs of preeclampsia developed at 28 weeks, but cleared following vaginal bleeding, presumably because the molar half of the single placenta was separated from the uterine wall by blood clot. The specimen weighed 1,420 g. On the fetal surface the amnion covered the mole as well as the normal placenta. Therefore, if the mole (absent fetus) represents half of a uniovular twin placenta, it is the rare monoamniotic variety.

Plate 119 Separation of the firm fibrinous covering on the maternal surface of the specimen shown in plate 118 revealed unusually large vesicles. Invasive mole or choriocarcinoma can develop after evacuation of a hydatidiform mole with coexistent fetus.

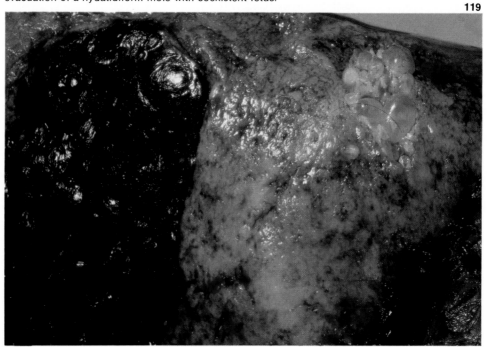

120

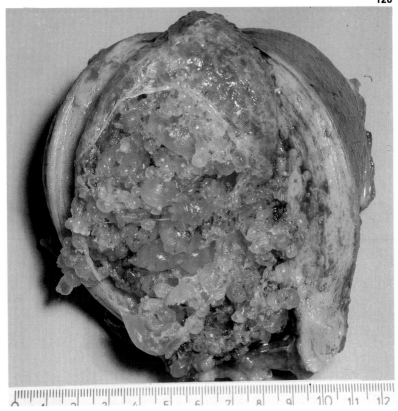

Plate 120 Subtotal hysterectomy specimen showing intact hydatidiform mole with large vesicles discoloured by formalin. In many moles the vesicles are small (rice grain size), photograph poorly, and can be overlooked as air bubbles unless blood clot is washed away from aborted tissue. The patient was a 42-year-old multipara who presented with vaginal bleeding and dyspnoea at 12 weeks' gestation. She had severe preeclampsia, disproportionate uterine enlargement and was in heart failure. Evacuation of the uterus by intrauterine injection of 50% dextrose and intravenous oxytocin infusion failed (this was in 1964 before introduction of the suction curette). The ovaries contained theca-lutein cysts and were conserved. After operation, the signs of preeclampsia rapidly resolved. There were no malignant sequelae.

Plate 121 The patient was a 46-year-old para 6 who presented at 20 weeks' gestation having passed a large vesicular mass after intermittent vaginal bleeding for 6 weeks. Because of age and parity (increased risk of malignant sequelae), primary treatment was abdominal hysterectomy. Urinary HCG excretion was 48,500 IU/24 hours after operation and 150 IU/24 hours 6 weeks later. The red velvety appearance of the posterior uterine wall is due to subserosal decidual reaction. These theca-lutein cysts (5 ×4 × 3 cm) were removed because of the patient's age but are benign and regress spontaneously. Occasionally they develop rapidly after evacuation of a hydatidiform mole. **121**

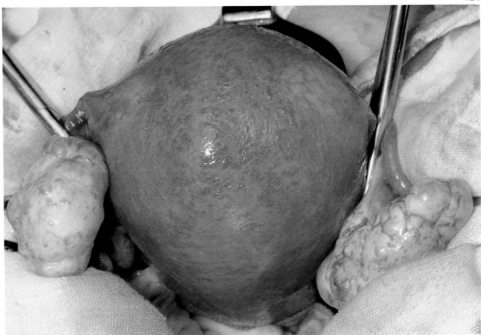

122

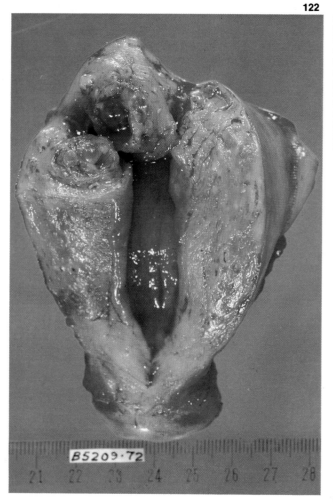

Plate 122 Hysterectomy specimen showing vesicles of invasive mole within the uterine wall. The patient was a 39-year-old para 4 who presented at 14 weeks' gestation with severe hyperemesis, vaginal haemorrhage, and uterus larger than dates. She was anaemic (haemoglobin value 9.5 g/dl) and the urinary HCG excretion was 5,264,000 IU/24 hours. Hydatidiform mole was confirmed by ultrasonography. After commencement of oxytocin infusion, 480 g of mole tissue was evacuated by suction curettage. Hysterectomy was performed 8 weeks later because of continued bleeding and persistently elevated HCG levels. There has been no recurrence in 7 years. In view of age and parity, primary prophylactic hysterectomy would have been proper initial therapy.

123

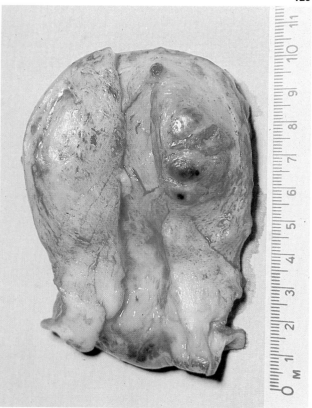

Plate 123 Invasive hydatidiform mole causing haemorrhagic nodules (4 × 3 cm) in the uterine wall. Metastases in the vagina characteristically show a similar appearance. The patient was a 25-year-old para 3 who presented initially with threatened abortion and severe hyperemesis, and again at 12 weeks' gestation with preeclampsia and rapid uterine enlargement to the size of a 20-week pregnancy. Curettage was performed after a vesicular mass was aborted by an oxytocin infusion. Hysterectomy was performed 5 weeks later because vaginal bleeding continued and the HCG titre remained elevated. There was no evidence of metastatic spread beyond the uterus. One course of methotrexate was given postoperatively. Follow-up for 8 years has revealed no evidence of recurrence. Had the patient been a nullipara, chemotherapy would have been a proper alternative to hysterectomy.

124

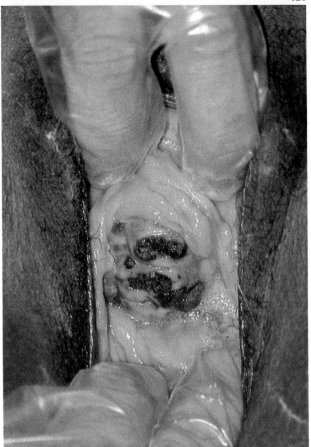

125

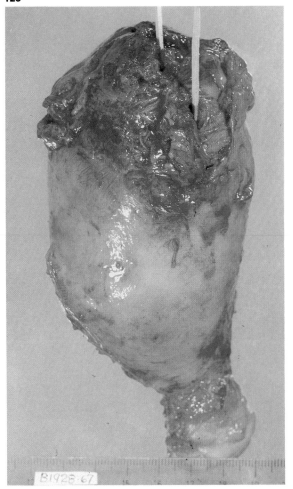

126

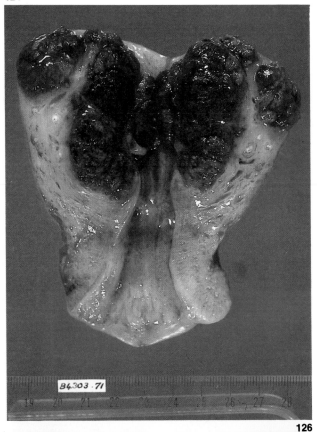

Plate 124 Choriocarcinoma. The patient was a 26-year-old para 3 who presented with menorrhagia and anaemia (haemoglobin value 8.2 g/dl) 10 months postpartum. Histology of bulky, friable curettings established the diagnosis. The urinary HCG excretion was 162,400 IU/24 hours. Pulmonary metastases responded to multiple courses of chemotherapy, but the HCG titre remained elevated, and pelvic arteriography revealed atypical vascularity consistent with residual tumour mass. Hysterectomy was performed and the specimen shows typical haemorrhagic lesions. Sadly the patient died from haemorrhage into cerebral metastases.

Plate 125 Choriocarcinoma. This uterus was removed as a life-saving procedure when a 17-year-old patient developed an acute haemoperitoneum during curettage for suspected incomplete abortion. The probes indicate where the growth had penetrated the uterine wall. As in 50% of cases there was no preceding hydatidiform mole (excluding those diagnosed by biochemical evidence alone — HCG levels in plasma or urine). The operative diagnosis was ruptured cornual pregnancy. X-ray then revealed multiple pulmonary metastases. Recovery was complete after treatment with methotrexate and actinomycin D.

Plate 126 Vaginal metastases from a choriocarcinoma. This 28-year-old multigravida, after no apparent pregnancy for 4 years, presented with heavy bleeding from these friable lesions on the anterior vaginal wall. Surrounding tissues were not indurated. The uterus was mobile and not enlarged. After biopsy, vaginal packing and transfusion were required. Histology revealed choriocarcinoma. Urinary HCG levels were elevated and chest radiography was clear. The vaginal lesions diminished in size after methotrexate therapy was instituted, but pulmonary metastases became evident, and the patient succumbed.

64

127

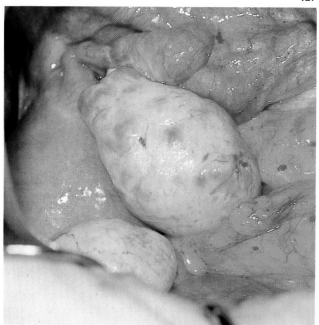

Plate 127 Polycystic ovaries in a 28-year-old para 3 lying behind and above the uterus and showing thickened tunica albuginea and numerous follicular cysts. These features are suggestive of the Stein-Leventhal syndrome, but the patient lacked the clinical features of infertility, hirsutes and oligo-amenorrhoea. The right Fallopian tube is bulbous due to past infection. Not all polycystic ovaries are due to the Stein-Leventhal syndrome!

Plate 128 Stein-Leventhal syndrome. Bilateral wedge resections from a 27-year-old patient who presented with primary infertility and secondary amenorrhoea. Bimanual palpation had revealed enlargement of both ovaries to an extent unusual in this syndrome. Note the multiple follicular cysts and smooth, white, thickened ovarian capsule. The rest of the ovarian cortex and medulla seems involved in the fibrotic process.

Plate 129 Posterior view of a normal-sized uterus and bilateral adnexal masses (640 g in all), removed from a 39-year-old para 2 who presented with lower abdominal pain and a tender abdominal mass. The operative diagnosis was endometriosis since there were numerous puckered haemorrhagic lesions on the pelvic peritoneum and tarry fluid escaped when the right ovary was freed from adhesions. Histology confirmed endometriosis in the right tuboovarian mass, but the 10 × 11 × 7 cm left-sided tumour was a benign cystic teratoma, as should have been suspected from its smooth outer wall.

128

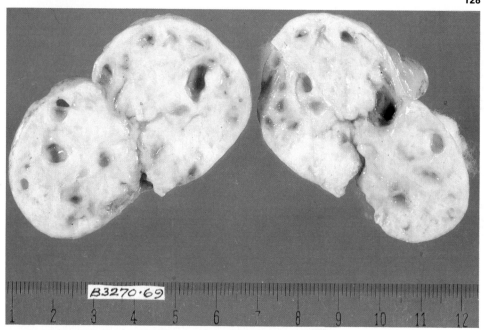

129

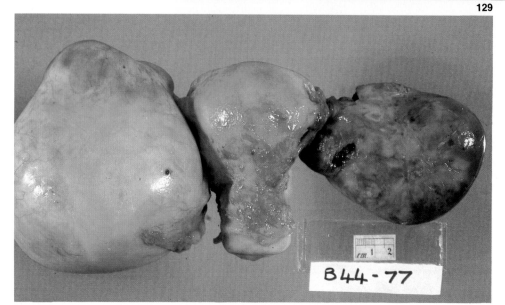

130

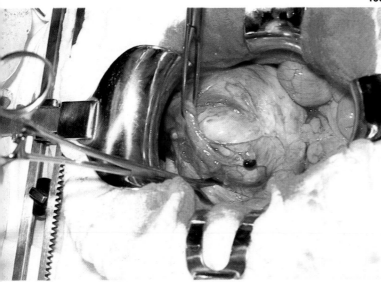

Plate 130 Endometriosis. The patient presented with infertility, deep dyspareunia and a mass filling the pouch of Douglas and extending above the level of the umbilicus. Tests for tubal patency and ovulation were normal. At laparotomy, the mass was immobile, cystic and attached to uterus and bowel.

131

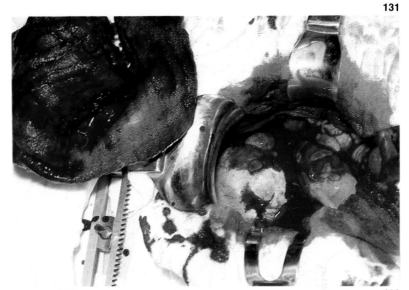

Plate 131 When freed from attachments, typical chocolate contents were released. The endometriotic cyst walls were removed and the ovary was reconstituted (Dr Ian Johnston). The right ovary had been removed 3 years earlier when cysts were seen in it at the time of appendicectomy! A McBurney's incision is inadequate for inspection and operation on the uterus and ovaries.

Plate 132 After ovarian reconstruction, hydrotubation was performed to help preserve tubal patency. Conception occurred 16 months later and the patient had a normal delivery of a living male infant at 38 weeks. The moral is that conservative surgery can promote fertility even when endometriosis is most extensive.

Plate 133 Five years later, placenta praevia necessitated Caesarean section for delivery of the patient's third son and allowed further inspection of the pelvic contents. There was an unusually well marked decidual reaction, giving a velvety appearance to the surfaces of the ovary, uterus and round ligament.

132   **133**

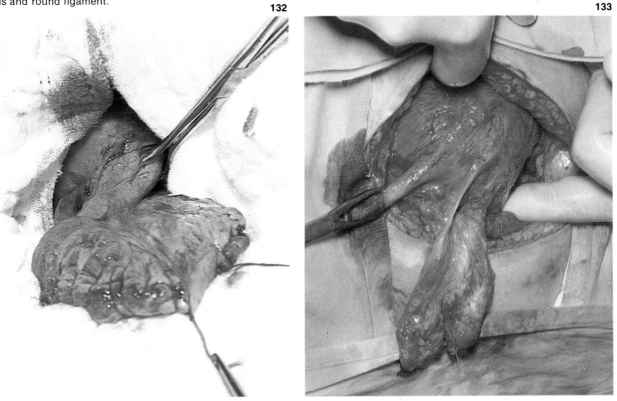

66

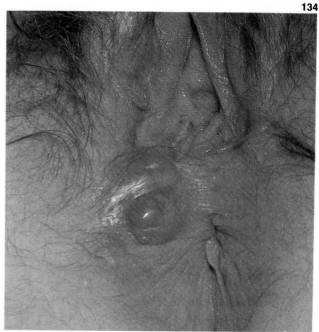

Plate 134 Perineal endometriosis. This patient had endometriosis of an episiotomy wound. She became pregnant and at 19 weeks decidual reaction had caused softening and enlargement of the ectopic endometrial tissue. Pregnancy cured her dyspareunia. (From Beischer, N.A. Obstet. Gynec. 28: 15, 1966).

Plate 135 Endometriosis. Uterus and ovaries removed from a 38-year-old patient with primary infertility and menorrhagia. In view of associated tubal pathology (demonstrated by hysterosalpingography and laparoscopy) and her husband's disappointing seminal analysis, treatment was abdominal hysterectomy and bilateral salpingo-oophorectomy. Note the lesions on the serosa of the posterior uterine wall, one of the common sites where foci of endometriosis are seen. This is often the site of dense adhesions of the rectosigmoid to the uterus and cervix.

Plate 136 Chronic inflammatory disease — uterus and densely adherent tuboovarian masses removed from a 34-year-old woman who became infertile after spontaneous abortion 18 years previously. She had recurrent episodes of irregular menstruation, abdominal pain and pyrexia for 15 years. Large, tender adnexal masses and yellow vaginal discharge persisted in spite of courses of antibiotics. Pelvic clearance to relieve pain was performed with difficulty, due to numerous adhesions to bladder and bowel.

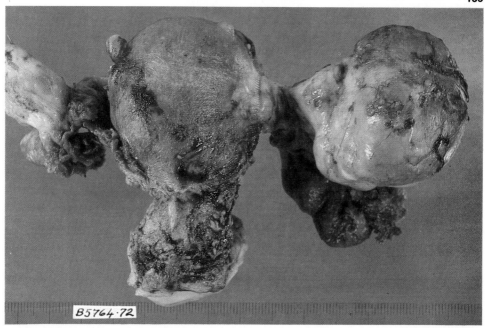

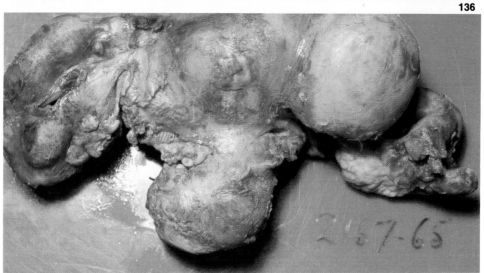

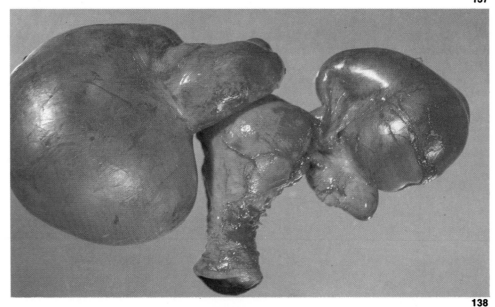

137

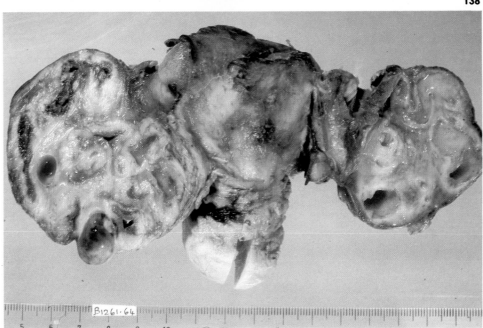

138

B1261·64

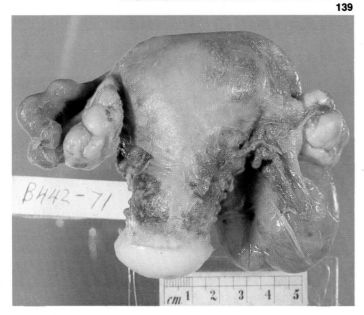

139

B442-71

Plate 137 Uterus and bilateral hydrosalpinges removed from a 42-year-old para 1. She had a history of chronic pelvic inflammatory disease, dysmenorrhoea and recent irregular vaginal bleeding. The tubes are trumpet-shaped due to occlusion of the fimbriated ends and distension with fluid.

Plate 138 Chronic tuboovarian abscesses. The patient was a 47-year-old para 1 who presented with yellow vaginal discharge and night sweats. She had an enlarged, fixed, retroverted uterus and bilateral adnexal masses, but minimal tenderness. Total hysterectomy and bilateral salpingo-oophorectomy was performed. The histology was suggestive of tuberculosis (caseation and giant cells), but cultures were negative.

Plate 139 Bilateral hydrosalpinges, ovaries and normal-sized uterus removed from 37-year-old para 1 who presented because of dyspareunia and lower abdominal pain, worse premenstrually. Antibiotics had been given for acute episodes of pelvic infection on 5 occasions in recent years. A tender left adnexal mass adherent to the uterus was noted on bimanual examination. The patient agreed to surgery rather than further conservative management. Oestrogen replacement therapy was commenced post-operatively to prevent menopausal symptoms.

68

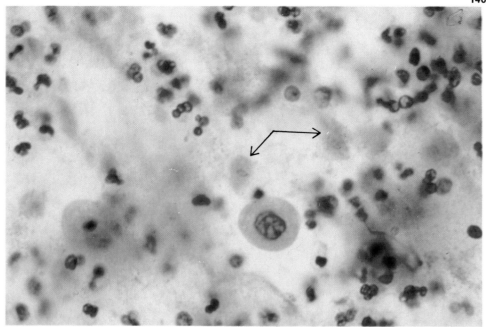

140

Plate 140 Papanicolaou stain of a vaginal smear from a patient with trichomonal vaginitis. The field contains numerous trichomonads, some of which are arrowed. These organisms have oval nuclei, are poorly defined by this stain, and are about twice the size of the numerous polymorphs. Note the nuclear changes in the vaginal cell in the middle of the field induced by trichomonal infection. Such appearance can be confused with dysplasia. When infection and an abnormal smear coexist, the infection should be treated and the smear repeated. (Magnification × 250).

Plate 141 Endocervicitis and associated trichomonal vaginitis in a 36-year-old para 8 who presented with lower abdominal pain. Like many women with obvious clinical evidence of vaginitis, she did not complain of discharge or itch. Note the bubbles typical of trichomonads, the presence of which was undiagnosed until examination under anaesthesia prior to cervical diathermy, when this photograph was taken.

141

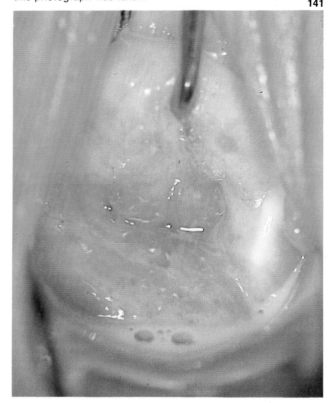

Plate 142 Trichomonal vaginitis in a 25-year-old para 2 at 29 weeks' gestation who complained of vaginal discharge and pruritus vulvae. The frothy, greenish-coloured discharge is seen on the edge of the Sims' speculum. Increased pelvic vascularity of pregnancy accounts for the purple colour of the vaginal epithelium. The infection responded promptly to metronidazole, 200 mg 3 times daily for 7 days. Monilial vaginitis (plates 26 and 143) is at least 3 times more common than trichomonal vaginitis during pregnancy.

142

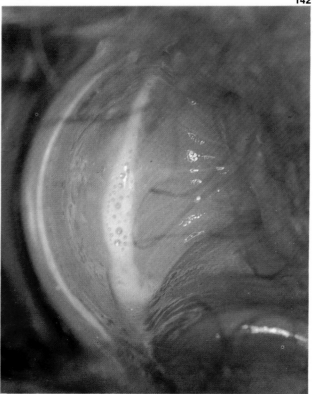

143

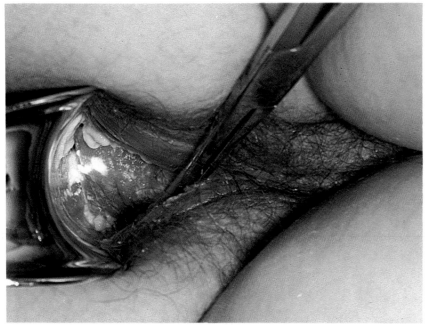

144

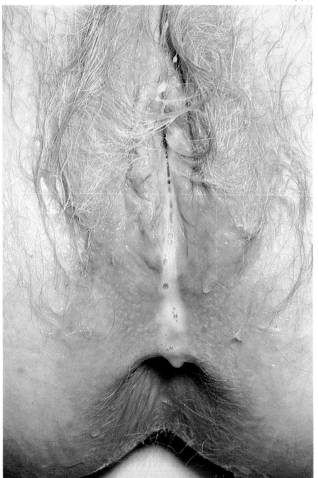

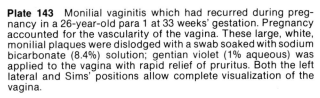

Plate 143 Monilial vaginitis which had recurred during pregnancy in a 26-year-old para 1 at 33 weeks' gestation. Pregnancy accounted for the vascularity of the vagina. These large, white, monilial plaques were dislodged with a swab soaked with sodium bicarbonate (8.4%) solution; gentian violet (1% aqueous) was applied to the vagina with rapid relief of pruritus. Both the left lateral and Sims' positions allow complete visualization of the vagina.

145

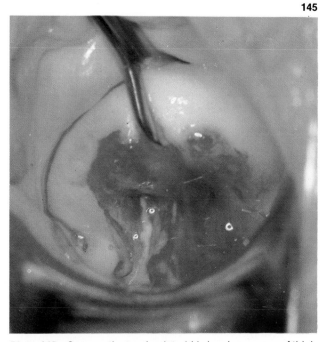

Plate 144 This 72-year-old para 1 presented with purulent vaginal discharge and episodes of vaginal bleeding. It is uncommon for senile vaginitis to be associated with such copious discharge and trichomonal and monilial vaginitis were excluded. Four years previously the patient had had a radical mastectomy for carcinoma and commenced continuous oestrogen therapy 2 years later when biopsy of supraclavicular lymph nodes showed metastatic disease. The uterus was mobile and irregularly enlarged probably due to oestrogen-induced enlargement of fibromyomas.

Plate 145 Same patient as in plate 144 showing escape of thick pus (pyometra) and fresh bleeding from the cervix following cervical dilatation. Careful curettage (to minimize risk of perforation) produced copious, friable tissue macroscopically suggestive of endometrial carcinoma. Histology revealed polypoid endometrial hyperplasia (oestrogen effect) without evidence of malignancy. Symptoms were controlled by cessation of oestrogen therapy. It may have been wiser to perform hysterectomy since oestrogen therapy had apparently controlled the breast cancer metastases.

70

146

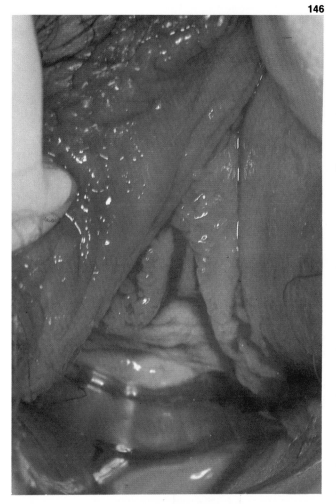

Plate 146 Multiple tiny condylomata acuminata of cervix, entire vagina and labia minora in a 45-year-old para 2 who presented with menorrhagia and recent history of vaginal discharge and pruritus vulvae. Such lesions are not easily seen (as in this picture) and are diagnosed by palpation at the time of bimanual vaginal examination, the vaginal walls and labial skin feeling like sandpaper. Patients seldom discover these lesions themselves. Usually there is trichomonal and/or monilial infection present and the condylomata rapidly disappear with appropriate treatment (metronidazole, nystatin) as occurred in this patient. Electrocautery is reserved for large lesions such as those in plates 147 and 148. Although caused by a virus, condylomata seldom develop in the absence of vaginitis due to another cause.

147

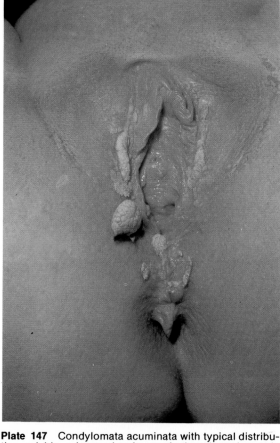

Plate 147 Condylomata acuminata with typical distribution on labia majora and perineum. As these hyperkeratotic lesions develop, they coalesce to form warty polyps that have frond-like papillary projections on the surface. The rest of the vulval skin is normal, contrary to what is seen in chronic vulval dystrophies (plates 218 to 220).

148

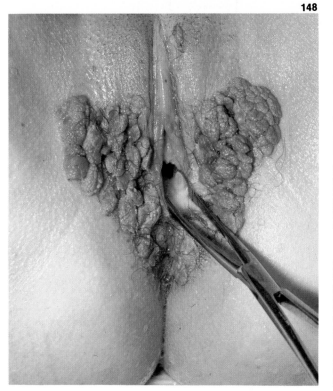

Plate 148 Large, multiple condylomata acuminata of the vulva in a single 24-year-old nullipara (1 termination of pregnancy). She presented with pruritus vulvae for 2 months, worse at night. The vulval warts had been steadily increasing in size for 2 years. She had a yellowish-green vaginal discharge displayed by the opened sponge forceps. The vaginal smear showed numerous trichomonads. The lesions were excised and the raw areas sutured. Metronidazole was prescribed. Postoperative pain necessitated an indwelling catheter for 3 days and hospitalization for 6 days. Serology for syphilis and gonorrhoea was negative. (Courtesy of Dr Kevin Barham).

149

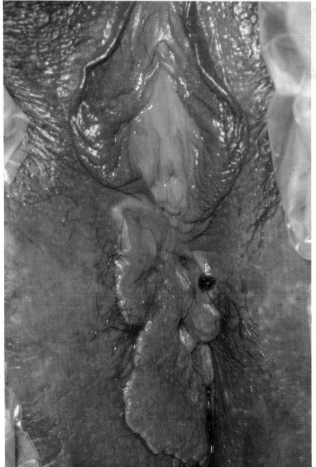

Plate 149 Wart virus disease of the cervix (papilloma virus of papovavirus group). The cytological features of this infection are seen in about 1% of cervical smears. Three cells show the typical double nuclei, characteristic perinuclear halo and thickened peripheral rim of cytoplasm ('balloon cells'). The field contains many polymorphs and squames of intermediate and superficial type. Wart virus-induced epithelial atypia was previously called mild dysplasia. The same or a similar virus is also responsible for condylomata acuminata of vagina and vulva. (Magnification × 300). (Courtesy of Dr Ruth Davoren).

150

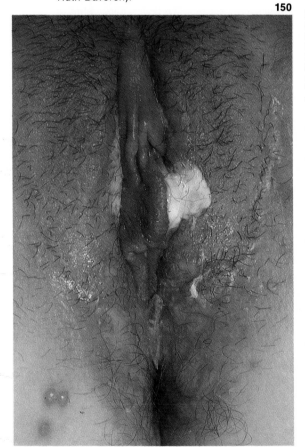

Plate 151 Granuloma inguinale (Donovanosis) involving peri-anal skin of perineum and buttock, showing the characteristic elevated surface of soft granulation tissue. This venereal disease extends through the skin and the perianal form is often seen in male homosexuals. Diagnosis is established by smears or biopsy showing the pathognomonic encapsulated inclusion bodies (Donovan bodies) within large mononuclear cells. Treatment with streptomycin and tetracycline is usually effective. (Courtesy of Dr Neil Astill).

151

Plate 150 Herpes vulvovaginitis in a 25-year-old nulli-para who presented with a 6-week history of pruritus vulvae and pain which became intolerable when secondary infection occurred. Typical vesicles and ulceration are evident. The white patches are anaesthetic cream. There was associated monilial vaginitis and condylomata acuminata. Tests for syphilis and gonorrhoea were negative.

72

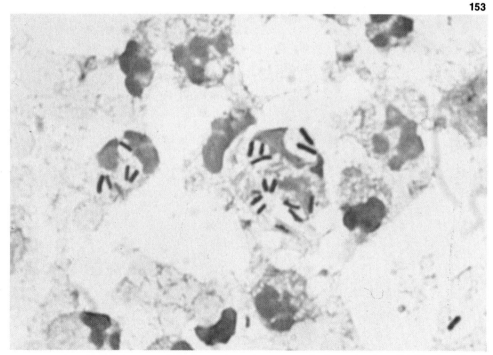

152

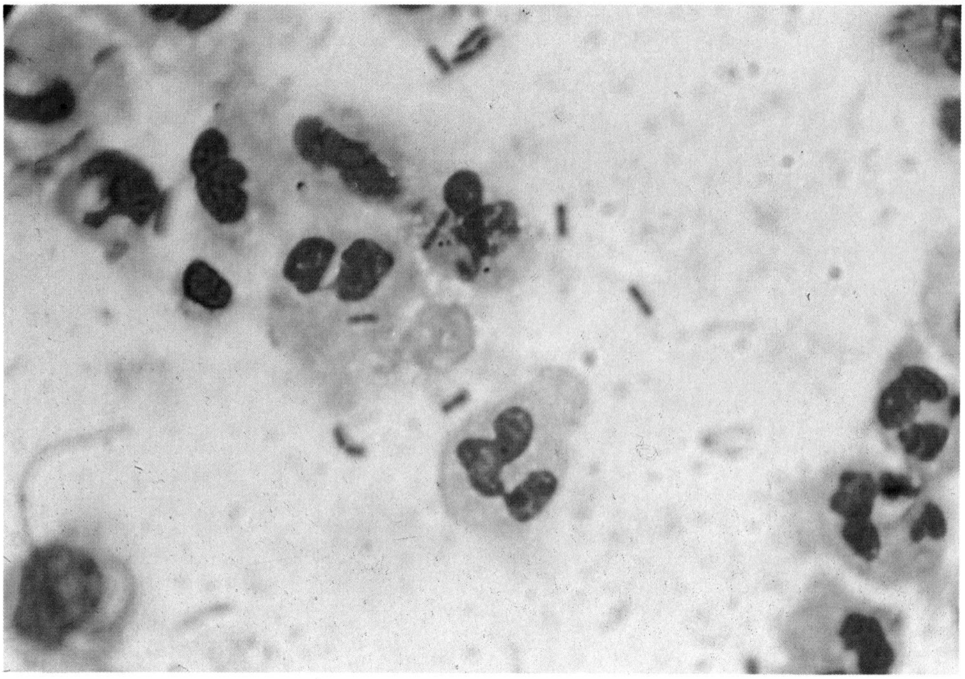

Plate 152 Photomicrograph of a stained direct cervical smear showing the typical appearance of Clostridium welchii (perfringens) organisms as Gram-positive bacilli. The polymorph leucocytes are well preserved as seen in infections with a nonvirulent strain. The bacilli are mainly extracellular, but when phagocytosis has occurred the polymorphs have not been destroyed. This type of smear can be obtained from a patient who has no clinical signs of infection. (Magnification × 3,000).

153

Plate 153 Direct cervical smear from the patient whose uterus is shown in plate 154. The bacilli are numerous and largely intracellular. The fragmentation of the polymorphs is diagnostic of a highly virulent strain. (Magnification × 3,000).

154

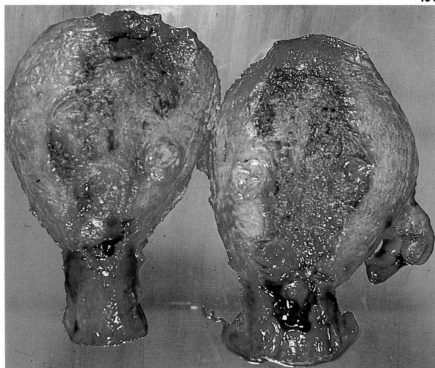

Plate 154 Postpartum uterine gangrene due to Clostridium welchii infection. The patient was a 38-year-old para 4 who came into labour following an accidental haemorrhage at 28 weeks' gestation. Severe uterine infection progressed to septicaemia resulting in death 3 days after delivery in spite of chemotherapy, antitoxin and hysterectomy. Note the oedematous uterine wall and extensive necrosis at the fundus. The entire organ was friable.

155

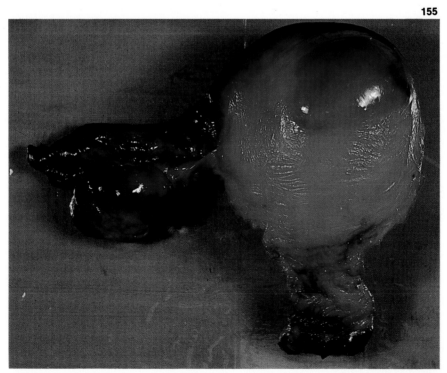

Plate 155 Gangrenous uterus, tube and ovary removed from a 27-year-old para 2 who presented with a septic incomplete abortion. She was deeply jaundiced, oliguric with port-wine urine, and had extreme pelvic tenderness and vulval oedema. During hysterectomy, extensive pelvic thrombophlebitis was noted. The cervical smear had shown evidence of severe Clostridial infection. Although moribund before operation, the patient survived. Examination of this specimen showed full thickness necrosis of the uterine wall.

156

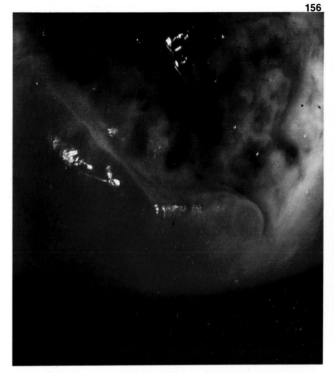

157

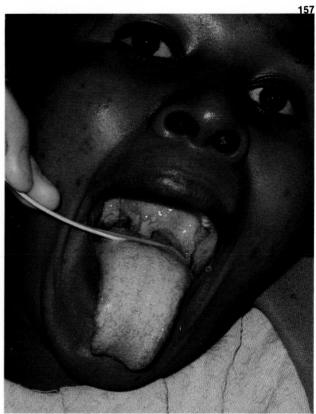

Plate 156 Primary chancre due to syphilis on the cervix as seen at colposcopy. These lesions are less conspicuous in the female, the usual sites being labia majora, labia minora and clitoris. Note the typical punched out edge of the ulcer and the grey necrotic tissue in its base. The patient was pregnant which accounts for the vascularity of the cervix. This lesion had been mistaken for carcinomatous ulceration. (Magnification × 12). (Courtesy of Dr William Chanen).

Plate 157 Snail-track ulcers of the palate seen as greyish lesions near right tonsillar area and uvula. This is one of the clinical manifestations of the secondary stage of syphilis, appearing 6 weeks to 6 months after the primary treponemal infection.

Plate 158 Typical maculopapular rash of secondary syphilis in a 22-year-old para 1 who was 18 weeks pregnant. She had generalized aches and pains, lymphadenopathy and was mildly jaundiced. During the pregnancy she was given 2 courses of procaine penicillin, each consisting of 1 million units per day for 10 days.

158

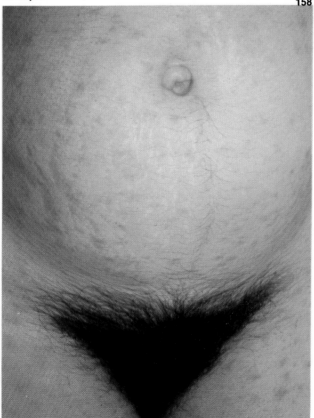

Plate 159 Multiple condylomata lata involving labia majora and perineum and associated vulval oedema. This is another manifestation of secondary syphilis and can be associated with a generalized rash and lymphadenopathy. These lesions have a greyish necrotic appearance and are usually multiple as in this patient. They are raised only slightly above the surrounding skin and lack the frond-like projections typical of condylomata acuminata (plates 147 and 148). Such condylomata are infectious and spirochaetes are readily recoverable from them.

159

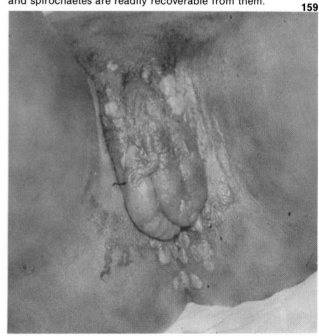

160

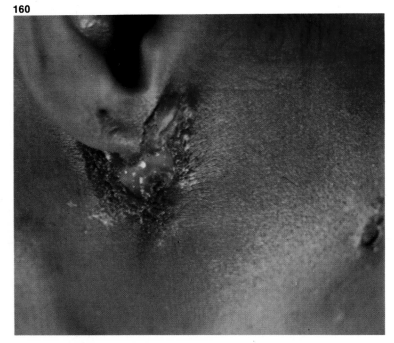

Plate 160 Tuberculous ulcer. This 25-year-old patient was admitted to an obstetric unit with rapid abdominal distension and pain and was thought to have either acute polyhydramnios or complication of a large ovarian cyst. After pregnancy was excluded by palpation, auscultation and abdominal radiography, the correct diagnosis was suspected when this typical tuberculous ulcer was observed beneath the ear. Abdominal paracentesis confirmed the presence of tubercle bacilli. Pelvic tuberculosis is now uncommonly seen in developed countries.

Plate 161 Pyosalpinges due to tuberculosis seen at laparotomy in a 35-year-old patient who presented with primary infertility and menorrhagia. The ovaries were involved in the fibrocaseous reaction, but there was no ascites or evidence of tubercles on the peritoneum. Total hysterectomy and bilateral salpingo-oophorectomy was performed. The patient was given a 12-month course of isoniazid, 100 mg orally 3 times daily, and streptomycin sulphate, 1 g by intramuscular injection twice weekly.

Plate 162 Tuberculous pyosalpinges and endometritis. It is unusual for the disease to involve the uterine wall so extensively in a premenopausal patient, since periodic shedding of the endometrium prevents invasion of the uterine wall. The disease usually extends from the tubes to endometrial cavity. Tuberculosis of the pelvis usually responds to chemotherapy alone, but occasionally surgery is indicated if tuboovarian masses persist, even in the absence of symptoms.

161

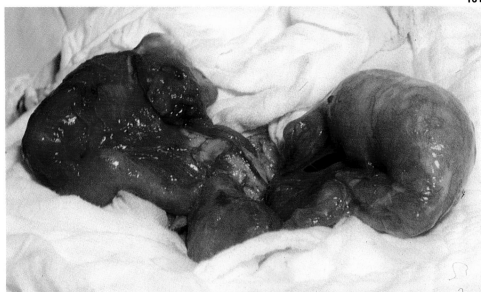

162

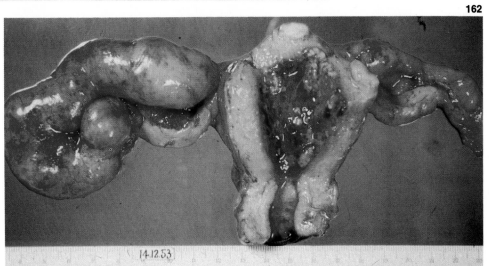

163

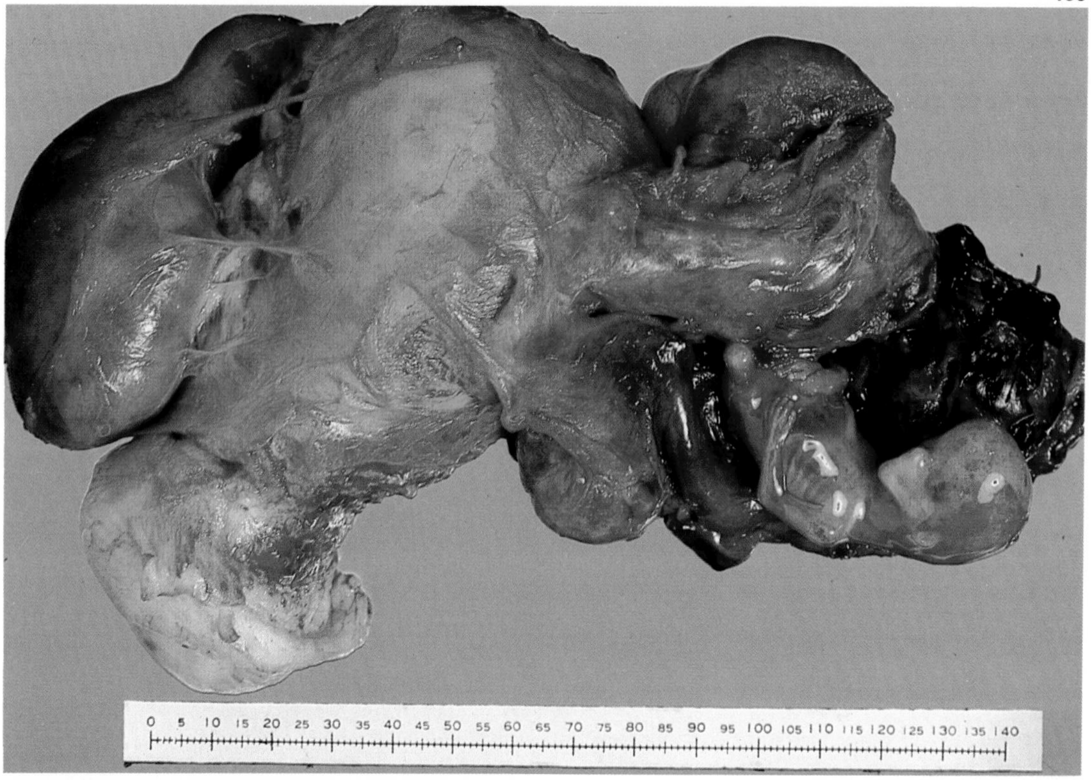

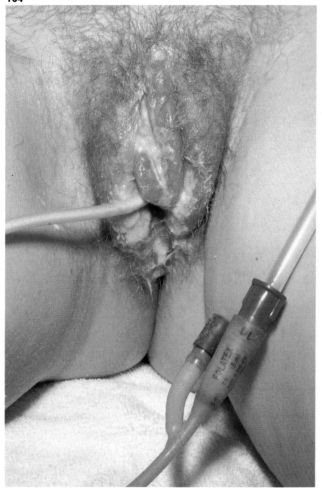

0 5 10 15 20 25 30 35 40 45 50 55 60 65 70 75 80 85 90 95 100 105 110 115 120 125 130 135 140

164

Plate 163 Chronic pelvic inflammatory disease resulting in hydrosalpinges, multiple adhesions to surrounding structures, and a tubal pregnancy. The patient was a 34-year-old nullipara who had had a long period of infertility subsequent to a termination of pregnancy. After several months of irregular vaginal bleeding and pelvic pain, total hysterectomy and bilateral salpingo-oophorectomy was performed. The patient had not suspected the possibility of pregnancy. A fetus of about 12 weeks' maturity is shown in the dilated left tube. It is uncommon for an ectopic pregnancy to reach this maturity unless situated in the peritoneal cavity (primary or secondary abdominal pregnancy), or interstitial portion of the tube (thicker muscle wall allows more expansion before rupture occurs). Replacement oestrogen/progestin therapy was commenced 2 weeks after the operation.

Plate 164 Acute vulvovaginitis in a 38-year-old para 3 who presented with acute urinary retention and a painful vulva for 3 days. Inguinal lymph nodes were enlarged and tender. Temperature was 38.5° C. The diagnosis was monilial vulvovaginitis with secondary bacterial infection. A similar picture is sometimes seen with gonococcal vulvovaginitis and when herpes vulvitis (plate 150) is complicated by secondary infection. The infection responded to erythromycin (the patient was allergic to penicillin) and nystatin cream, but a catheter was required for 6 days.

165

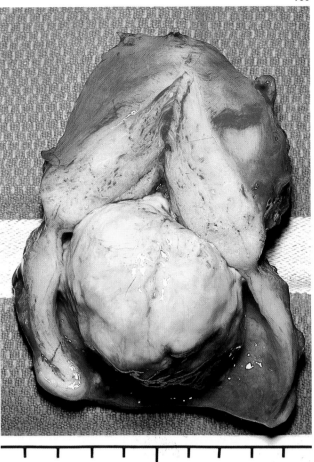

CM 5 1

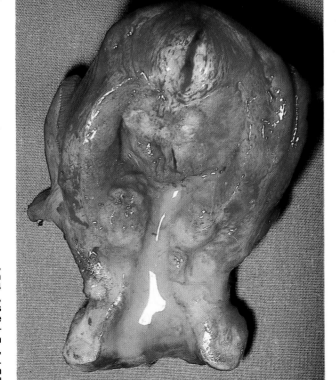

Plate 165 Large, ballvalve, submucus fibromyomatous polyp causing expansion of the endocervical canal and external os; it is covered with a thick coat of matted pus. It was visible through the cervix of a 33-year-old para 2 who had had abdominal pain and continuous vaginal bleeding for 7 weeks. Abdominal hysterectomy with conservation of ovaries was performed. The operation was more vascular than usual due to the infection.

Plate 166 Total hysterectomy specimen showing a pyometra, small incised fundal fibromyoma, and a large fungating growth involving the lower part of the body of the uterus. Curettage 14 days earlier had revealed copious, friable, yellowish tissue, confirmed by histology to be an adenocarcinoma. The ovaries were removed separately at the beginning of the operation since 10% contain metastases which could result in peritoneal contamination if left attached to the uterus during its removal. When endometrial cancer involves the lower part of the uterine body, lymphatic spread is lateral as for a primary lesion of the cervix. The patient was a 75-year-old para 2 who presented with intermittent bleeding for 1 year. She weighed 90.6 kg. Radical hysterectomy preceded by radiotherapy would have been the preferred treatment had the patient been younger and thinner.

78

167

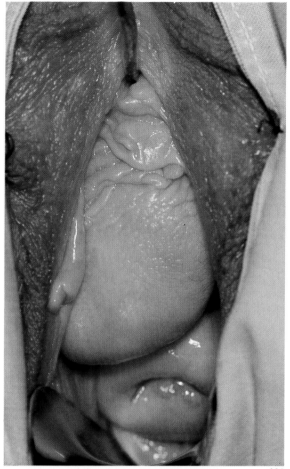

168

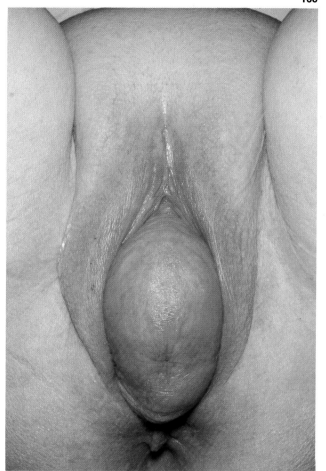

169

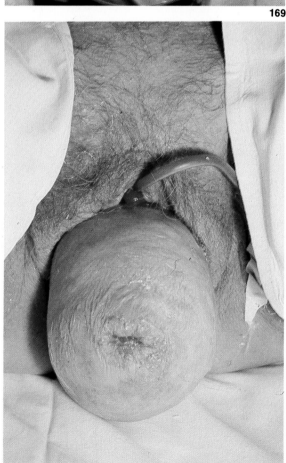

Plate 167 Large cyst of Gartner's duct in a 40-year-old para 2 who had noted the mass for 5 years. Her presenting symptom was frequency of micturition. Note that the mass is typically antero-lateral to the healthy patulous cervix and lacks the symmetry of a cystocele. Treatment was excision which can be a formidable task when the cyst extends into the broad ligament. The sound identifies the external urinary meatus. Such cysts are usually much smaller and have a bluish colour due to the retained mucus seen through the thin cyst wall (plates 61 and 240).

Plate 168 Large uterovaginal prolapse in an elderly postmeno-pausal patient. Note atrophic vaginal epithelium and absence of cervix due to previous Manchester repair. The mass consists of large cystocele, small atrophic uterus and enterocele. The term procidentia by derivation means prolapse, but is used to describe any large prolapse protruding outside the introitus. It is also used to signify third degree uterine prolapse (when the uterine fundus lies at or below the level of the introitus); in these patients the vagina is usually completely everted (plate 170).

Plate 169 Huge procidentia in a 73-year-old patient who presented with acute retention of urine — hence the indwelling catheter. Vaginal eversion is incomplete and the urethra became kinked where the lower anterior vaginal wall remained normally supported. A cherry-red urethral caruncle is also visible. Note the keratinization of the long-exposed vaginal epithelium. When replacing such a prolapse push back enterocele contents first, then uterus and finally cystocele; this is the reverse order of descent of such a prolapse when the patient strains (or stands).

170

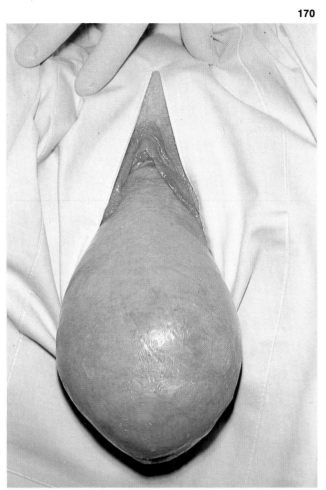

Plate 170 This, the largest procidentia we have seen, was an incidental finding in a 69-year-old para 2 diabetic admitted to a medical ward with hypertensive cardiac failure and peripheral vascular disease causing gangrene of the left foot! The mass has been irreducible for many years. The plasma urea was 60 mg per 100 ml (10 mmol/l) before vaginal hysterectomy and repair was performed. The mass consisted of a vast cystocele (ureters kinked outside the body), third degree uterine prolapse and an enormous enterocele containing loops of intestine.

Plate 171 Huge procidentia in a 75-year-old diabetic grand multipara living in the west of Ireland. The mass had been present for 30 years and shows gross keratinization and ulceration. Usually ulceration involves the cervix but this huge enterocele was the lowest part of the mass and most prone to injury. Such ulceration must be distinguished from carcinoma (biopsy if healing fails to occur after reduction of mass with vaginal pack). Note complete eversion of vagina. (Courtesy of Dr Christopher Targett).

Plate 172 Large uterovaginal and rectal prolapse in a patient at the Mater Misericordiae Hospital, Dublin. These neglected lesions are not a sign of lack of medical or hospital facilities, but are testimony to the equanimity and acceptance of disabilities by the aged. Many elderly women with large prolapses refuse surgery, claiming that 'the lump is no bother at all'. Others ultimately consent to surgery when urinary symptoms develop or ulceration causes haemorrhage.

171

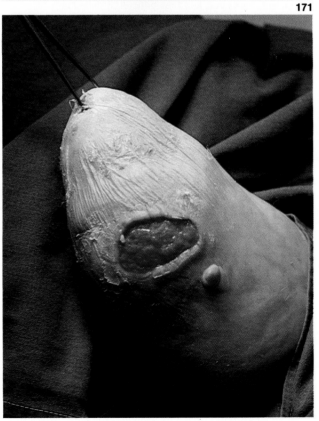

172

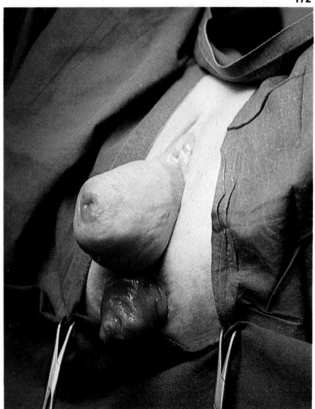

80

173

174

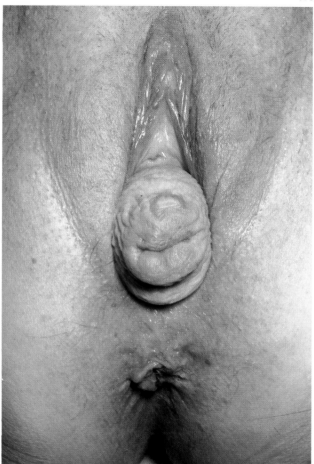

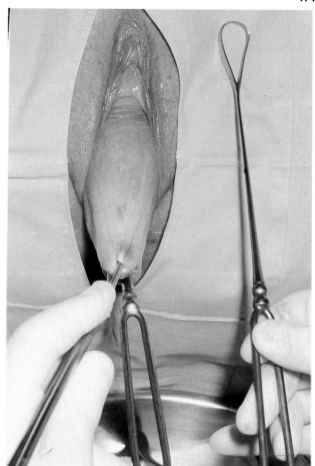

Plate 173 Procidentia in a 74-year-old para 4 with severe acromegaly. The prolapse had been present for many years. The mass is seen "at rest" with the patient anaesthetized and in the lithotomy position preparatory to draping for vaginal hysterectomy and repair. Note the large cystocele and enterocele.

Plate 174 Same patient shown in plate 173 illustrating the extent of the cervical hypertrophy and elongation; 18 cm length of curette lies within the patient whose uterus has *not* been perforated! Bimanual palpation revealed a small retroverted uterus which was soft and thus difficult to delineate.

Plate 175 Anterior colporrhaphy has commenced, the urethra and fascia overlying the cystocele being exposed by dissection of a triangular-shaped flap of anterior vaginal wall epithelium.

175

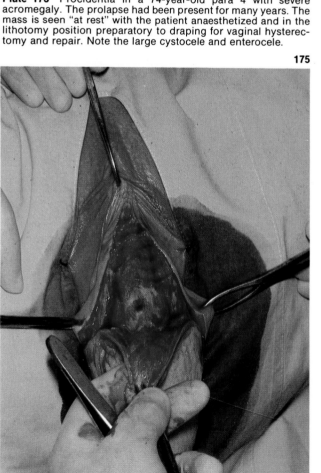

Plate 176 The anterior incision in the vaginal epithelium has been continued posteriorly and the uterus thus freed from vaginal attachment. The upper part of posterior vaginal wall will be removed with the uterus and will result in a shortened vagina unless the incision is closed vertically. The large pouch of Douglas (enterocele) has been opened. The next step in vaginal hysterectomy is clamping of uterosacral and transverse cervical ligaments. Organs are smaller outside the body due to loss of blood and tissue turgor; the operative specimen weighed 95 g, the dimensions being uterine body 9.5 cm, endocervical canal 4 cm.

Plate 177 Large enterocele or hernia of the pouch of Douglas in a 54-year-old para 3. The prolapse developed within 6 months of vaginal hysterectomy. The neck of such a hernial sac is large, and once the herniation is initiated, enlargement is rapid. Enterocele develops because of an abnormally deep pouch of Douglas and/or damage to the rectovaginal septum and levatores ani muscles caused by childbirth. The common type is a traction enterocele where the pouch of Douglas is drawn down the vagina as part of a genital prolapse. This picture shows the less common pulsion enterocele, where the elongated sac protrudes into the upper vagina, pushing the posterior vaginal wall ahead of it. Repair entails isolation and high ligation of the sac and closure of the space between the uterosacral ligaments and levatores ani muscles. (Courtesy of Dr Robert Zacharin).

176

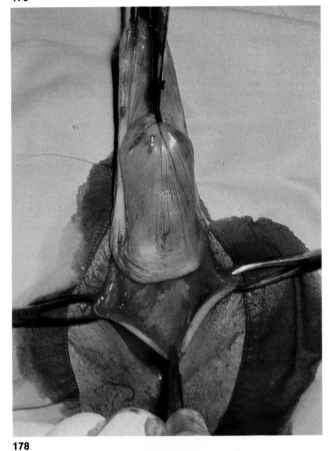

177

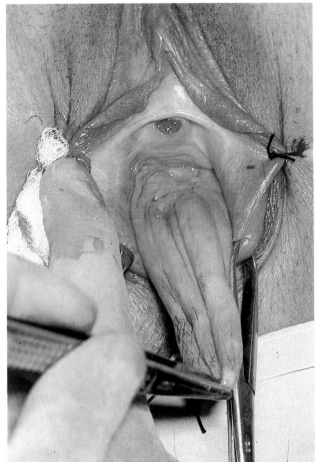

178

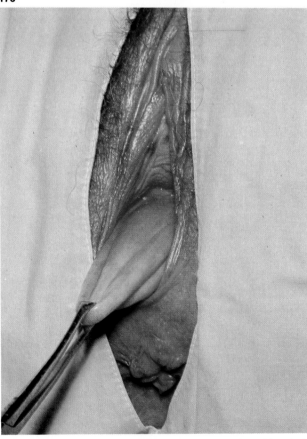

179

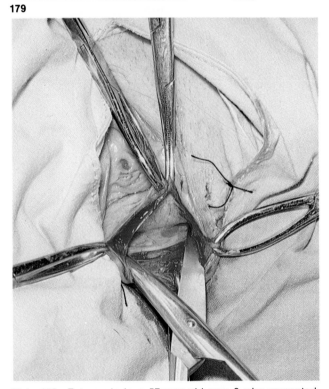

Plate 178 Huge rectocele demonstrated by traction with volsellum. The patient was a 55-year-old para 7 who presented because this lump was 'hanging outside and causing a dragging pain'. Treatment was vaginal hysterectomy and repair with excision of redundant posterior vaginal wall epithelium. There was no enterocele.

Plate 179 Enterocele in a 57-year-old para 2 who presented with a lump and bearing down sensation 13 years after vaginal hysterectomy. The vaginal vault was incised transversely and scissors demonstrate the pale, glistening peritoneum of the pouch of Douglas; the enterocele sac was separated from bladder and rectum and excised. Posterior colporrhaphy was then performed, the vaginal incision being closed vertically to allow a calibre adequate for continued coitus. (Courtesy of Dr Charles Barbaro).

82

180

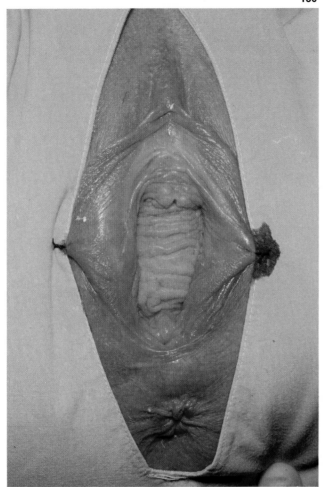

Plate 180 The following series of illustrations demonstrate the features of a procidentia treated by vaginal hysterectomy and repair. The patient was a 48-year-old para 3 who stated that she had noted a vaginal lump for 12 months which had become much larger in recent months. She had lower abdominal pain, intermittent bleeding and chafing from the lump, and stress incontinence of urine. The hyperkeratotic epithelium of the anterior vaginal wall is shown. Note that the uterine prolapse is not apparent.

181

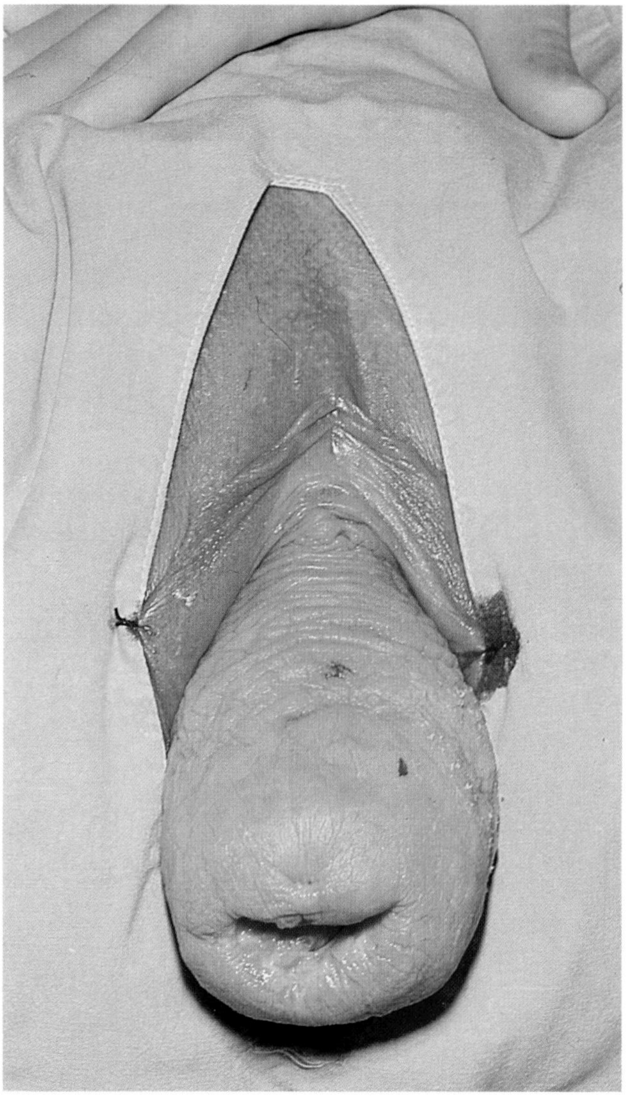

Plate 181 The uterus has been pulled down by traction on the cervix. There is enormous cervical hypertrophy which largely accounts for the size of the mass. The hyperkeratosis of ectocervical and vaginal squamous epithelium shown here only occurs where the area protrudes outside the introitus.

182

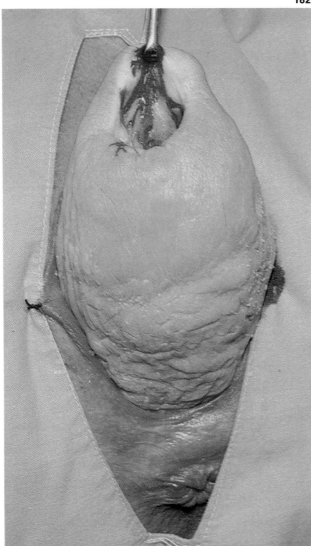

Plate 182 The cervix is grasped with a volsellum and held forwards to display the posterior vaginal wall. There was a moderate-sized enterocele and rectocele. The extent of an enterocele is often difficult to assess until the pouch of Douglas is opened.

183

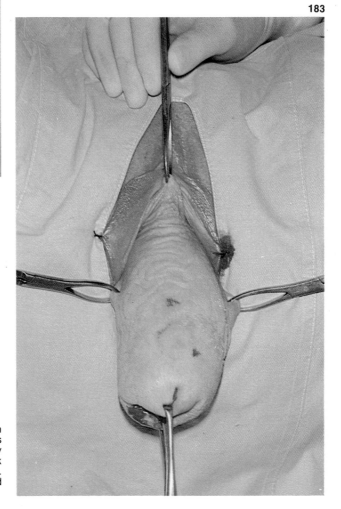

Plate 183 The 4 Morrison forceps outline the area of epithelium which will be excised from the anterior vaginal wall. The incisions run parallel to the introitus and extend to the external urinary meatus (plate 175) so that an adequate repair of the bladder neck area can be effected to restore the posterior urethrovesical angle. The uterus weighed 200 g; histological examination revealed adenomyosis and cystic hyperplasia of the endometrium.

184

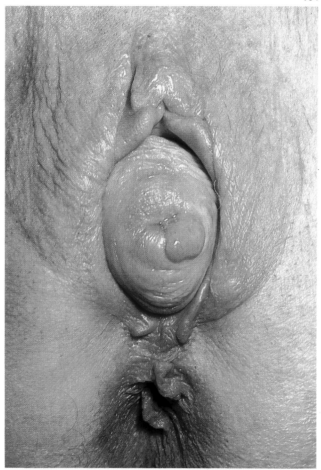

185

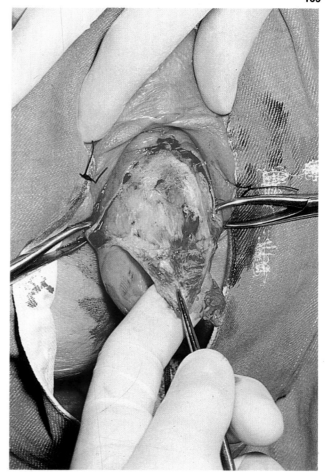

186

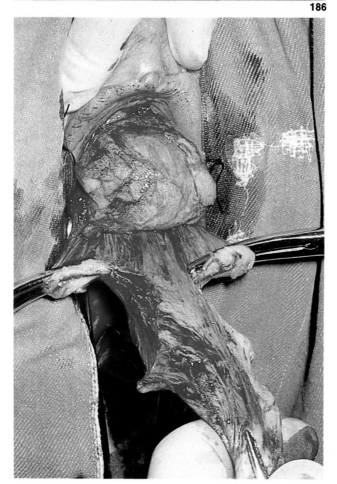

Plate 184 Third degree uterine prolapse with cystocele and rectocele in a hypertensive 89-year-old para 2 who presented because of urinary frequency and a vulval lump. A small endocervical polyp is shown protruding through the external os.

Plate 185 Manchester repair. Dilatation and curettage was performed to exclude endometrial carcinoma and facilitate reconstruction of the cervix. A triangular flap of epithelium has been dissected from the anterior vaginal wall exposing pubocervical fascia overlying the cystocele.

Plate 186 The bladder has been separated from the cervix by gauze and sharp dissection until the vesicouterine pouch of peritoneum was seen. The transverse cervical ligaments with descending branches of the uterine arteries have been clamped and divided on each side. Next the redundant cervix was amputated by cutting between the clamps.

Plate 187 A suture (posterior Sturmdorf) has been placed in the midline of the posterior vaginal wall flap and this will be used to cover the cervical stump which is held anteriorly. The pedicles of the transverse cervical ligaments are often ligated at this stage and attached to the cervical stump. There was no enterocele in this patient.

Plate 188 The posterior Sturmdorf suture has been completed. Sutures placed laterally and anteriorly will cover the stump, the anterior stitch being placed so as to act as a Fothergill stitch.

Plate 189 The Fothergill stitch fixes the transverse cervical (cardinal) ligaments to the anterior aspect of the cervical stump, elevating and anteverting the uterus, and creating the main support of the new vaginal vault.

Plate 190 The cervix has been reconstituted and mattress sutures in the vesical fascia have inverted the bladder wall and reduced the cystocele. Interrupted sutures are now inserted in the fascia between the vagina and bladder. The edges of the vagina are not undermined because excessive bleeding outweighs any advantage gained from wide lateral dissection.

187

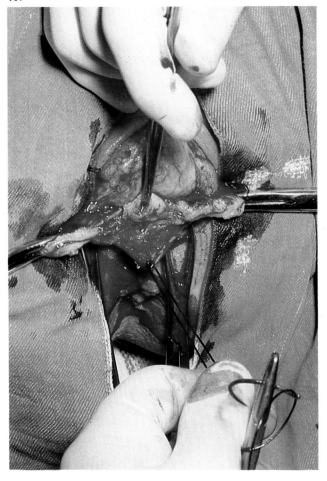

188

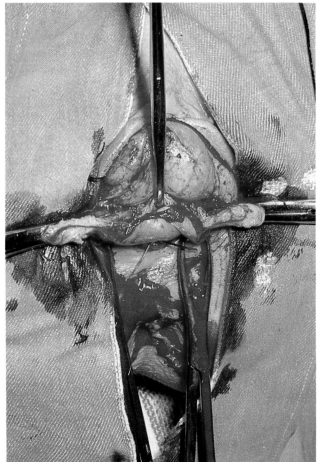

189

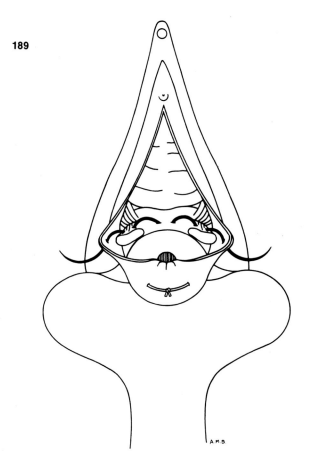

190

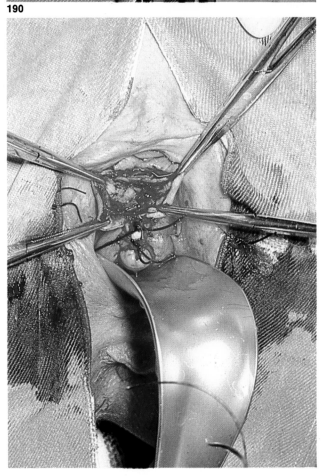

191

192

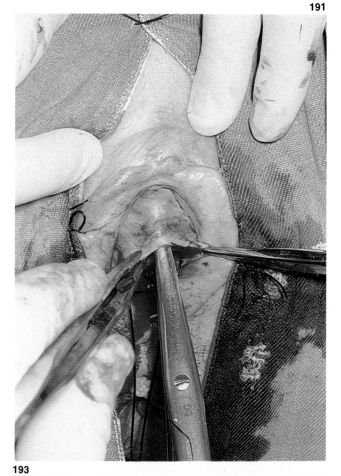

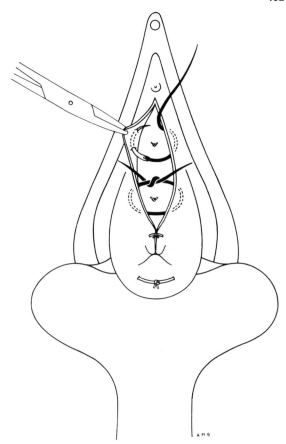

193

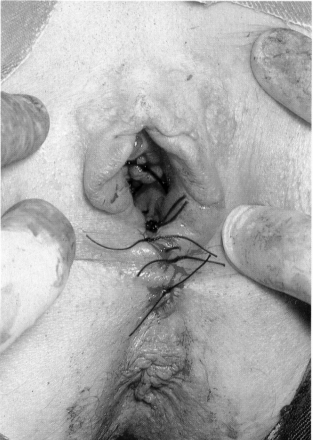

Plate 191 The apex of the anterior vaginal wall incision is extended to the external urinary meatus exposing the urethra. A suture is placed on either side of the bladder neck (as shown in plate 192) to elevate this area to maintain or restore a normal posterior urethrovesical angle and minimize the risk of stress incontinence of urine.

Plate 192 Two mattress sutures in vaginal fascia are shown. The technique, described by Dr George Gibson in Northern Ireland, is to hold the vaginal wall under tension with tissue forceps and insert the needle beneath the cut edge in a lateral direction and parallel to the surface of the vaginal epithelium. The stitch being inserted in paraurethral vaginal fascia will, when tied, elevate the urethrovesical junction. The 2 knots in the midline indicate where bladder has been inverted by sutures in vesical fascia.

Plate 193 Appearance after completion of the Manchester repair. A vaginal pack and indwelling urinary catheter are now inserted. Details of posterior colpoperineorrhaphy are shown in plates 390 to 392 and 410 to 415.

194

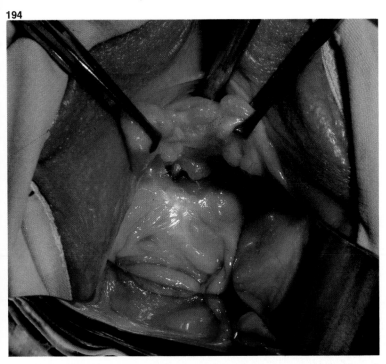

Plate 194 Vesicovaginal fistula which occurred as a complication of an Aldridge sling operation for treatment of stress incontinence of urine. Two failed attempts at closure of the fistula account for the dense scar tissue visible on the anterior vaginal wall, at the level of the urethrovesical junction. The anterior lip of cervix is visible at the edge of the Auvard speculum. Allis tissue forceps retract the vagina at the edges of the fistula. A metal catheter displays the external urinary meatus and its tip is visible in the base of the fistula. A successful repair was effected using a Martius graft (pedicle of fat from labium majus which covers the repaired fistula and lies between it and the vaginal epithelium).

196

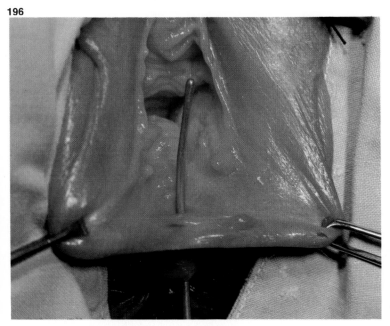

Plate 196 Rectovaginal fistula which occurred, as do 90% of cases, due to failure of healing after repair of a third degree tear at childbirth. Less common causes are posterior colpoperineorrhaphy and haemorrhoidectomy. The probe has been passed through the anus to emerge through the fistula, low on the posterior vaginal wall. Repair was effected by incision through the vaginal epithelium and external anal sphincter to lay open the fistula, with closure of rectum, suture of sphincter with reformation of the perineal body, and then closure of the vaginal epithelium. Such cases require neither grafting nor preliminary colostomy. (Courtesy of Dr Robert Zacharin).

195

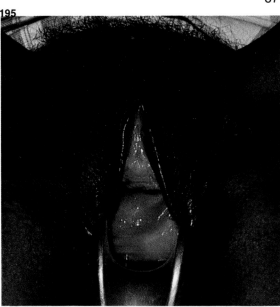

Plate 195 Vesicovaginal fistula. This large fistula, involving almost the entire anterior vaginal wall, was due to neglected obstructed labour in a patient who had not sought medical assistance at that time. Shown is the fistulous opening with the bladder mucosa clearly visible. The ureteric orifices could be seen at the posterior edge of the fistula. The urethra and urethrovesical angle were not damaged. This fistula was successfully repaired by the vaginal route.

Plate 197 Rectovaginal fistula in a 30-year-old para 4 whose last delivery, 6 years previously, of a 5,000 g infant, resulted in a third degree tear, which apparently was not repaired. She presented with intermittent dyspareunia. Note absent perineal body and retracted ends of torn external anal sphincter. Tissue forceps show vagina and rectum separated by only thin rectovaginal septum. During repair the vaginal epithelium and rectal mucosa were separated and the anterior rectal wall was restored. The levatores ani muscles were then sutured together anterior to the anal canal to reform the perineal body. Separated ends of the external sphincter were then sutured together and finally the perineal skin was sutured.

197

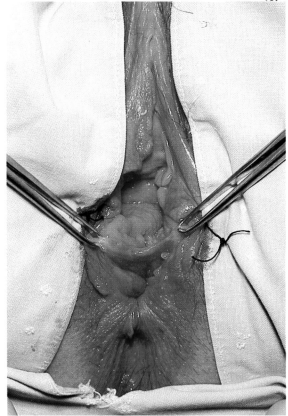

88

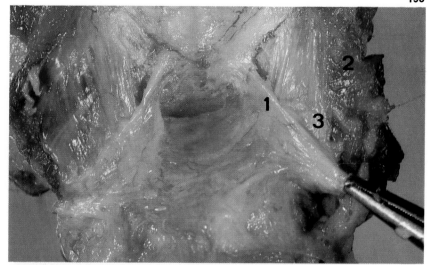

198

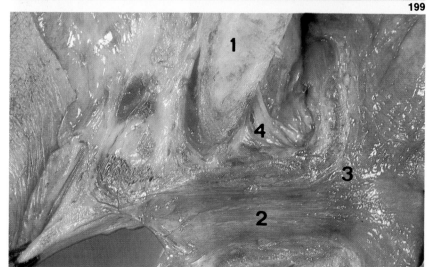

199

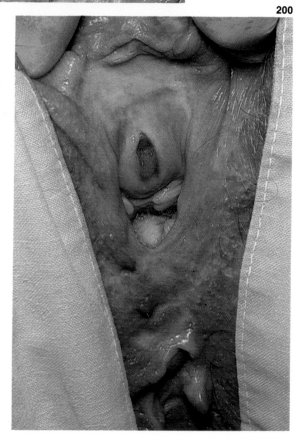

200

Plate 198 Pelvic surface of the pubic symphysis viewed from above. The posterior pubourethral ligaments (1), levatores ani muscles (2) and their fascia (3) are shown. Tension by the forceps emphasizes the expansion from the posterior pubourethral ligament which crosses the levator ani fascia.

Plate 199 The suspensory mechanism of the urethra, best described by Zacharin, whose abdominoperineal operation for stress incontinence of urine elevates the urethra by suturing aponeurotic strips, cut from the anterior abdominal wall, to the paraurethral attachment of the posterior pubourethral ligaments (Zacharin, R. F. Obstet. Gynec. 50:1 1977). This suspensory mechanism provides support of the upper urethra and bladder neck as the levatores ani muscles and pelvic cellular tissue maintain the position of the vagina and uterus. This magnified sagittal view of the pelvis shows symphysis pubis (1), urethra (2) and urethrovesical junction (3). The right posterior pubourethral ligament (4) is shown attaching to the upper third of the paraurethral tissue. This ligament has an expansion which passes below the symphysis to fuse with the anterior pubourethral ligament, which is a prolongation of the suspensory ligament of the clitoris.

Plate 200 Urethral caruncle in a 78-year-old para 4 who presented with vaginal spotting for 12 months. Urinary frequency had been present for years. Note that the cherry-red lesion is situated at the posterior aspect of the external urinary meatus. This common condition occurs after the menopause, is often asymptomatic, but can cause dysuria, dyspareunia and postcoital bleeding. Treatment was initially dienoestrol vaginal cream, but when bleeding persisted the caruncle was excised, the base cauterized, and uterine curettage performed (to exclude endometrial carcinoma). Caruncles are rarely malignant, but tend to recur after surgery. Local oestrogen therapy for associated senile vaginitis often provides symptomatic relief. This patient also has anal skin tags.

201

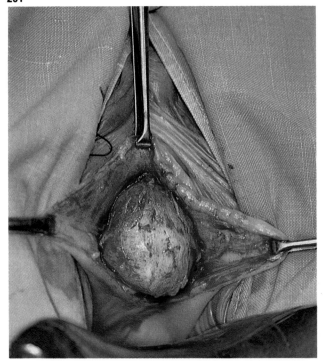

202

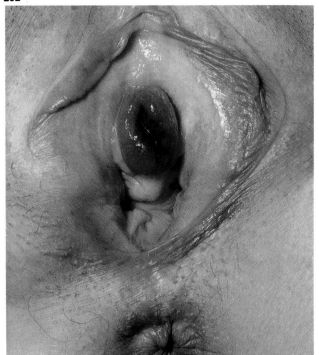

Plate 201 Urethral diverticulum. This condition is uncommon and notoriously difficult to diagnose unless urethroscopy as opposed to cystoscopy is performed. This patient was a 30-year-old para 2 who presented with recurrent 'bladder' infections. Palpation of the lump caused pus to appear at the external urinary meatus. Often it is necessary to lay open the urethra to determine the full extent of the lesion, which is then excised. Here the anterior vaginal wall has been incised in the midline and reflected to expose the sac of the diverticulum.

Plate 203 Huge urethral prolapse simulating cervix, in a 67-year-old para 1 who had noticed a vulval mass for 12 months. Hysterectomy had been performed for carcinoma of the endometrium 8 years previously and there was no evidence of recurrence. The prolapse was excised flush with the vestibule and the urethral mucosa sutured to the circumference of the external urinary meatus. Urethral prolapse can be so extreme in paraplegics, due to tissue laxity, that urinary diversion (ileal conduit) is required.

Plate 202 Prolapse of the urethral mucosa. Note the characteristic postmenopausal atrophy of the vaginal epithelium. Urethral prolapse is uncommon and is distinguished from a caruncle by the presence of the urethral orifice in its centre. The lesion is due to straining when there is urethritis and loss of tone in the urethral wall (due to lack of oestrogen). Sometimes (as seems to be the case in this patient) thrombosis of a vein forms the apex of the prolapse which is really an intussusception of the urethral wall.

Plate 204 Carcinoma of urethra. This fungating lesion was diagnosed as a carcinoma of the vulva, but at panendoscopy it was seen to be arising from the lower urethra. The patient was 50 years of age, but refused radical surgery, and response to excision of the tumour and local irradiation was excellent. The optimum treatment would have been radical vulvectomy with removal of inguinal, femoral and external iliac lymph nodes.

203

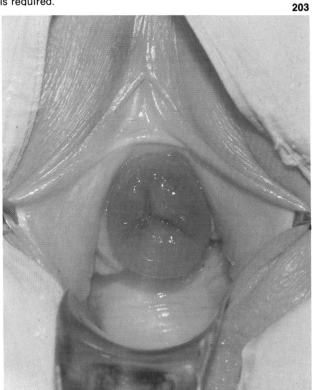

204

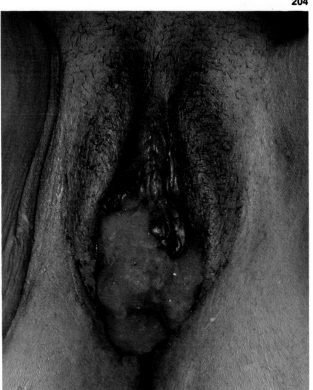

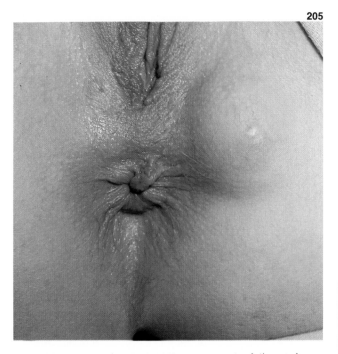

Plate 205 Unusually large sebaceous cyst of the perineum posterolateral to the fourchette, but not extending into the labium majus and hence obviously not a cyst or abscess of Bartholin's gland or duct (plate 211). Note the punctum of the obstructed sebaceous duct on the summit of the cyst. The overlying skin was incised, the cyst removed intact and the cavity oversewn. Small sebaceous cysts are very common in the labia minora and majora and often become infected.

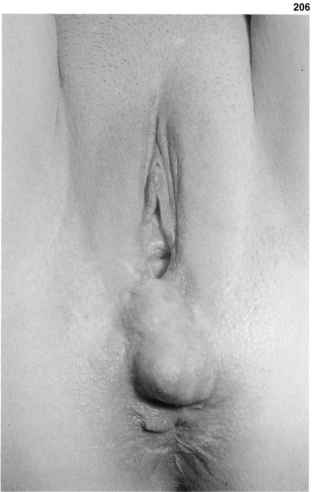

Plate 206 Inclusion dermoid due to desquamation of cells from epithelium invaginated at repair of an episiotomy incision. The patient was a 33-year-old para 2 whose children were aged 10 and 7 years, respectively. Her first episiotomy was large, broke down and required resuture. Small inclusion cysts are often seen when cutting through old episiotomy scars at subsequent deliveries, but large lesions such as this are rare.

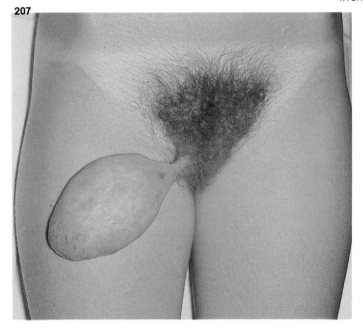

207

Plate 207 Neurofibroma of the vulva in a single, 17-year-old virgin. One might wonder where she hid the tumour when she sunbathed in her bikini! She weighed 48.3 kg. The lump had grown during the past 12 months and had been painful for 2 months; it was attached by a 1 cm base to the right labium majus and was 15 cm in length and ulcerated in 2 areas. There was an intact annular hymen. The pedicle was transfixed, ligated and divided.

208

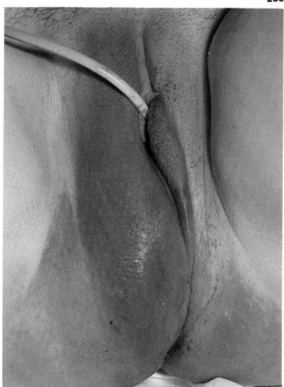

Plate 208   Vulval haematoma extending into buttocks and right labium majus. The patient was unable to void and hence the indwelling catheter. She required a 4-unit blood transfusion. Treatment was conservative and the clot discharged 9 days later. Some physicians favour immediate evacuation of the clot, mainly to relieve pain, but this can result in difficulty in achieving haemostasis. This patient had had a difficult forceps delivery and third degree tear. The same condition can be due to falling astride, or follow a normal delivery, with or without an episiotomy.

209

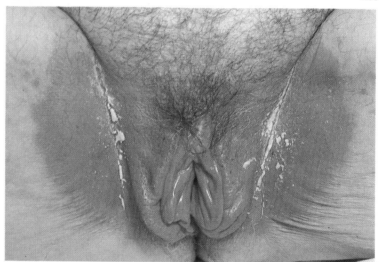

Plate 209   Classical diabetic vulvitis in an obese (80 kg) 69-year-old para 3. This typical brick-red appearance and labial oedema subsided with control of her diabetes (fasting blood sugar 16 mmol/l). She had presented with pruritus vulvae which had defied treatment by her local practitioner for 4 months. Monilial infection alone does not account for this clinical picture.

210

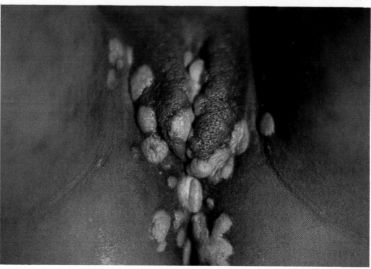

Plate 210   Secondary syphilis. These multiple condylomata lata of the vulva and perineum show pregnancy-induced hypertrophy. Some of the lesions show the characteristic central depression. Note that the lesions extend onto the patient's thighs (plate 159).

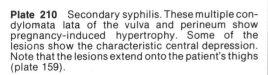

92

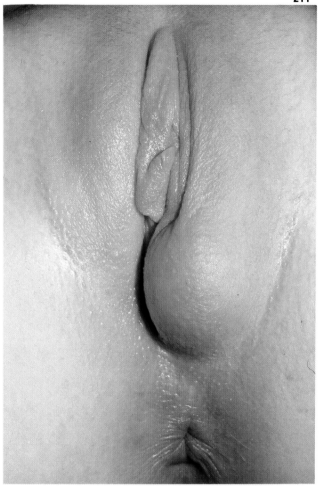

211

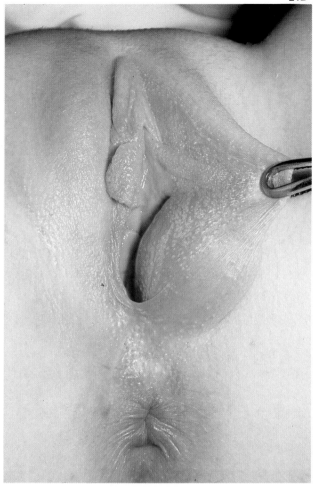

212

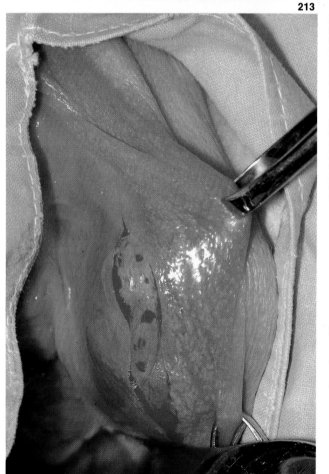

213

Plate 211 Bartholin's cyst in a 22-year-old para 1 who presented because of the vulval lump and superficial dyspareunia which developed 12 weeks after her confinement. Incision of a labial cyst had been performed 18 months previously. This 'cyst', although only slightly tender, was in fact an abscess, since after excision it was found to contain thick pus which grew E.coli. Often the ductal obstruction that causes cyst or abscess formation is due to gonococcal infection.

Plate 212 Vulval skin pulled to the left to display the abscess in the typical location in the posterior half of the labium majus. The vulval tissues are readily distensible (cyst, abscess, blood) and a Bartholin's cyst of moderate dimensions can be overlooked unless the area is palpated between finger in vagina and thumb on perineum. When there is associated cellulitis there is acute pain and treatment should be chemotherapy and marsupialization rather than excision.

Plate 213 Excision of Bartholin's cyst. The incision is made parallel to the long axis of the labium majus just below the hymeneal remnant where vagina joins vulva. If sited on the vulva, the resulting scar can cause dyspareunia. Vaginal epithelium, unlike labial skin, contains glycogen and stains black with Lugol's 5% iodine solution which can be used to delineate the correct site for the incision.

214

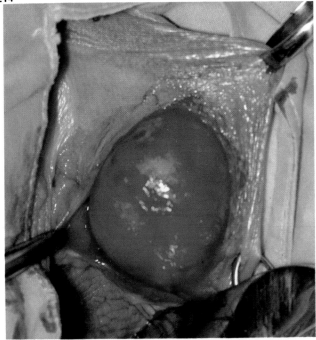

215

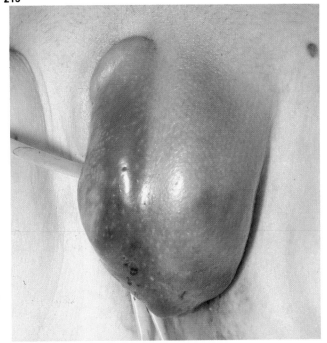

Plate 214 The cyst has almost been enucleated. The vulva is very vascular and excision of a Bartholin's cyst may turn out to be a major procedure. Hence the recent popularity of marsupialization of cyst or abscess, where only an elipse of the medial wall is excised, and the edges of cyst wall and vagina are sutured together to allow drainage. This operation is easier and retains the function of the gland, but the persistent pouch disappoints some patients (plate 216).

Plate 215 Although interrupted sutures were used to obliterate the depths of the cavity, and a drain was inserted, this patient developed a large vulval haematoma. This was treated conservatively, although some surgeons favour immediate evacuation of the clot and resuture. The patient was unable to void because of pain and required an indwelling catheter. This photograph was taken 6 days after surgery; 2 days later the dependent, gangrenous skin sloughed and the clot discharged. Healing was complete after 12 days' hospitalization.

Plate 216 Late result of marsupialization of a left Bartholin's cyst in a 37-year-old para 1 presenting with secondary infertility. The forceps displaces the left labium majus, showing the blind pouch which simulates a double vagina; the vaginal wall that was stretched over the cyst appears as a vaginal septum (plate 35). The patient had (surprisingly) no coital problems due to the pouch or 'septum'. There are few reports of long term results of marsupialization of Bartholin's cysts or abscesses. The operation is simple and relatively bloodless, but the final result is less aesthetic even when function of the gland is maintained. **216**

Plate 217 Incomplete rupture of the hymen in a 28-year-old, 4-year married nullipara, who complained of recurrent postcoital urethrotrigonitis (frequency and scalding), in spite of voiding immediately after coitus. This persistence of 'honeymoon urethritis' is due to introduction of bacteria into the urethra when the meatus is pulled open and directed into the vagina as the introitus is dilated during penetration. This occurs because the hymen is attached to the anterior vaginal wall. It happens even in the absence of dyspareunia, because the hymen is distensible as in this patient. The condition is not uncommon and can destroy a marriage. Treatment is division of the anterior bridge of the hymen on either side of the external urinary meatus. **217**

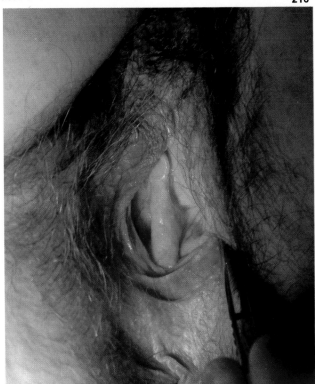

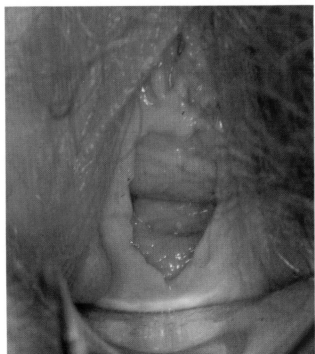

94

218

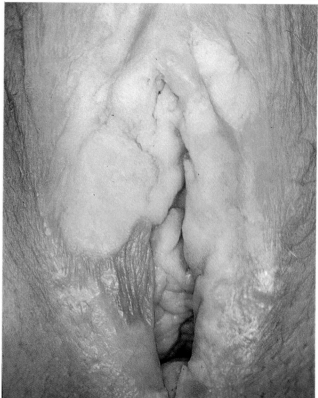

219

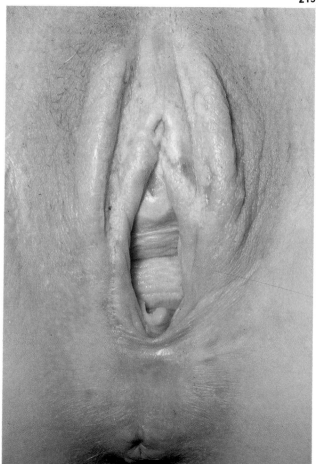

220

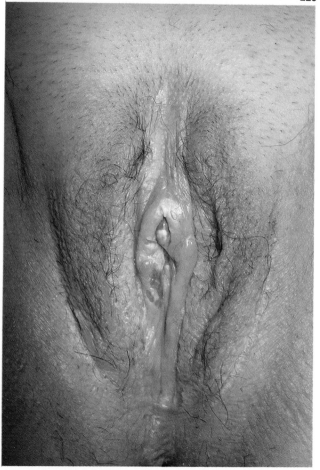

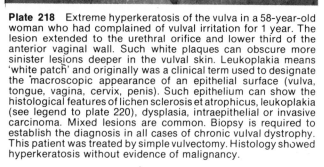

Plate 218 Extreme hyperkeratosis of the vulva in a 58-year-old woman who had complained of vulval irritation for 1 year. The lesion extended to the urethral orifice and lower third of the anterior vaginal wall. Such white plaques can obscure more sinister lesions deeper in the vulval skin. Leukoplakia means 'white patch' and originally was a clinical term used to designate the macroscopic appearance of an epithelial surface (vulva, tongue, vagina, cervix, penis). Such epithelium can show the histological features of lichen sclerosis et atrophicus, leukoplakia (see legend to plate 220), dysplasia, intraepithelial or invasive carcinoma. Mixed lesions are common. Biopsy is required to establish the diagnosis in all cases of chronic vulval dystrophy. This patient was treated by simple vulvectomy. Histology showed hyperkeratosis without evidence of malignancy.

Plate 219 Leukoplakia of the vulva in a 48-year-old multipara who presented with severe pruritus. Whitening of the skin had been present for 20 years, but had recently become more marked and cracks had occurred. Radioactive phosphorus uptake did not suggest abnormal mitotic activity characteristic of dysplasia or carcinoma. Biopsy revealed hyperkeratosis with a mixed hyper-trophic/atrophic pattern (mixed chronic vulval dystrophy) and no nuclear atypia.

Plate 220 Chronic mixed vulval dystrophy (hypertrophic and atrophic areas) involving mainly labia minora and perineum in a 62-year-old para 1 who presented with urinary frequency, urgency and strangury and also pruritus vulvae. She had atrophic vaginal epithelium and marked narrowing of the introitus (previously called kraurosis vulvae). Radioactive phosphorus testing showed no area of increased uptake, but even so all such lesions warrant biopsy to exclude carcinoma. The condition had progressed over 7 years and fissures occurred at the posterior fourchette on occasions. Biopsy showed hyperkeratosis, epithelial hyperplasia, elongation of rete pegs and hyalinization of the subepithelial layer (histological criteria of leukoplakia), with other areas showing atrophic epithelium and underlying fibrosis (histological criteria of lichen sclerosis et atrophicus). Symptoms improved with application of 1% hydrocortisone cream to vulva and dienoestrol cream to vagina. Androgen cream is also effective in this condition. Glucose tolerance was normal. Simple vulvectomy was planned if symptoms returned. Continued surveillance is mandatory because of the risk of carcinoma.

221

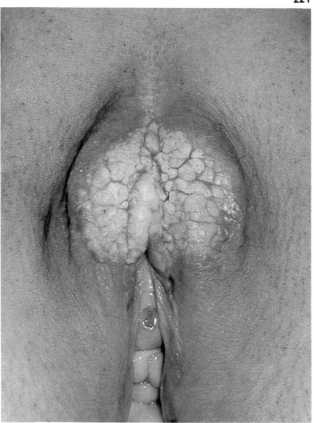

Plate 221 Leukoplakia localized to the anterior aspect of the vulva involving the clitoris, labia majora and labia minora. Note that the remainder of the vulval skin is atrophic. Treatment was local excision of the white area with continued surveillance of the rest of the vulva.

Plate 222 Hidradenoma of left labium majus in a 50-year-old para 6 who had noticed the lump for several years and presented when it became painful and bled. It had rolled edges and a friable centre; umbilication is typical of this lesion which arises from sweat glands. Histologically the dermis was packed with papillary projections covered by regular columnar epithelium. The tumour is uncommon, always benign, although misdiagnosed as adenocarcinoma in the past. Excisional biopsy provided diagnosis and curative treatment.

Plate 223 Fibrolipoma of the vulva in an 84-year-old para 2 with Parkinson's disease. She was a strong-minded old lady and insisted that this lump, which had been present for many years, did not bother her. She consented to its removal (a simple 5-minute procedure with excision across the pedicle and suture of skin) only when ulceration resulted in haemorrhage. As explained in the legend to plate 172, the aged do not complain and indeed often refuse surgical treatment that is clearly indicated. This patient also had an asymptomatic cystocele, enterocele and rectocele of moderate dimensions.

222

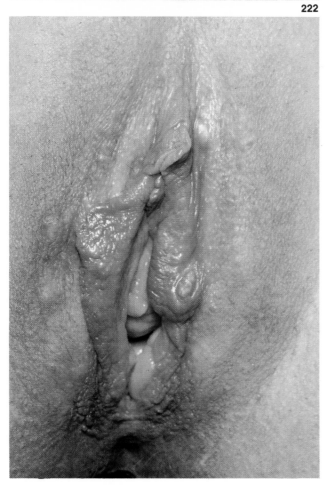

223

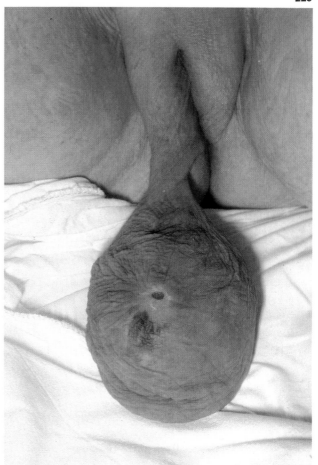

224

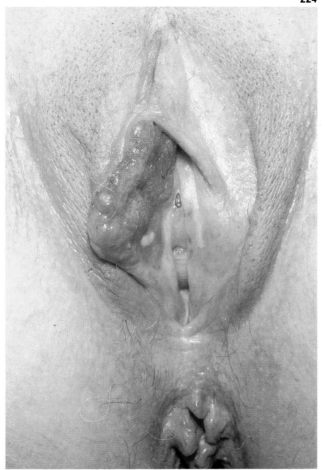

225

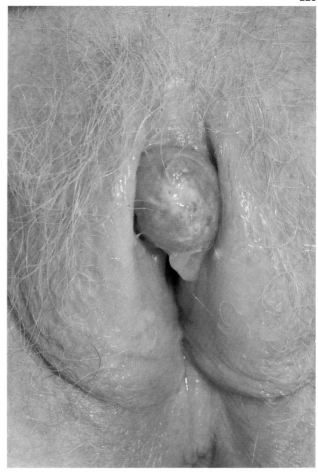

226

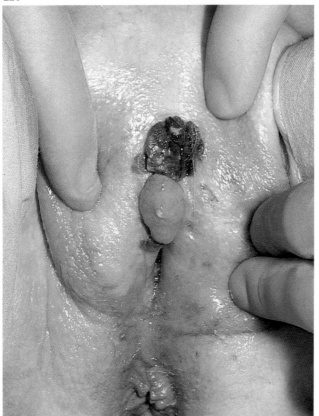

Plate 224 Carcinoma of the vulva in a 60-year-old, para 2 diabetic. She had noticed a lump in the right labium majus, slowly increasing in size for 9 months, with recent contact bleeding. The anterior vulval skin shows leukoplakia. Excisional biopsy (4 × 2 × 1 cm) showed a well differentiated squamous cell carcinoma; radical vulvectomy was performed 12 days later. There was no tumour in the operative specimen, which included relevant lymph nodes. The patient remains well 7 years after surgery without evidence of recurrence.

Plate 225 Carcinoma of the clitoris in a 71-year-old patient who had had 3 heart attacks and was in cardiac failure. She presented with a 6-month history of a painful vulval swelling and recent bleeding. Biopsy showed a well differentiated squamous carcinoma. Simple vulvectomy was performed and the patient died with metastatic disease 3 months later.

Plate 226 Malignant melanoma of the vulva in a 76-year-old nullipara. The tumour is characteristically pigmented and has infiltrated lymphatics near the clitoris causing it to become oedematous and erect. The patient was unfit for radical surgery (hemiplegia due to previous stroke) so excisional biopsy (5 × 3 × 2 cm deep), removing mass and clitoris, was performed. Histology showed a cellular mass of melanin-containing spindle naevus cells with extensive invasion of the dermis. The patient survived for 3 years then returned with multiple lymph node metastases in the groins and succumbed without further treatment. (Courtesy of Dr Michael Somerville).

227

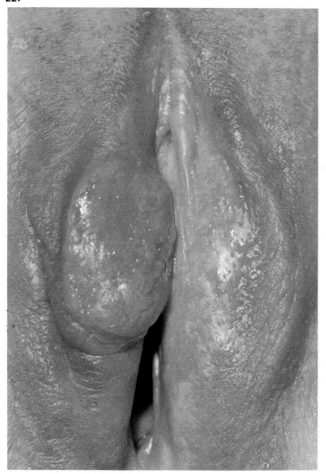

228

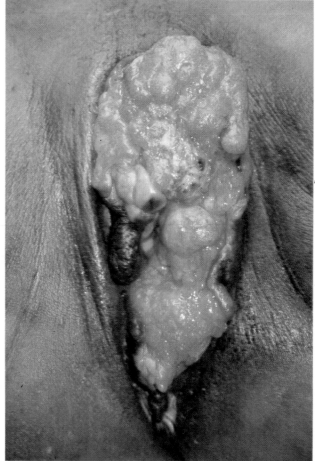

229

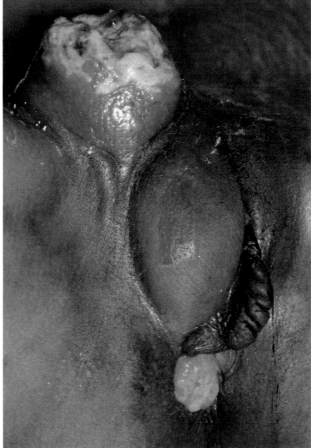

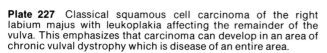

Plate 227 Classical squamous cell carcinoma of the right labium majus with leukoplakia affecting the remainder of the vulva. This emphasizes that carcinoma can develop in an area of chronic vulval dystrophy which is disease of an entire area.

Plate 228 Carcinoma of the vulva. This exophytic vulval lesion was seen in a 65-year-old patient who had noted the presence of a lump on the vulva for only 3 months. Diagnosed on biopsy as a squamous cell carcinoma, it involved the lower urethra and vagina, and extended over the perineum to the anterior margin of the anus. Treatment was radical vulvectomy with removal of the lower third of the urethra and vagina, and external anal sphincter as well as groin and pelvic lymphadenectomy. Healing, following primary closure of the operative defect, was satisfactory, and the removed lymph nodes were histologically clear of carcinoma.

Plate 229 Too late presentation of carcinoma of the vulva with ulcerating inguinal lymph node metastases in a 72-year-old patient. The relatively small primary growth of this squamous cell carcinoma is seen fungating from the posterior fourchette where it arose at the junction of vagina and perineum. The right labium majus is oedematous and displaced by a huge mass of tumour plus lymphoedema due to associated secondary infection. The patient died before treatment could be commenced.

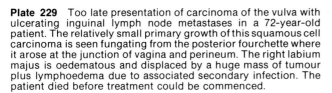

98

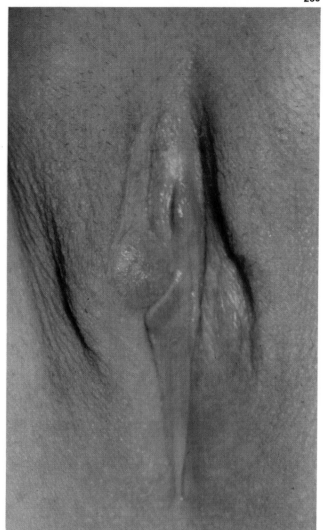

Plate 230 Squamous cell carcinoma of right labium majus in a 65-year-old para 1 who had had a stroke and femoral embolectomy. She had noticed the lump enlarging for 3 months; it was tender and bled on contact but was not ulcerated. In view of her debility, treatment was excisional biopsy. The patient died 6 years later.

231

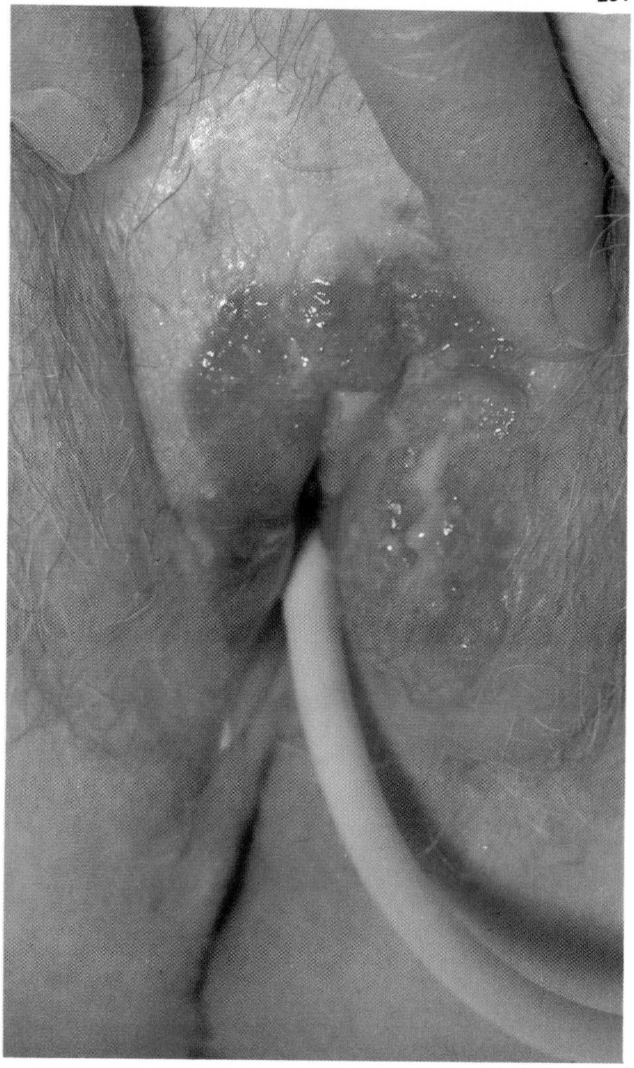

Plate 231 Well differentiated squamous cell carcinoma of left labium majus extending onto clitoris, right labium majus and lower 2 cm of vagina. The patient was an 85-year-old para 3 who presented with progressively severe dysuria for 4 months and a painful lump for 6 weeks. Treatment was radical vulvectomy, inguinal lymphadenectomy and removal of the lower one-third of vagina. Although the lymph nodes were free of tumour, a local recurrence developed 11 months later and finally caused her demise 26 months after her initial presentation.

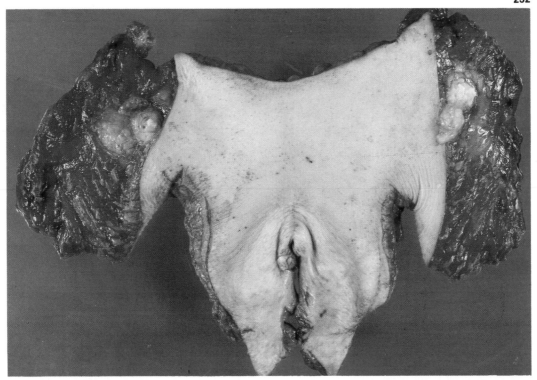

Plate 232 Radical vulvectomy specimen showing bilateral involvement of inguinal lymph glands from a squamous cell carcinoma of the clitoris in an 83-year-old nullipara who presented with a lump in the vulva of 6 weeks' duration. Four months later masses were palpable on the lateral pelvic walls and she died 14 months after operation.

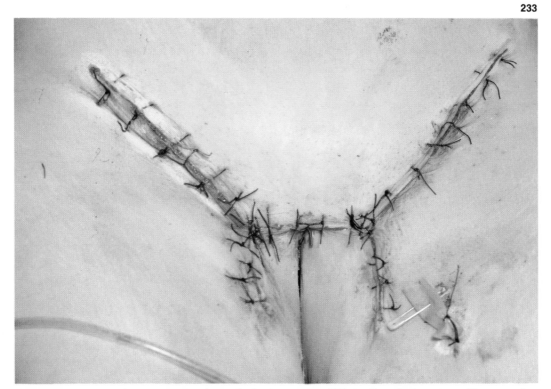

Plate 233 Postoperative appearance after radical vulvectomy and bilateral lymphadenectomy. The suture line around the new introitus cannot be seen (plate 419). These patients are often obese and primary skin closure is possible as here. The patient was aged 60 years and had a 2.5 cm diameter, ulcerating squamous cell carcinoma of the left labium majus when she presented with postmenopausal bleeding. She is alive and well 16 years after surgery.

234

235

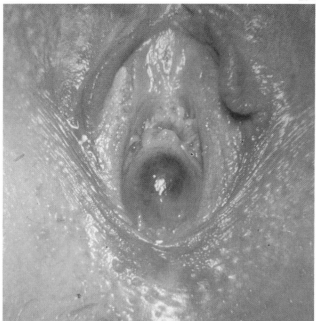

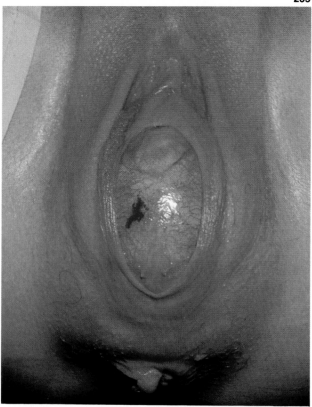

Plate 234 Cryptomenorrhoea due to a transverse vaginal septum in a 15-year-old girl who presented because of vague abdominal pain for 6 months. A haematocolpos caused a symmetrical abdominal mass that extended to the level of the umbilicus. A bulging blue membrane was situated above the hymen which is seen at the circumference of the occluding membrane and was pushed downwards by it. Rectal examination revealed a fluctuant mass filling the pelvis. The septum was excised and 600 ml of thick brown fluid drained away. An intravenous pyelogram was normal. Histology of the septum showed squamous epithelium on the lower surface and columnar epithelium on the upper surface — the latter cells had the appearance of endocervical epithelium. Usually a transverse vaginal septum has squamous epithelium on both surfaces.

Plate 235 Imperforate hymen bulging downwards with the pressure from haematocolpos above; view under anaesthesia before excision of the membrane and drainage of retained menstrual blood. The patient was aged 16 years and presented with urinary frequency, pelvic discomfort and primary amenorrhoea. She had noticed fullness in the perineum for 6 months. Signs of puberty had been present for 3 years.

Plate 236 Tarry fluid blood escapes under pressure after a scalpel has incised the bulging transverse vaginal septum (above level of hymen) in a 15-year-old girl who presented with amenorrhoea and an abdominal mass extending to the umbilicus that her local practitioner thought was an ovarian cyst. This case is similar to that shown in plate 234. The mass was entirely due to the haematocolpos which contained 1,200 ml of blood. Retained blood balloons the vagina and sometimes the tubes (haematosalpinges), but the uterus, with its thicker muscle wall, is less distensible. Blood in the tubes can result in inflammation, tubal occlusion and sterility, and reflux can cause endometriosis. These cases would not occur if it was routine practice to take the temperature of all female infants at birth with a thermometer inserted into the vagina. The septum was excised. (Courtesy of Dr Graeme Ratten).

236

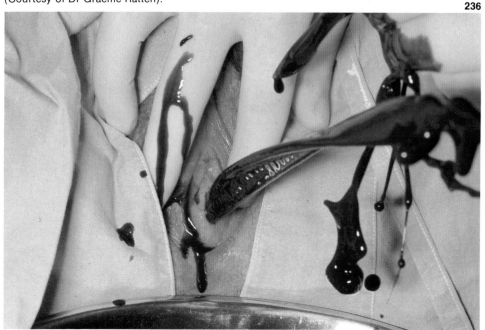

237

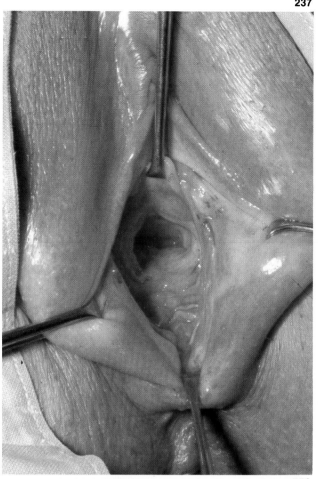

Plate 237 Vaginal stenosis due to excessive excision of vaginal epithelium at posterior colporrhaphy. The patient had had 3 vaginal repairs for correction of stress incontinence of urine. Considerable experience is required to master the technique of posterior colporrhaphy. Hence this operative complication, which causes severe dyspareunia, (the presenting symptom in this patient), is called a 'registrar's ring'.

Plate 238 Repair was achieved by incising the vagina vertically and suturing the wound transversely. A similar but less extensive procedure is performed to relieve superficial dyspareunia due to a tight perineum, when other means of dilatation have failed. This view shows the remaining scar tissue in the midline that must be incised to reach the level of the ring at the junction of the upper and middle thirds of vagina. Note how retraction of the cut edges of vagina has widened the introitus.

Plate 239 Skin from the left side of the vulva was rotated as a broad-based flap (to avoid sloughing due to impairment of blood supply) to fill the defect in the posterior vaginal wall. This view shows the flap sutured in position, with 2 drains to avoid haematoma formation. The vagina now has an adequate capacity. (Courtesy of Dr Robert Zacharin).

238

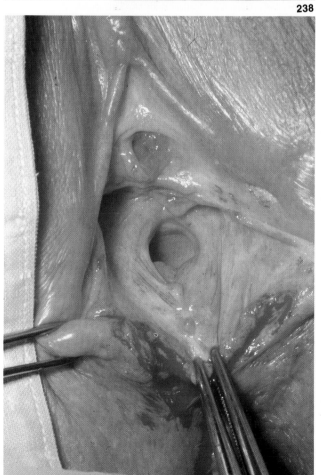

239

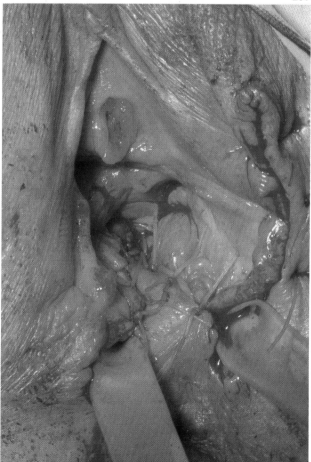

240

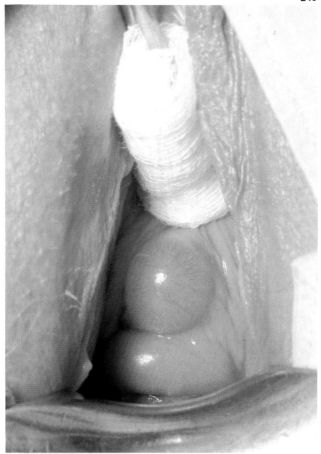

241

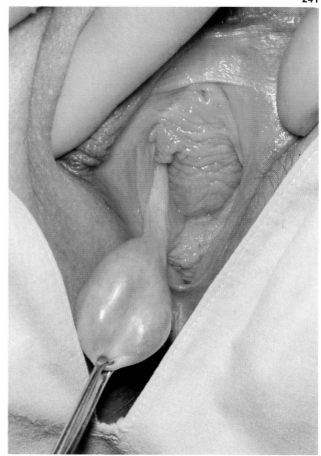

242

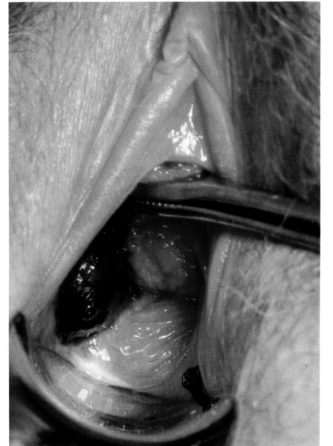

Plate 240 Cyst of Gartner's duct. The swab displaces the anterior vaginal wall to display the bluish, benign, translucent cyst, typically anterolateral to the cervix. These lesions are usually small as in this patient, but can be large and multiple (plates 61 and 167). Although often asymptomatic, the patient may complain of a vaginal lump or dyspareunia. Gartner's duct (mesonephric or Wolffian duct) runs from the mesosalpinx via the broad ligament to cervix, thence in an anterolateral position throughout the whole length of the vagina. Occasionally, malignant tumours arise from the duct causing adenocarcinoma of cervix or vagina.

Plate 241 Benign vaginal fibroma with myxomatous degeneration. The patient was a 43-year-old para 5 who stated that the mass had steadily enlarged over an interval of at least 5 years. She had regular periods. The pedicle of the tumour was clamped, divided and ligated.

Plate 242 Multiple primary malignant melanomas of the vagina in a 72-year-old multipara. She presented with postmenopausal bleeding. Note that the lesions are characteristically black due to melanin production. The larger lesion extends half-way up the right lateral vaginal wall. Treatment was excisional biopsy. More radical treatment (vaginectomy, vulvectomy with groin and pelvic lymph node dissection) was unacceptable, and unreasonable in view of the patient's age and the biology of this tumour. Two years later the patient developed liver secondaries and died (plate 226). (Courtesy of Dr William Chanen).

243

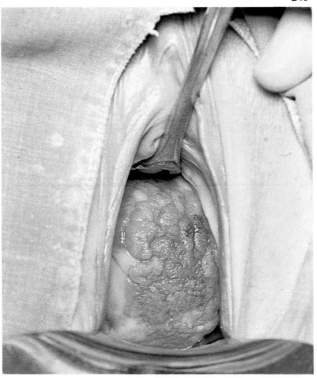

244

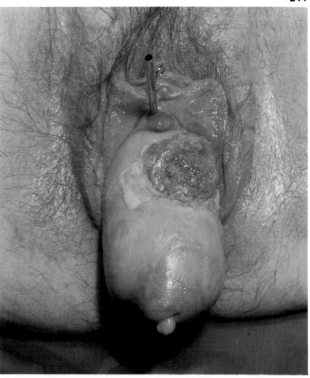

Plate 243 Intraepithelial carcinoma of the anterior vaginal wall as seen 14 months after total abdominal hysterectomy performed for carcinoma in situ of the cervix in a 50-year-old para 5. The lesion disappeared after radon application and subsequent vaginal biopsies showed normal epithelium. The message is that continued surveillance is required after definitive treatment of intraepithelial carcinoma of the cervix (plate 295).

Plate 244 Large necrotic ulcerating squamous cell carcinoma of lower anterior vaginal wall in an 85-year-old woman who had had a large procidentia for 20 years. These lesions were usually associated with prolonged use of a rubber pessary which had not been changed, but there was no such history in this patient. The metal catheter displays a polypoid urethral caruncle and a cervical polyp is also shown. Treatment was local excision and the vagina healed completely! She died of unrelated causes 12 months later.

245

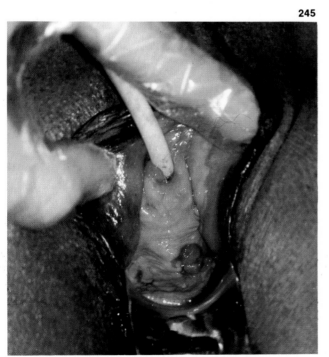

Plate 245 Primary, clear-cell adenocarcinoma of the vagina arising in the mesonephric remnant that runs in the anterolateral vaginal wall from cervix to external urinary meatus (plates 61, 167 and 240). The patient was aged 65 years and presented with vaginal bleeding from this soft, haemorrhagic tumour, which was invading the anterior vaginal wall at the junction of middle and upper thirds. Tumour was visible through the external urinary meatus, and involvement of the bladder base, with fistula through to the vagina, was apparent at cystoscopy. Intrauterine exposure to diethylstilboestrol can predispose to the development of this tumour, but had not occurred in this patient. Anterior pelvic exenteration was planned, but the patient refused such radical surgery. (Courtesy of Dr David Abell).

246

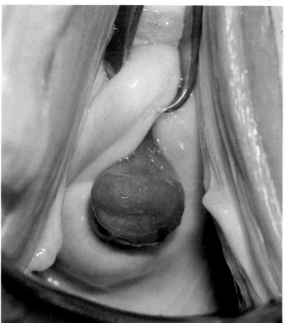

Plate 246 Endocervical polyp in a 69-year-old Italian woman who presented with a 3-year history of post-menopausal bleeding which had been profuse for 6 months. The haemorrhagic polyp, seen extruding through the dilated external os, contrasts sharply with the atrophic vaginal epithelium. Treatment was polypectomy and curettage (to exclude coexistent endometrial cancer), although many would advocate hysterectomy in a patient of this age. Histology showed cystically dilated glands without evidence of malignancy.

Plate 248 Endometrial polyp. The patient was a 41-year-old para 6 who presented with a 6-month history of non-irritating, offensive vaginal discharge and intermenstrual bleeding. Note dilated external os and patulous external urethral meatus. The polyp appears infected and hence the discharge and bleeding; it was removed vaginally and contained endometrial glands and stroma. Clinically, because of its position, it was thought to be arising from the endocervix.

247

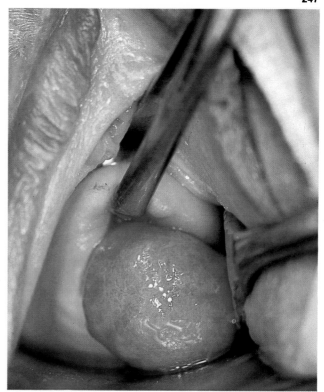

Plate 247 Cervical polyp in a 54-year-old patient who presented with postmenopausal bleeding of 4 weeks' duration. The anterior lip of the cervix has been grasped with a volsellum forceps and the polyp protrudes through the expanded external os. There were no currettings. A cervical polyp can have a carcinoma of the endometrium above, just as bleeding haemorrhoids can have a carcinoma of the rectum above!

Plate 249 Pedunculated endocervical polyp (5.5 × 2.5 × 1.5 cm) in a 55-year-old para 3 who presented with heavy post-menopausal bleeding of 1 day's duration. The polyp was twisted off and histology revealed cystic glands and inflammatory changes — hence the bleeding. Curettage was carried out to exclude endometrial carcinoma and there were no curettings.

248

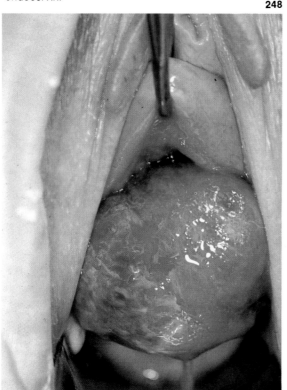

249

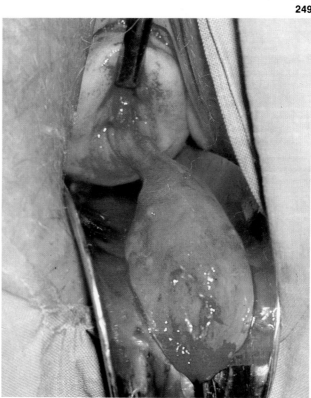

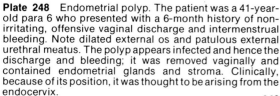

250

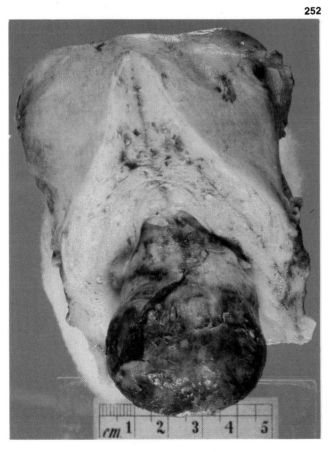

Plate 250 Chronic inversion of the uterus. The patient was an obese 24-year-old para 5, confined 8 weeks previously who required manual removal of the placenta. Note the glistening red surface of the endometrium and central canal simulating the external os and indicating that the inversion was incomplete. A ring pessary was inserted and a spontaneous cure resulted.

251

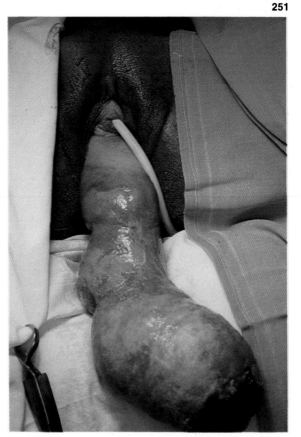

Plate 251 Large chronic complete inversion of the uterus and vagina due to a large submucous fibromyoma in a Papua New Guinean. She was para 3 and had noted a large lump protruding from the vulva for 10 months. The 10 cm submucous polyp had a broad base, attached to the fundus of a completely inverted uterus. The cervix could be palpated at the junction with vagina, and lay well outside the introitus. An intravenous pyelogram showed that the lower ureters and the bladder lay beyond the introitus. The patient was emaciated and severely anaemic. After a 7-unit blood transfusion, laparotomy was performed and the internal iliac arteries were ligated. Then, the polyp was excised from below, and the uterus and cervix were incised vertically along the posterior aspect and repositioned after incising, from above, the posterior aspect of the ring through which the right ovary and tube had passed. Abdominal hysterectomy was performed after the pelvic viscera were replaced to their normal position, the vault being suspended to the round ligaments to prevent future prolapse. (Courtesy of Dr Peter Henderson).

252

Plate 252 Uterus (190 g) incised in lower anterior wall showing a broad-based submucous fibromyomatous polyp (6 × 4 × 3 cm) attached to the posterior uterine wall and protruding through the cervix. The end of the polyp was haemorrhagic, necrotic, ulcerated and painted blue. The patient was a 49-year-old para 4 who presented with dysmenorrhoea, menorrhagia and offensive vaginal discharge of 4 months' duration. Her haemoglobin value was 8.3 g/dl. Three months previously, a curettage had been performed when it was noted that the cervix was dilated 10 mm. The polyp must have been missed and subsequently enlarged. The patient's symptoms continued until hysterectomy was performed. Vaginal myomectomy would not be considered in a patient of this age and parity.

106

253

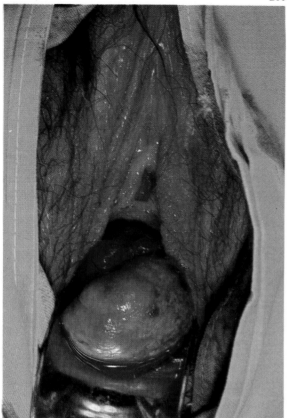

254

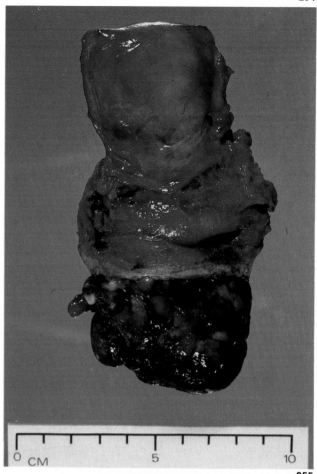

255

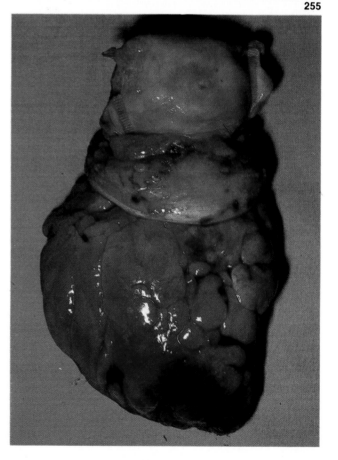

Plate 253 Sarcoma botryoides. Appearance during speculum examination under anaesthesia of a 14-year-old girl who presented with a 4-month history of blood-stained vaginal discharge. Her menarche had occurred 12 months previously. This soft, grey mass was vesicular and necrotic and distended the upper vagina. The cervix and uterus could not be delineated. This tumour is one of the mixed sarcomas of Mullerian origina (see plates 255 and 258 which illustrate other members of this group of mixed mesodermal tumours). Biopsy showed groups of very pleomorphic cells with areas of cartilage blending with surrounding spindle cells. The infantile type of this tumour also arises from cervix or upper vagina and histologically sarcomatous elements, (usually rhabdomyosarcoma) predominate.

Plate 254 Following histological diagnosis, radical hysterectomy with removal of the upper vagina and pelvic lymph nodes was performed. The ovaries were conserved. Bonney's blue swabbing of the vagina preoperatively has discoloured the tumour. The patient returned to school, but 15 months later noted slight vaginal bleeding. There was an 0.5 cm nodule on the lower anterior vaginal wall. Excisional biopsy was performed. Histology showed pleomorphic cells similar to those of the primary tumour. (Courtesy of Dr Ian MacIsaac).

Plate 255 Malignant mesodermal mixed cell tumour of the cervix in a 56-year-old para 6 who presented because of a foul discharge and passage of necrotic tissue vaginally. She had had intermittent vaginal bleeding for 4 years. The vagina was distended by an ulcerated, infected tumour mass. Antibiotics were commenced and abdominal hysterectomy, with bilateral salpingo-oophorectomy and excision of the upper vagina, was performed. The uterine body was friable (note that the clamp had torn through the right side of the uterus) and sat upon the tumour (8 × 6 × 7 cm) which arose from the cervix and expanded the vaginal vault. The tumour appeared gelatinous and polypoid. Histologically it showed sarcomatous and carcinomatous elements, with pleomorphic spindle cells and areas of well differentiated cartilage. The patient had no evidence of metastases and has survived, although wound sepsis necessitated hospitalization for 3 weeks.

256

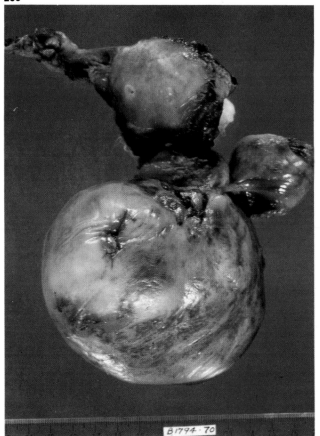

257

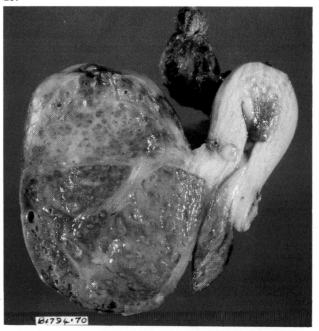

Plate 257 Externally this tumour resembled a fibromyomatous polyp (plate 252), but this picture shows its origin from cervix. The cut surface is fleshy and vascular around the edges, quite different from the whorled appearance of a fibromyoma. Previously called a papillary adenofibroma, this tumour has been recategorized by Östör and Fortune as a variant of mixed Mullerian tumour of the uterus with low grade malignancy. The characteristic histological feature is dual participation of both epithelium and stroma in the neoplastic proliferation.

Plate 256 Mesodermal mixed cell tumour of the cervix in a 48-year-old multipara who presented to her local practitioner in a country centre because of difficulty with voiding. Unwisely, because facilities for major surgery were unavailable, the tumour was biopsied (note wound on its surface). Profuse haemorrhage resulted and the patient was transfused and referred to a major hospital where total abdominal hysterectomy was performed. At laparotomy the uterus sat like a hat atop the tumour which was readily removed, although a large incision in the expanded vaginal vault was required. The patient remains in good health 10 years later.

Plate 258 Endometrial adenosarcoma in a 68-year-old para 1 who presented with heavy vaginal bleeding for 3 days. Thick friable tissue was obtained at curettage; histology revealed sheets of small cells with pleomorphic nuclei. The cervix was ligated to lessen the risk of dissemination and total hysterectomy and bilateral salpingo-oophorectomy was performed. Plates 253-258 illustrate different members of the mixed mesodermal group of adenosarcomas. These are the commonest sarcomas of the genital tract and can arise from cervix, uterine body or endometrium. The other genital tract sarcomas also exhibit a wide range of malignancy and are the leiomyosarcomas (arising from myometrium or fibromyomas), stromal sarcomas (arising in endometrium or areas of endometriosis) and lymphosarcomas.

258

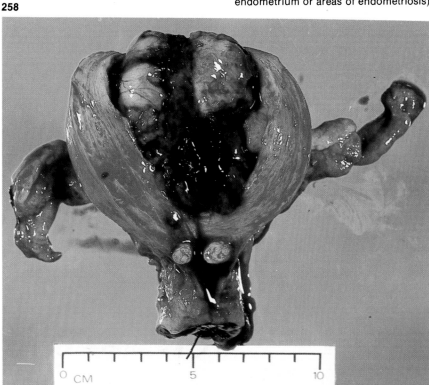

259

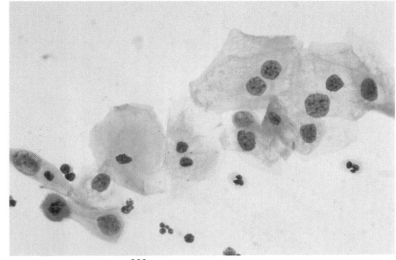

Plate 259 Mild dysplasia as seen in a cervical smear stained by a modification of the Papanicolaou method, giving brighter colours. The atypical squames have abundant cytoplasm, the abnormal features being enlargement of the nucleus, irregular nuclear outline and clumping of nuclear chromatin. There is a group of abnormal cells on the right side, and 2 on the left. Also shown are normal intermediate and superficial squames in the middle of the picture, and several polymorphs. (Magnification × 630).

260

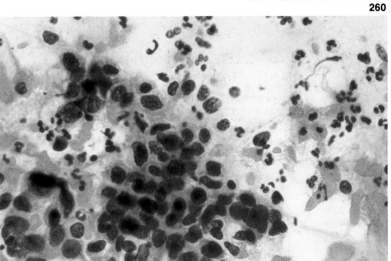

Plate 260 Papanicolaou smear of severe dysplasia of the cervix. The nuclei show many of the features seen in malignant cells (enlargement and irregularity of nuclei), but the cytoplasm is more plentiful. The abnormal cells are seen as a cluster, mainly in the centre of the picture. Numerous polymorphs are shown. (Magnification × 250).

261

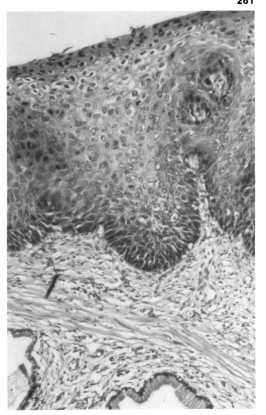

Plate 261 Severe dysplasia of the cervix. Although there is some surface differentiation of cells, the deeper layers show marked nuclear irregularity. The basement membrane is distinct and there is no stromal invasion. Muscle fibres run in the stroma between basement membrane and normal endocervical gland showing columnar cells. Note the dermal papillae where vessels approach the surface of the epithelium, giving the abnormal vascular pattern recognized at colposcopy. (Magnification × 120).

262

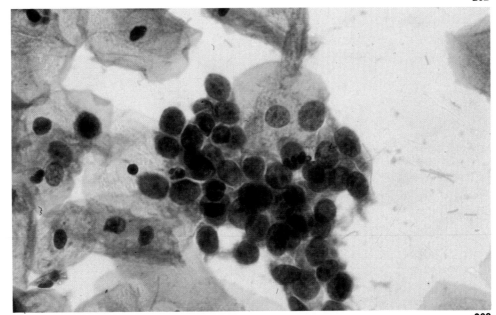

263

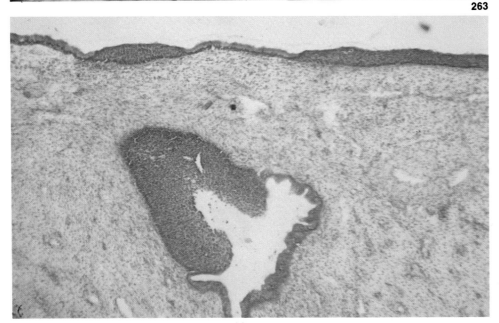

264

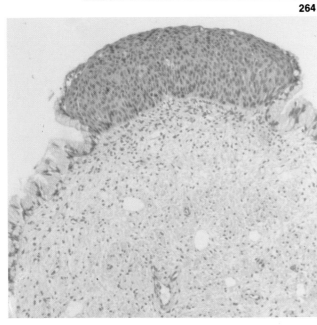

Plate 262 Papanicolaou smear of intraepithelial carcinoma of the cervix. Note the highly abnormal group of malignant cells that reflect the epithelial pattern seen in plate 263. The cells are uniform and have a high nuclear:cytoplasmic ratio. The nuclei are round to oval and show marked hyperchromasia. Cytoplasm is sparse and inconspicuous. Most of the malignant cells in the section are massed centrally. There is a background of normal intermediate and superficial squames. (Magnification × 300).

Plate 263 Intraepithelial carcinoma of the cervix with partial involvement of an endocervical gland by direct extension. This must not be confused with metastatic involvement of a lymph node by an invasive carcinoma. Note the typical basophilia of the epithelium due to the high nuclear:cytoplasmic ratio. There is no transgression of the basement membrane. The epithelium shows full thickness replacement by undifferentiated cells. (Magnification × 50).

Plate 264 Intraepithelial carcinoma of the cervix showing lack of differentiation with the disordered cellular pattern involving the full thickness of the epithelium. Note how the normal columnar endocervical cells on either side have been lifted up and displaced by the advancing edge of the intraepithelial carcinoma. There is no stromal invasion. This lesion was situated either within the endocervical canal or on part of a cervical eversion (ectopy). (Magnification × 100).

110

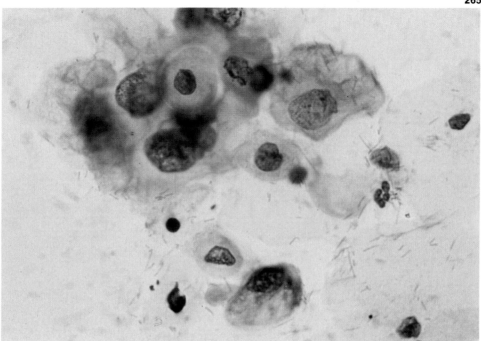

Plate 265 Moderate dysplasia. This and the following 3 plates show a changing pattern of nuclear: cytoplasmic ratio and degree of nuclear irregularity, as dysplasia merges into intraepithelial carcinoma. There is no clear, unarguable line of cytological demarkation between these conditions. The same is true of histological interpretation of degrees of cervical neoplasia. The group of abnormal cells have irregular, large nuclei with chromatin clumping, but cytoplasm is abundant. To the right of the picture is the lobed nucleus of a polymorph and just below mid-field there is the small, pyknotic nucleus of a normal squame. (Magnification × 630).

Plate 266 Severe dysplasia. The cells shown here are further advanced along the spectrum of abnormality between normal and malignant. Numerous abnormal cells are shown with polymorphs scattered in between. The cytoplasm is reduced and nuclei occupy a greater proportion of the cells. Chromatin clumping and nuclear irregularity is evident. (Magnification × 630). (Courtesy of Dr Michael Drake).

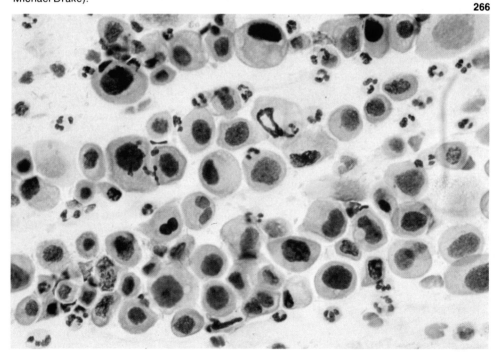

267

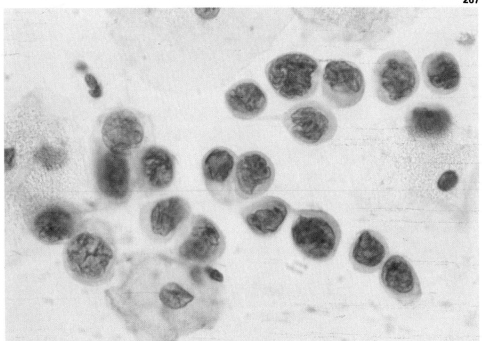

Plate 267 Intraepithelial carcinoma. The cells are uniformly abnormal with a high nuclear: cytoplasmic ratio. The degree of chromatin clumping and nuclear irregularity is suggestive of malignancy. Note the contrast with the relatively normal intermediate cell, with plentiful cytoplasm, at bottom left of the field. (Magnification × 630).

Plate 268 Intraepithelial carcinoma. Most cytologists would not choose to distinguish between the degree of malignancy in this smear, and that shown in plate 267. Both photomicrographs were taken at the same magnification, illustrating that malignant cells vary in size from patient to patient, and within the same smear as shown here. To the right is a normal squame with pyknotic nucleus. There are many polymorphs and this is common in cervical smears, even when there is no clinical evidence of infection or ulceration. Although the nuclei of the abnormal cells vary in size, they lack the marked pleomorphism characteristic of invasive carcinoma. (Magnification × 630).

268

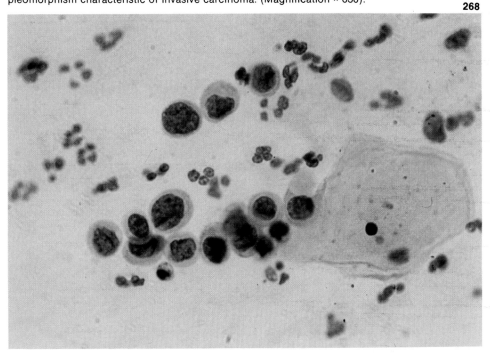

269

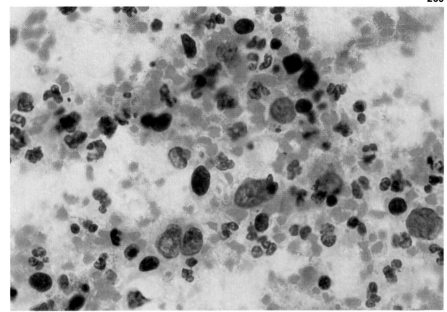

Plate 269 Invasive squamous cell carcinoma of the cervix. This smear shows scattered malignant cells, with minimal cytoplasm, and great variation in density of the nuclei, many of which show a homogeneous purple colour. There is a background of red blood cells and cellular debris as well as polymorphs. This is characteristic of an invasive lesion with ulceration. These scattered cells with nuclear pleomorphism are indicative of a poorly differentiated squamous cell carcinoma. (Magnification × 630).

270

Plate 270 The spindle cell typical of invasive squamous cell carcinoma. There is a background of red blood cells, polymorphs and cellular debris, the latter probably resulting from disintegration of tumour cells. The spindle cell has an elongated nucleus and dense, pink-staining cytoplasm due to excessive keratin content. A blob of keratin is shown at one end of this cell. (Magnification × 630).

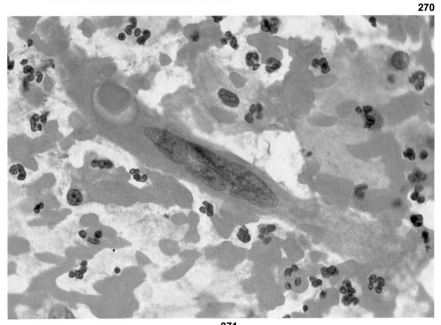

271

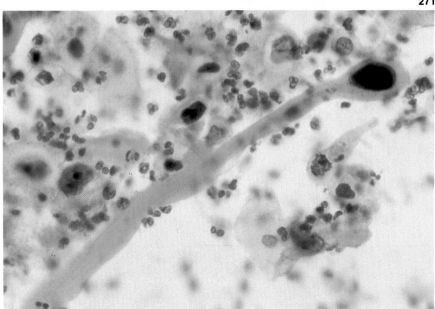

Plate 271 The tadpole cell, although regarded as pathognomonic of invasive squamous cell carcinoma, is so uncommon (less than 5% of cases) that it is seldom helpful in establishing a diagnosis. Note the large dense nucleus of this cell, the bizarre shape and high keratin content of the cytoplasm. The field also contains other malignant cells similar to those shown in plate 269, in addition to much cell debris. (Magnification × 400).

272

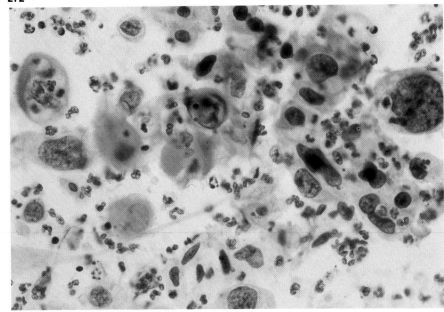

Plate 272 Invasive squamous cell carcinoma. This smear shows malignant cells with marked variation in size and staining qualities. Note the huge nucleus in the cell at top right of the picture. The equally large but poorly staining cell at top left contains polymorphs in the cytoplasm and was probably about to disintegrate. The smaller bizarre-shaped nuclei are probably those of degenerated malignant cells. It is not known whether polymorph ingestion by tumour cells is a manifestation of host response. Its presence or absence in smears is of no known prognostic significance. There is no correlation with histological evidence of small round cell and plasma cell aggregation at the edge of the tumour mass invading cervical stroma. The presence of ingested polymorphs suggests degeneration of the cancer cell and is a common finding. Several eosinophilic squames are present but blurred due to being out of focus. (Magnification × 630).

273

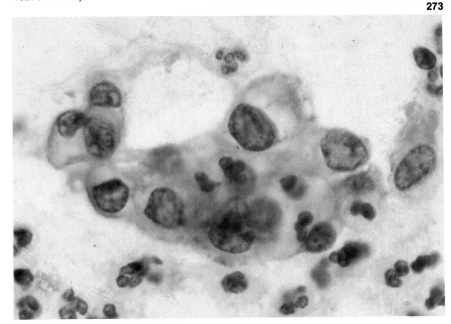

Plate 273 Adenocarcinoma of endometrium. This smear shows a clump of 12 malignant cells with variation in size and shape of nuclei. The prominent cytoplasmic vacuoles are typical of adenocarcinoma. They reflect the secretory activity of the cells and allow discrimination from malignant squamous cells. Cervical cytology is positive in about 40% of endometrial cancers. The pick-up rate is higher if the endocervical canal or posterior fornix pool is sampled. (Magnification × 630).

274

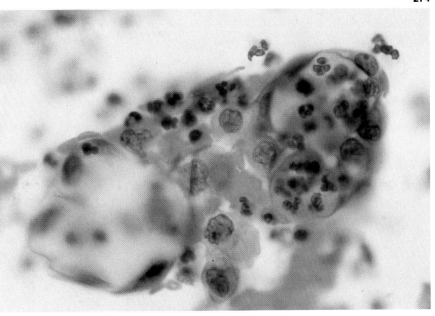

Plate 274 Adenocarcinoma of endometrium. This smear shows the typical cluster of cells shed from an adenocarcinoma. Also shown are huge cytoplasmic secretory vacuoles containing engulfed phagocytes. There is a background of pink degenerating blood and scattered polymorphs. The cell with the huge secretory vacuole on the left of the field is poorly defined and was probably about to disintegrate. (Magnification × 630).

275

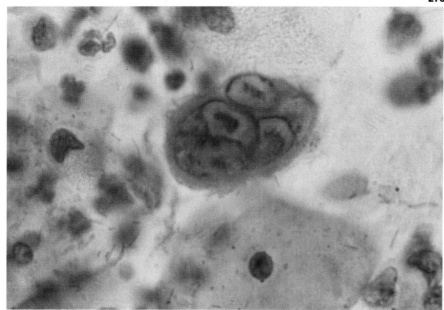

Plate 275 Herpes simplex infection of the cervix. This smear shows the multinucleate cell (from cervical or vaginal epithelium) typical of herpes infection in mid-field, lying above a normal squame with eosinophilic cytoplasm and round, pyknotic nucleus. The multiple nuclei seem moulded around each other. A central, intranuclear inclusion body is shown. The sharp outline of the nuclear border is characteristic, the chromatin having dispersed away from the intranuclear inclusion body. All the nuclei contain inclusion bodies but only one is in sharp focus. (Magnification × 1,000).

276

Plate 276 Smear showing numerous multinucleate cells at lower magnification. Note the characteristic glassy appearance of the chromatin in the nuclei. This evidence of herpes infection is seen in 1 in 1,000 smears and often the patient has no clinical evidence of infection. Type 1 (usually above the waist) and type 2 (usually below the waist) herpetic lesions have the same cytological features. There are no intranuclear inclusions in the multinucleate cells in this smear. The significance of this finding is uncertain, but it does not distinguish between primary and recurrent infections. Numerous polymorphs are scattered among the multinucleate cells which are poorly preserved. Because neonatal herpes infection is often fatal, and can cause brain damage in survivors, proven herpes cervicitis is an indication for Caesarean section (plate 150). (Magnification × 630).

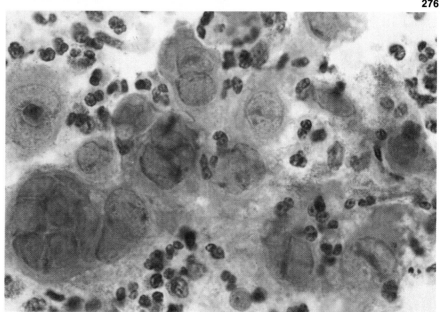

277

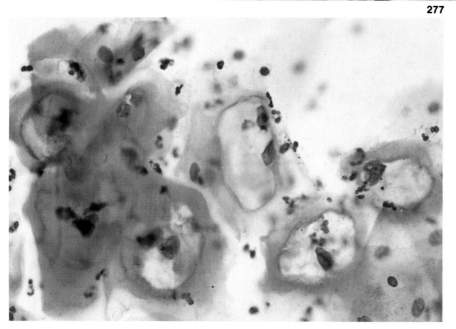

Plate 277 Wart virus disease of the cervix. The features of this infection are seen in 1% of routine cervical smears which is an incidence 10 times greater than that of herpes cervicitis. Note the typical balloon cells with perinuclear halo, and aggregation of densely staining cytoplasm, (usually a fuchsia or magenta colour), at the peripheri of the cells. Several cervical cells also show the double nuclei typical of this infection. The importance of this disease is the possibility that the papilloma virus that causes it may result in cellular atypia that in some patients proceeds to invasive carcinoma (plate 149). (Magnification × 630).

278

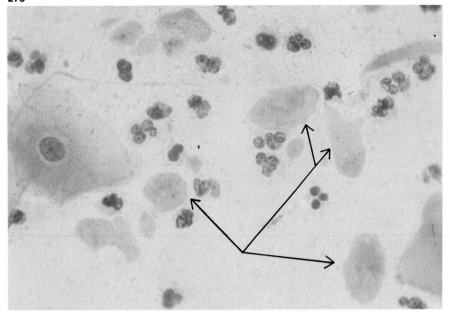

Plate 278 Trichomonal infection as seen in a Papanicolaou smear. There is an intermediate type squame with a vesicular nucleus to the left of the field, showing a perinuclear halo, which is a change induced by the presence of trichomonads, 4 of which are indicated by arrows. These organisms have approximately twice the diameter of polymorphs, many of which are shown with distinct lobed nuclei and poorly-stained cytoplasm. (Magnification × 630).

279

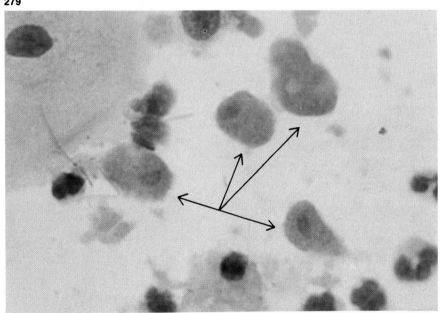

Plate 279 Trichomonad organisms shown in greater detail at higher magnification (arrows). Note that these protozoa have an eccentric nucleus and the cytoplasm contains reddish-coloured granules. The organism at lower right shows the typical pear shape. Several polymorphs and a squame are also shown. (Magnification × 1,000).

280

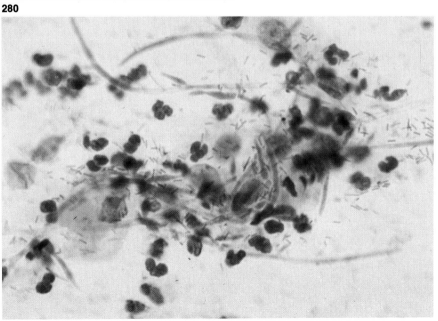

Plate 280 Monilial infection as seen in approximately 2% of cervical smears stained by the Papanicolaou method. Several threads of pseudohyphae are shown against a background of polymorphs and a few intermediate squames. There is also nuclear debris representing cytolysis of cells, and numerous Doderlein's bacilli, which are a common finding in a Papanicolaou smear. (Magnification × 630).

116

281

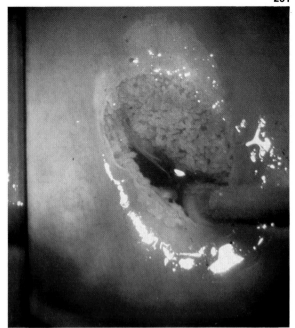

Plate 281 Colposcopic view (magnification × 12) of a normal cervix after application of 3% acetic acid which is a mucolytic agent and causes the surface epithelium to swell. The greater the nuclear density in the epithelium the whiter it will appear (as in metaplasia, dysplasia, intra-epithelial and invasive carcinoma where nuclear-cyto-plasmic ratios are relatively large). Columnar epithelium, either when in the endocervical canal, or on the ectocervix (ectropion), has this grape-like appearance on colpo-scopy. The columnar epithelium is undergoing metaplastic transformation to mature squamous epithelium under the stimulus of the acid pH of the vagina. The pale area (12 o'clock) is one of completed metaplasia and the dots within it are the mouths of Nabothian follicles formed by entrap-ment of mucus-secreting columnar glands by the meta-plastic squamous epithelium.

Plate 283 'Real' view of the cervix of a 17-year-old nulli-para after insertion of a bivalve speculum. The squamo-columnar junction can be seen on the ectocervix, near the centre of the picture where the slit of the external os is apparent. The original squamocolumnar junction would have been situated 1 cm caudad. The transformation zone shows white patches of metaplastic squamous epithelium and small Nabothian follicles (plates 40, 88 and 89).

282

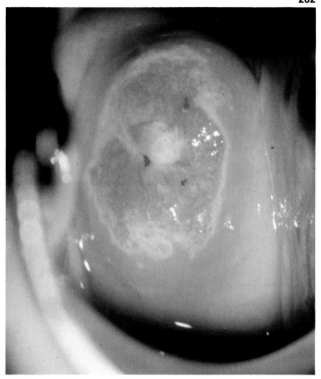

Plate 282 Cervix of an asymptomatic 56-year-old postmeno-pausal woman. The white line marks the upper extent of the transformation zone (area between the original squamocolumnar junction and upper (cranial) limit of columnar epithelium under-going squamous metaplasia). Postmenopausal atrophy of the cervix often causes the squamocolumnar junction to "retreat" into the endocervical canal. The columnar epithelium shown here is thin, and so the underlying vascular pattern is more obvious. This epithelium was exposed by pouting of the endocervix induced by the speculum.

Plate 284 View of the same cervix shown in plate 283 after separation of the blades of the bivalve speculum. This is the view most commonly seen and demonstrates how columnar epi-thelium can appear to occupy a much larger area on the ectocervix, since the endocervical canal is now more exposed. Insertion of a Sims' speculum also everts the cervix, which accounts for the apparent frequency of small ectropions. Note the clear, glistening mucus in the endocervical canal.

283

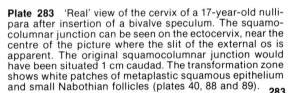
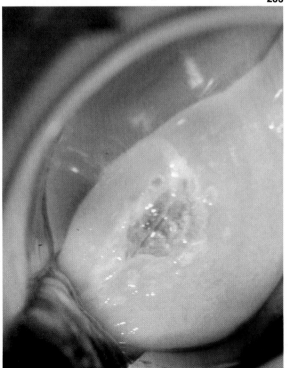

284

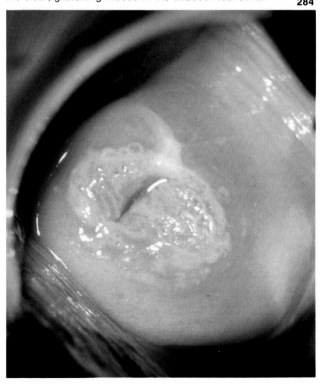

285

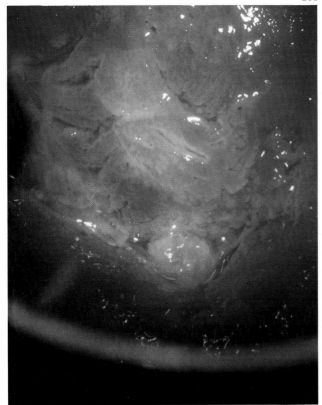

286

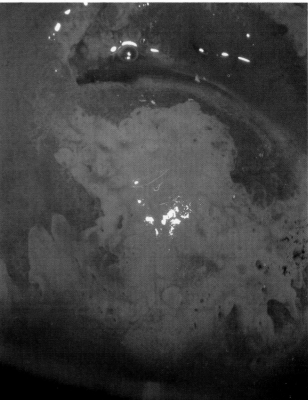

287

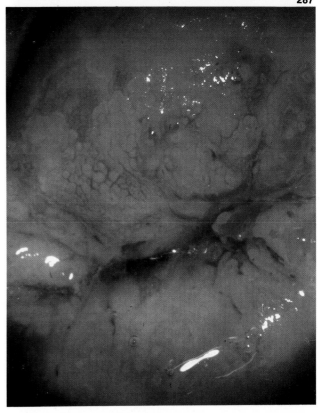

Plate 285 Squamous metaplasia occurring on the transformation zone on the anterior lip of the cervix. A white plug of mucus occupies the endocervical canal below the middle of the picture. The bulbous ends of columnar epithelium are seen adjacent to the white areas of metaplasia. The histological appearance of squamous epithelium derived by metaplasia is indistinguishable from original or native squamous epithelium. The whiteness is due to the high nuclear-cytoplasmic ratio of actively growing tissue. The squamocolumnar junction moves caudally in the neonatal period, at puberty, and during the first pregnancy, due to hormone-induced increase in the bulk of the cervix, causing eversion of the endocervix. This gives the appearance of the endocervical epithelium extending onto the ectocervix. The endocervical columnar epithelium does *not* replace original squamous epithelium.

Plate 286 Moderate dysplasia seen as an irregular area of whitened epithelium on the posterior lip of the cervix. Colposcopy, like cytology, recognizes a range of atypicality, extending from dysplasia through intraepithelial carcinoma to invasive carcinoma (legend to plate 265). Metaplasia only occurs in the transformation zone which can extend caudally as far as the vaginal fornices, and cranially high in the endocervical canal, beyond the view of the colposcope. Neoplasia arises as an area of atypical metaplasia within this zone. Note that here the atypical area does not reach the slit of the external os. Treatment was conservative, by electrocoagulation diathermy, after target biopsy.

Plate 287 Intraepithelial carcinoma. The white areas are more dense, heaped up, and the surface more irregular than that seen in plate 286. There is a greater prominence and abnormality of blood vessels (the colposcopic hallmark of neoplasia) as demonstrated by the punctate and mosaic pattern. These patterns are produced by dermal papillae containing capillaries extending close to the surface of the abnormal squamous epithelium, probably under the influence of angiogenesis factor and other similar products produced by the rapidly dividing cells. Note that the lesion extends up the endocervical canal. Cone biopsy, to exclude invasive carcinoma, is indicated if the endocervical speculum (plate 289) does not render the upper extent of the abnormal epithelium accessible to inspection and target biopsy.

118

288

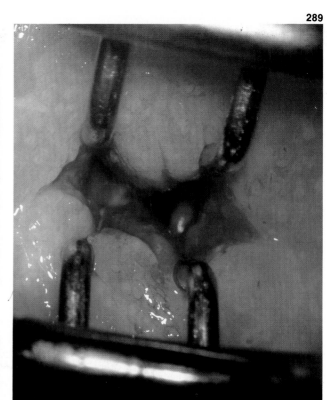

289

290

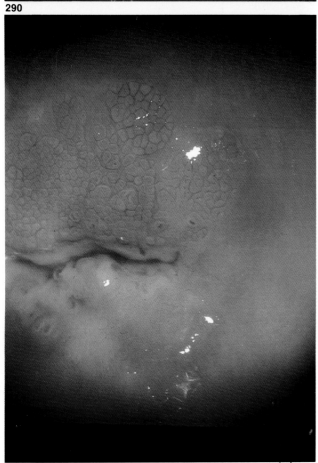

Plate 288 Intraepithelial carcinoma confined to a small area on the anterior lip of cervix. The diagnosis was confirmed by target biopsy which was followed by electrocoagulation diathermy. Velvety columnar epithelium visible cranial to the abnormal area indicates that all of the abnormal area was within view of the colposcope. Fortunately, the pathology of cervical neoplasia is such that a cervical lesion does not have another associated intraepithelial or invasive area further up the endocervical canal (skip lesion) if there is a complete cranial ring of normal columnar epithelium. Hence, the great value of colposcopy in reducing the cone biopsy rate to less than 30% of patients with an abnormal smear.

Plate 289 Use of the Chanen endocervical speculum to assist evaluation of abnormal cytological smears with the colposcope. It allows inspection of the endocervical canal and helps delineate the uppermost limits of dysplasia or intraepithelial carcinoma in those patients in whom it extends into the endocervical canal. It has allowed further reduction in the incidence of diagnostic cone biopsy. This picture shows the features of an intraepithelial carcinoma which does not extend beyond the view of the colposcope. Treatment was electrocoagulation diathermy. At follow-up there was a normal cervix on colposcopy and negative cytology.

Plate 290 Intraepithelial carcinoma showing a classical mosaic pattern in the whitened abnormal area on the anterior lip of cervix. The lesion extended beyond range of the colposcope, and cone biopsy was performed to exclude invasive carcinoma. As in approximately 70% of patients with intraepithelial carcinoma having cone biopsies, the follow-up cytology was negative. Cone biopsy is not preferred to electrocautery as definitive treatment of intraepithelial carcinoma because of the high incidence of complications (primary and secondary haemorrhage, infection, cervical stenosis or incompetence).

291

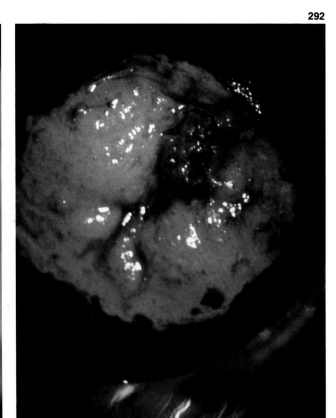

292

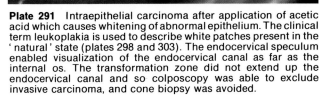

293

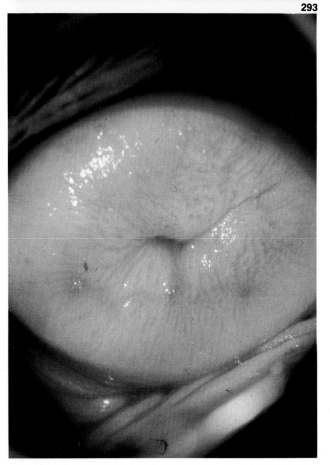

Plate 291 Intraepithelial carcinoma after application of acetic acid which causes whitening of abnormal epithelium. The clinical term leukoplakia is used to describe white patches present in the 'natural' state (plates 298 and 303). The endocervical speculum enabled visualization of the endocervical canal as far as the internal os. The transformation zone did not extend up the endocervical canal and so colposcopy was able to exclude invasive carcinoma, and cone biopsy was avoided.

Plate 292 Schiller's test. To delineate the extent of the lesion shown in plate 291, Lugol's iodine solution was applied and gave a good correlation with the colposcopic assessment of the cervical limits of the lesion. The uptake of iodine by glycogen-containing squamous cells is not specific in terms of cancer detection or elimination. Normal columnar epithelium (no glycogen — no stain) cannot be distinguished from atypical squamous epithelium, and conversely, invasive carcinoma can contain glycogen and give a false staining reaction. Now that colposcopy is available, there is little value in Schiller's test to select a biopsy site.

Plate 293 Typical postdiathermy radial capillary pattern of the cervix in a 49-year-old para 3. For 3 years she had had atypical cervical smears interspersed with normal smears. This can be a sampling error (false negative) and merits repetition of the smear. Colposcopy revealed a 5 mm area of intraepithelial carcinoma obscured by a large Nabothian follicle. After histology of the target biopsy confirmed the colposcopic diagnosis, curettage and then radical electrocoagulation diathermy was performed under general anaesthesia. Cryosurgery is reported to be equally effective as electrocoagulation in destroying intraepithelial neoplasia. With either modality, the risk of recurrence is less than 10% if the entire transformation zone is treated. In a series of 1,500 patients with histologically proven cervical intraepithelial neoplasia, 90% of those under 30 years of age were suitable for treatment by electrocoagulation diathermy (Dr William Chanen, Royal Women's Hospital, Melbourne). After such treatment, normal squamous epithelium generates from the stem cell believed to be in the dermis, provided an acid pH medium is maintained in the vagina (Aci-gel or Sultrin cream).

120

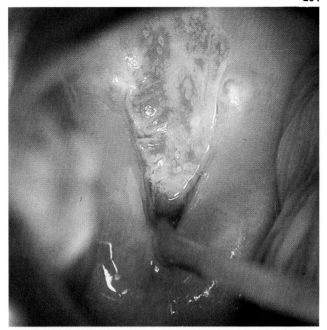

Plate 294 Late recurrence of intraepithelial carcinoma of the anterior lip of cervix following treatment by laser. The advantages of laser are that general anaesthesia is not required and healing is completed within 1 week. The triangular area of atypical epithelium does not extend up the endocervical canal. Nabothian follicles are shown on either side of the area of cervical neoplasia. The message is that continued surveillance is necessary after treatment of cervical intraepithelial neoplasia by any modality (cone biopsy, electrocoagulation, cryotherapy, laser, cervical amputation, hysterectomy).

Plate 296 Colpophotograph showing unusually well-marked mosaic appearance of intraepithelial carcinoma, with an oval-shaped area at 12 o'clock suspicious of invasive carcinoma. Note that the lesion was confined to the anterior lip of cervix and did not extend into the endocervical canal. The patient was a 32-year-old para 2 who planned to remarry. The bleeding area indicates the area of target biopsy; histology revealed microinvasion (in this case less than 1 mm penetration of stroma). Treatment was cone biopsy; histology of this specimen confirmed the presence of microinvasion (Stage 1a). Cervical cytology and colposcopy has remained negative on follow-up. (Courtesy of Dr William Chanen).

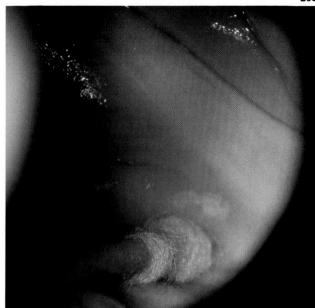

Plate 295 Recurrent or residual intraepithelial carcinoma of the right lateral vaginal vault after abdominal hysterectomy. Colposcopy was not performed preoperatively. The swab stick indicates an area of intraepithelial carcinoma. dumb-bell in shape, that was clearly seen after application of 3% acetic acid. This examination was performed when a vaginal smear taken 6 months after operation was suggestive of persistent or recurrent intraepithelial carcinoma. Under general anaesthesia, the abnormal area was excised, and nearby epithelium was diathermied. Without colposcopy, a much more radical and blind approach would have been necessary to eradicate the area responsible for the positive smear.

Plate 297 Colposcopic appearance of Stage 1b invasive squamous cell carcinoma of the cervix. Four months previously, this 34-year-old para 3 had a laparoscopic tubal diathermy performed. At that time the cervix appeared normal macroscopically, and cytology was negative. She presented because of postcoital and intermenstrual bleeding of 2 weeks' duration. Although it is believed that nearly all invasive cancers of the cervix pass through a preinvasive phase, detectable by cytology (and colposcopy), rapid progression in a matter of weeks or months does occur. This patient was treated with radiotherapy and radical hysterectomy.

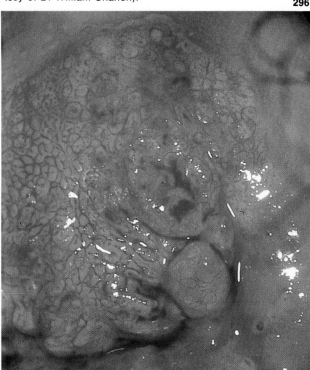

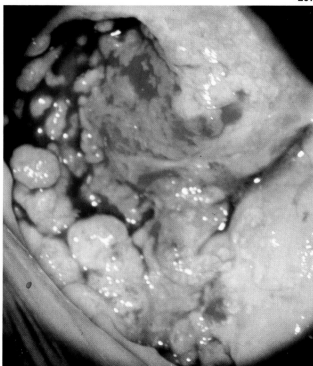

298

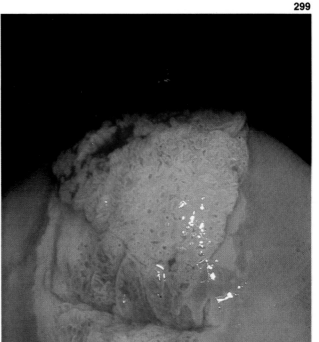

299

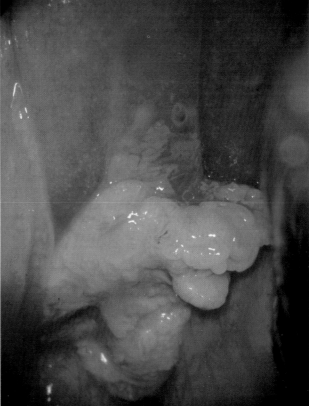

300

Plate 298 Leukoplakia of the posterior lip of the cervix in the transformation zone. These white patches were obvious with the naked eye without application of acetic acid. Histology showed hyperkeratosis without underlying cervical intraepithelial neoplasia. However, this appearance can be associated with dysplasia, intraepithelial or invasive carcinoma (plates 303 and 420). Colposcopy and biopsy are indicated in such a patient even if cytology is negative.

Plate 299 Condylomata of the anterior lip of cervix. This colposcopic appearance can be mistaken for frank neoplasia. Macroscopic inspection of the cervix showed clinical leukoplakia. Target biopsy histology showed hyperkeratosis without evidence of neoplasia. The condylomata are superimposed upon a transformation zone showing squamous metaplasia. This appearance can coexist with cytologic evidence of wart virus disease (plates 149 and 277) and presumably the wart virus causes the condylomata. Possibly the same papova virus causes the macroscopic condylomata of vagina and perineum (plates 146 to 148).

Plate 300 Another example of wart virus disease of the cervix caused by the papilloma virus (a member of the papova group of viruses). Swabbing of the cervix with acetic acid has rendered these condylomata more prominent. Such lesions occur mainly in the transformation zone. This infection is present in a high proportion (up to 20%) of patients with abnormal cytology. The cervical epithelium is often opaque and shows atypical vessels which can be confused with dysplasia or carcinoma in situ. The colposcopic pattern is often gyriform or brain-like, unlike that seen in intraepithelial carcinoma. The infection is sexually transmitted. Treatment is biopsy (to exclude intraepithelial neoplasia) and electrocoagulation diathermy when the lesions are large or persistent. Often the lesions are macroscopically invisible and regress spontaneously. Associated abnormal cytology requires the usual management (ruling out the presence of invasive cancer, and preventing further progression of intraepithelial neoplasia).

301

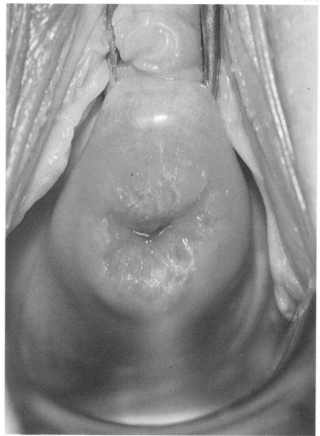

302

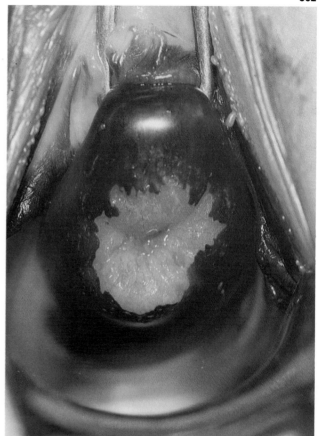

303

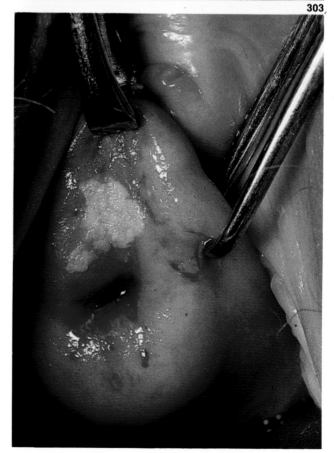

Plate 301 Cervical dysplasia in a 20-year-old patient whose postnatal cervical smear was found to be abnormal. The cervix is hypertrophied and shows a mild ectropion.

Plate 302 Schiller's test using Lugol's iodine solution (5% aqueous) stains glycogen-containing cells black and fails to stain metaplastic and columnar epithelium, and most areas of dysplasia and carcinoma in situ. Invasive lesions may contain glycogen and stain positively and so modern investigation is based largely on cytology to detect the presence of neoplasia, and colposcopy to delineate the appropriate area for target biopsy (plates 304, 420 and 421).

Plate 303 Leukoplakia of the cervix in a 40-year-old para 1 found at the time of routine cervical cytology which was indicative of severe dysplasia and intraepithelial carcinoma (carcinoma in situ). Cone biopsy was performed. Histology revealed carcinoma in situ at the site of the white plaque, together with surrounding dysplasia which stopped short of the edge of the cone. Follow-up cytology was normal and surveillance continues.

304

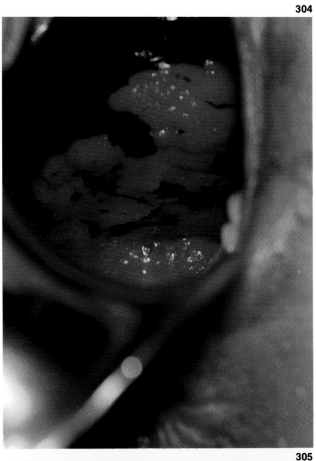

Plate 304 Positive Schiller's test in a 40-year-old para 3 with postcoital bleeding and a lesion extending from the cervix down the anterior vaginal wall. Biopsy revealed carcinoma in situ of the vagina and invasive squamous cell carcinoma of the cervix. She was treated with irradiation followed by radical surgery and is alive and well 13 years later.

Plate 305 Stage 1 carcinoma of the cervix in a 38-year-old para 2 who presented with postcoital bleeding and dyspareunia for 6 months. There was a yellow vaginal discharge. The cervix appeared friable and bled on contact. Biopsy showed a well differentiated, invasive squamous cell carcinoma. Treatment was irradiation followed by Wertheim hysterectomy and lymphadenectomy. There was no residual tumour in the uterus and lymph nodes were clear. The patient has survived for 16 years.

Plate 306 Ulcerating squamous cell carcinoma of the cervix, Stage 2a (vaginal involvement), in a 39-year-old para 3 who was 22 weeks' pregnant. She was treated by radical hysterectomy and postoperative irradiation to the pelvis (6,000 rads or 60 Grays). She developed radiation-induced bowel necrosis and vesico-vaginal fistula, requiring colostomy and ileal conduit with ureteric transplantation. She died 7 years after initial presentation due to bowel obstruction. At autopsy, no residual tumour was present. Cure of the malignancy was achieved but the sequelae of radiation therapy led to death.

305

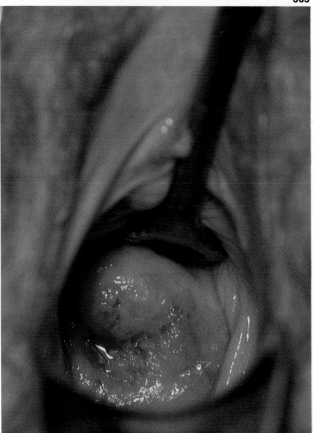

306

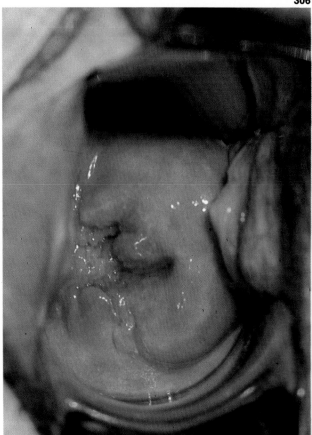

124

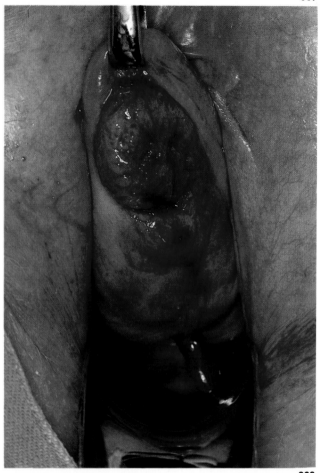

307

Plate 307 Stage 1b (clinically apparent lesion confined to cervix) squamous cell carcinoma in a 77-year-old para 3 who presented with vaginal bleeding of 7 days' duration. Because the cervix protruded through the introitus (second degree uterine prolapse) the lesion, which covered the anterior lip of cervix and extended to the posterior lip, was readily photographed, unlike many cervical carcinomas that appear as excavating lesions replacing the cervix at the vaginal vault. Megavoltage therapy followed by intracavitary irradiation not only cured the carcinoma, but also the uterine prolapse (irradiation-induced fibrosis).

Plate 308 Stage 2, poorly differentiated, squamous cell carcinoma arising from the cervix of a 74-year-old woman who presented with vaginal bleeding. This tumour is ulcerative and has replaced the cervix, giving the appearance of a primary vaginal carcinoma. The tumour has penetrated into the uterine cavity which is shown exposed at the upper right side of the growth. Note the indurated, sloughy base and thickened, rolled edge of the tumour, as seen in epitheliomas of the skin. Polypoid prolapsed urethral mucosa is also shown.

Plate 309 Recurrent adenosquamous carcinoma involving cervix and upper two-thirds of vagina in a 61-year-old obese diabetic. Diagnosis of a Stage 2 lesion was made 7 months earlier. Megavoltage therapy gave a good initial response, but then the tumour recurred. Intraarterial pelvic perfusion chemotherapy was commenced.

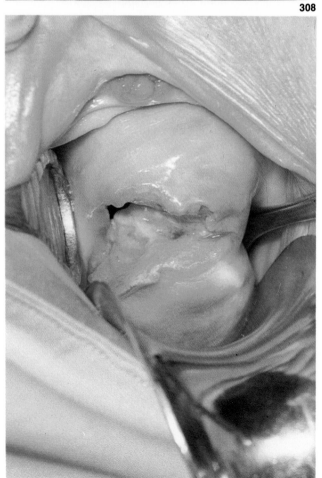

308

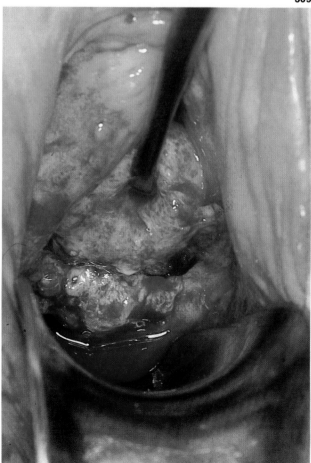

309

310

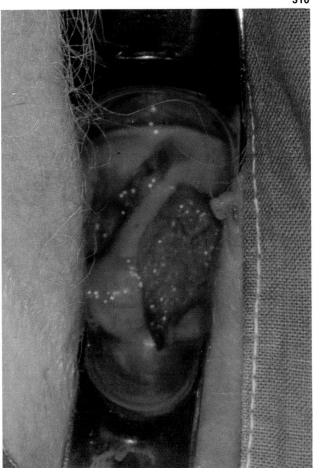

Plate 310 Vaginal metastasis from carcinoma of the cervix seen as a polypoid tumour on the left side of the upper one-third of vagina in a 58-year-old para 1 who presented with postmenopausal bleeding and yellow vaginal discharge of 2 months' duration. The uterus was small, irregular and mobile. No adnexal thickening was palpable.

Plate 311 At examination under anaesthesia the ectocervix was reddened and bled on contact, the appearance being that of a benign papillary ectropion in a premenopausal woman. The vaginal wall between cervix and the lesion shown in plate 310 appeared healthy and was not indurated. Biopsies of the cervix and vaginal tumour showed poorly differentiated squamous cell carcinoma.

Plate 312 A pyometra had developed due to cervical stenosis and infection. It was revealed by escape of thick yellow pus when a uterine sound was passed preparatory to cervical dilatation and careful curettage. This view was a bonus, the photographer being present to record the unusual vaginal lesion shown in plate 310! Treatment of this Stage 2a carcinoma of cervix (spread limited to upper one-third of vagina) was irradiation (caesium in uterus and upper vagina), followed 6 weeks later by radical hysterectomy with pelvic lymphadenectomy and excision of upper one-half of vagina. The patient remains free of recurrence.

311

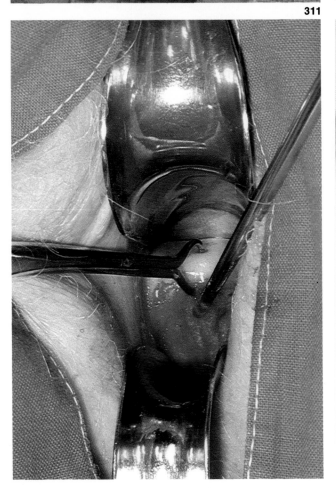

312

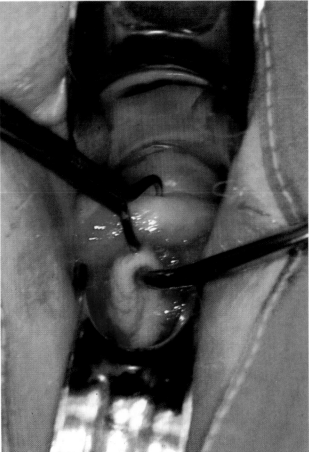

313

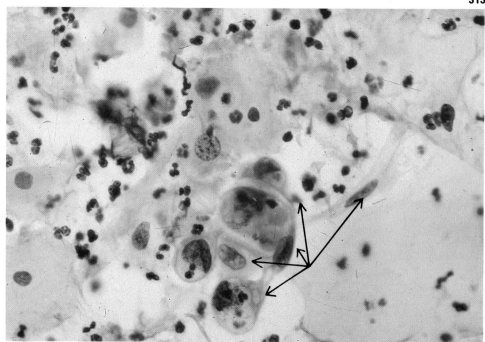

Plate 313 Papanicolaou smear of invasive squamous carcinoma of the cervix. Note the difference in size and shape (pleomorphism) of the clump of clearly abnormal cells (arrows). Polymorphs are scattered around the field and some have been ingested by the cancer cells which are large and multinucleate; the nuclei of the latter are irregular and show hyperchromatic change. Note the typical malignant spindle-shaped cell to the right of the main cell clump. Also shown are normal squames with faint pink cytoplasm and regular vesicular nuclei (see also plates 269-272). (Magnification × 400).

314

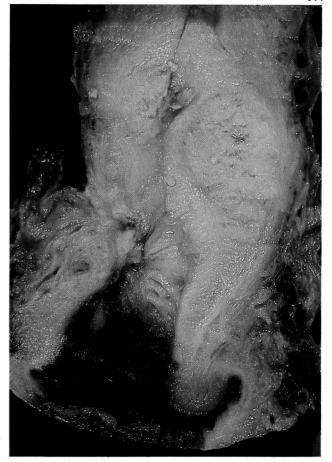

Plate 314 Endocervical, well differentiated, keratinizing, squamous cell carcinoma in a radical hysterectomy specimen from a 32-year-old patient treated by intracavitary caesium 6 weeks previously. The ectocervix and upper vagina are stained blue as a result of preoperative swabbing and appear normal. The upper endocervical canal is distorted by a softened, yellow tumour mass, 3.5 cm in diameter, which extends through the entire width of the substance of the cervix. These endocervical barrell-type growths are often extensive before ulceration results in symptoms. Further sectioning showed the growth to be completely spherical, involving the entire endocervix, but bulging anteriorly.

315

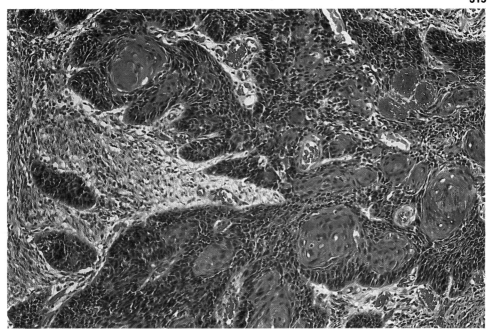

Plate 315 Moderately well differentiated squamous cell carcinoma of the cervix. The patient was a 61-year-old para 2 who presented with a history of postmenopausal bleeding for 2 weeks. Her cervix was replaced by a tumour which extended onto the posterior vaginal fornix. There was nodular extension along the right uterosacral ligament and along the right cardinal ligament to the lateral pelvic wall (Stage 3). This section taken from the cervical biopsy shows connective tissue heavily infiltrated and largely replaced by irregular sheets of pleomorphic cells, some of which are forming keratin and appear as epithelial 'pearls'. Note that most of the cells at the edges of the tumour, where it infiltrates the stroma, have elongated, hyperchromatic nuclei and relatively scanty cytoplasm (plate 269). The patient was treated with megavoltage to the pelvis and received a total dose of 6,000 rads. Three years later, vaginal bleeding recurred and examination revealed tumour recurrence at the vaginal vault. The patient was treated with chemotherapy (vincristine, actinomycin D and cyclophosphamide) and has survived, although the vaginal vault remains indurated and granular. (Magnification × 140).

Plate 316 Poorly differentiated squamous cell carcinoma of the cervix. The patient was a 60-year-old para 1 who presented with postmenopausal bleeding for 1-2 years, lower abdominal pain for 3 months and recent swelling of the right leg and urinary incontinence. Examination revealed a large, lower abdominal mass, arising from the pelvis and enlarged supraclavicular lymph nodes. The cervix was replaced by an ulcerating tumour which extended down the posterior vaginal wall to its middle one-third. Combined rectal and vaginal examination showed that the tumour extended to the pelvic walls and was continuous with the immobile mass in the lower abdomen. This section taken from the cervical biopsy shows irregular masses of pleomorphic cells invading the stroma. Needle biopsy of the nodes in her neck showed tissue composed of pleomorphic cells with numerous irregular mitoses, an appearance consistent with metastatic squamous carcinoma (Stage 4). The patient was treated with megavoltage irradiation to the pelvis and cytotoxic drug therapy. (Magnification × 140).

316

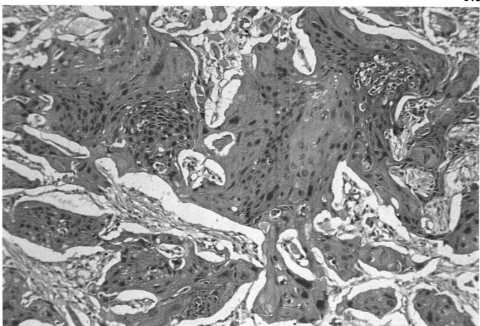

128

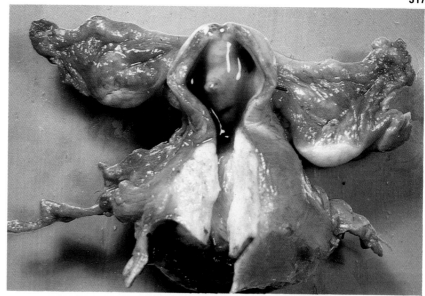

Plate 317 Extensive Stage 1 squamous cell carcinoma of cervix from a 61-year-old woman who presented with postmenopausal bleeding for 5 weeks. Radical hysterectomy and pelvic lymphadenectomy were performed without preoperative irradiation. Bonney's blue discolours the cervix and upper one-third of vagina. The tumour is seen as a white mass replacing the entire cervix; there is minimal ulceration or fungation. Some cervical stenosis is evident from the dilatation of the uterine cavity above. The lymph nodes were clear and the patient survived.

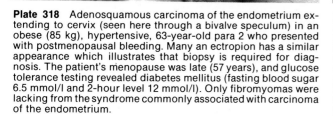

Plate 318 Adenosquamous carcinoma of the endometrium extending to cervix (seen here through a bivalve speculum) in an obese (85 kg), hypertensive, 63-year-old para 2 who presented with postmenopausal bleeding. Many an ectropion has a similar appearance which illustrates that biopsy is required for diagnosis. The patient's menopause was late (57 years), and glucose tolerance testing revealed diabetes mellitus (fasting blood sugar 6.5 mmol/l and 2-hour level 12 mmol/l). Only fibromyomas were lacking from the syndrome commonly associated with carcinoma of the endometrium.

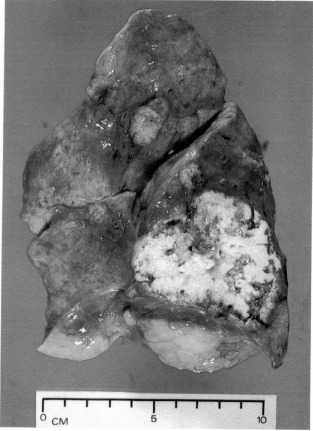

Plate 319 Huge cavitating lesion simulating an abscess at the base of the right lung from a 58-year-old para 2 who developed a pathological fracture of a thoracic vertebra and multiple metastases in the skull, 5 years and 8 months after treatment of an extensive Stage 2, poorly differentiated, squamous cell carcinoma of the cervix (by irradiation, radical hysterectomy and pelvic lymphadenectomy). After the fracture occurred, chest radiography showed multiple pulmonary metastases, although the pelvis was free of recurrence. She obtained symptomatic relief with chemotherapy (methotrexate, vincristine), but died 7 months later from cerebral secondaries. The moral is that cancer can recur years after apparent cure, without evidence of local disease. In this patient, chemotherapy destroyed the cancer cells in her lungs, but to be curative, early detection of metastases is essential.

320

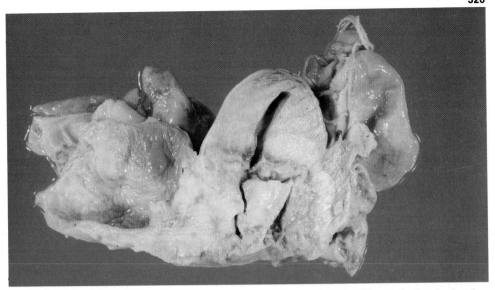

Plate 320 Gruesome autopsy specimen of Stage 4 carcinoma of cervix with massive local extension into parametrium, bladder and rectum. The patient was a 43-year-old para 2 who presented 9 months before death with severe, irregular vaginal bleeding (haemoglobin value 6g/dl) for 12 months. She was treated with megavoltage therapy (6,000 rads to the pelvis) and died from renal failure due to ureteric obstruction. At autopsy the tumour was confined to the pelvis; hence the rationale for exenterative procedures in locally advanced carcinoma of the cervix.

321

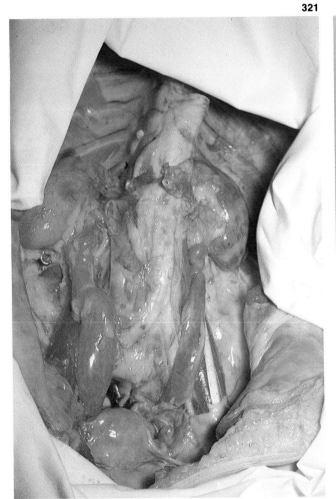

Plate 321 Death from uraemia in a 60-year-old para 12 who presented with heavy vaginal bleeding for 4 months. She had an extensive carcinoma of the cervix and refused treatment. She returned moribund (haemoglobin value 3g/dl) 4 years later and died. Note that the grossly dilated ureters are wider than the aorta as they cross the pelvic brim. Although there was extensive lateral infiltration, no tumour was found outside the pelvis.

322

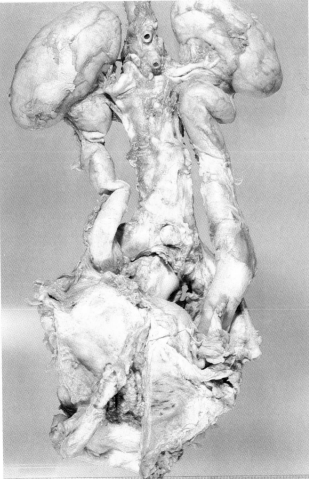

Plate 322 Death from squamous cell carcinoma of the cervix in a 36-year-old woman who refused treatment and died from haemorrhage 12 months later. The tumour extended massively to the lateral pelvic walls, causing bilateral ureteric obstruction and hydronephrosis. The rectum was involved but not the bladder. The tumour was limited to the pelvic cavity and is shown as an ulcerated mass replacing cervix and upper vagina.

323

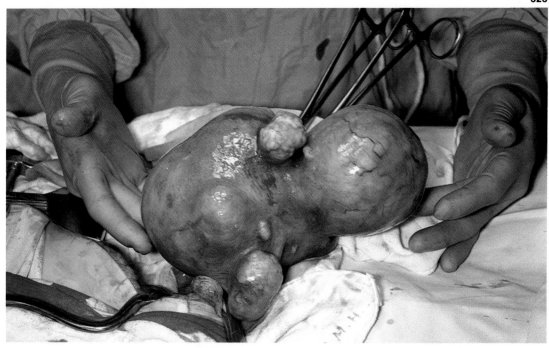

Plate 323 Multiple fibromyomas, ranging in size from 2 mm to 9 cm in diameter, seen during abdominal hysterectomy. The tumours were subserosal, intramural and submucosal in position. The patient was aged 45 years and had never conceived although married for 25 years. She presented because of menorrhagia of 3 weeks' duration. Although associated with sterility, fibromyomas of moderate proportions are present in 1% of pregnancies.

324

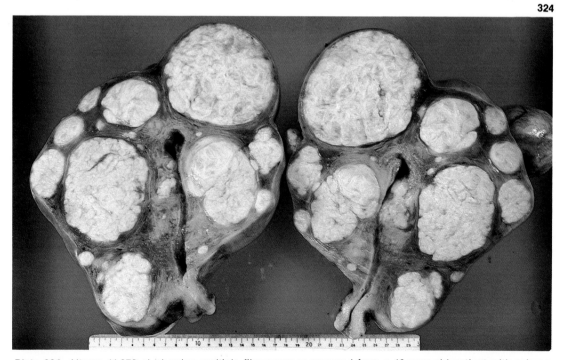

Plate 324 Uterus (4,070 g) showing multiple fibromyomas removed from a 46-year-old patient with primary infertility. She had noticed an abdominal mass for 12 months, but as her periods were regular did not present until abdominal soreness had been present for 2 weeks. The mass was the size of a 28-week pregnancy. It was hard, irregular, arose from the pelvis and moved with the cervix. Radiography revealed no calcification and renal function was normal. The fibroids show the typical whorled cut surface and pseudocapsule. They were submucous (hence menorrhagia due to ulceration), intramural and subserous, involving supravaginal cervix and uterine body.

325

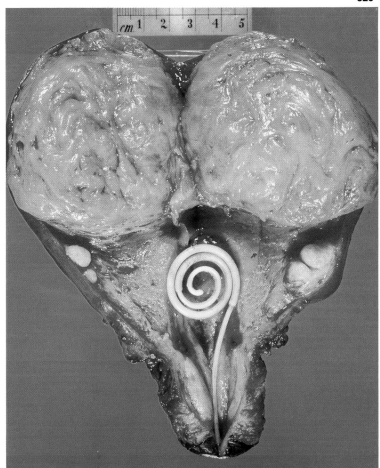

Plate 325 Uterus (440 g) removed from a 46-year-old para 2 (last child born by Caesarean section 18 years previously) with menorrhagia and a Gynekoil in situ for 6 years. She had noticed an abdominal mass for 6 months. The uterus has been incised anteriorly and Gynekoil, lower segment scar and multiple fibromyomas are shown. The cervix is blue due to preoperative swabbing of the vagina with Bonney's blue.

326

Plate 326 Red degeneration of a solitary, large, fundal fibromyoma. This typically occurs in the second trimester of pregnancy and is due to ischaemic necrosis. The patient was a 35-year-old para 1 who had had 4 spontaneous abortions (at 10, 18, 8 and 23 weeks). Her final pregnancy was complicated by vaginal bleeding and abdominal pain which began at 22 weeks and resulted in rupture of the membranes and premature delivery. Hysterectomy was performed 7 weeks later, the patient having decided against myomectomy and the possibility of another unsuccessful pregnancy. The uterus has been incised anteriorly and shows the pseudocapsule of areolar tissue that allows easy enucleation of such tumours. The cavity of the uterus is much larger than usual due to the distension caused by the tumour.

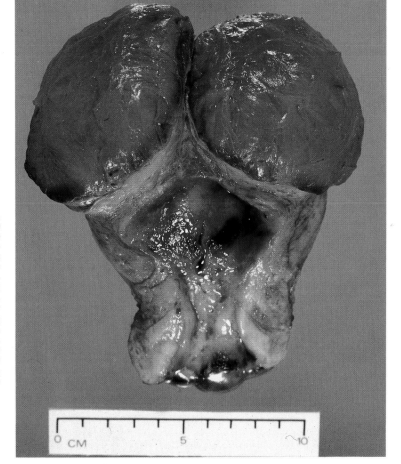

132

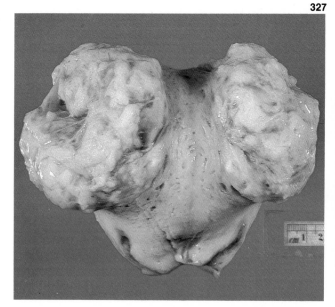

327

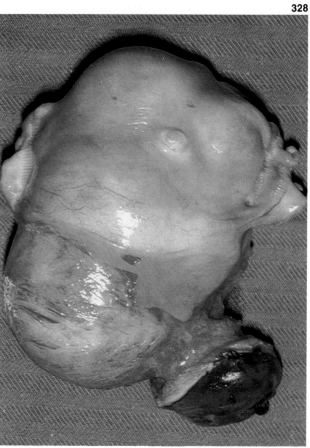

328

Plate 327 Hysterectomy specimen (475 g) showing hyaline change and cystic degeneration within a large fundal fibromyoma encroaching upon the uterine cavity. Note how tissue turgor causes the uterus to spring open when incised anteriorly as though part of its wall had been cut away — the less elastic fibroid has almost enucleated itself (plate 326). The patient was a 29-year-old quadriplegic with menorrhagia who had decided not to have children. In the 5 months before operation the uterus had enlarged from the size of a 12-week pregnancy to that of a 26-week pregnancy, which was suggestive of sarcomatous degeneration.

Plate 328 Hysterectomy specimen (12 × 8 × 6 cm) from a 45-year-old para 3 with regular menses who presented with abdominal pain. There was a hard, irregular mass attached to the cervix and extending into the left lower abdomen. It filled the pelvis and had limited mobility. There were submucous, intramural and subserous fibromyomas, but the largest arose from the supravaginal cervix and extended into the right broad ligament. Note the uterovesical fold of peritoneum reflected above this tumour.

329

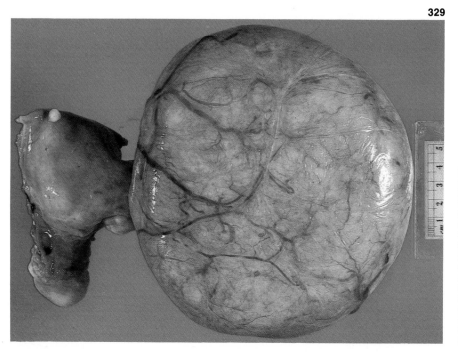

Plate 329 Hysterectomy specimen (1,335 g) showing a huge, pedunculated, subserous fibromyoma (15 × 14 × 8 cm) and several smaller tumours, one of which was calcified. The patient was a 47-year-old nullipara who presented with dysmenorrhoea and abdominal swelling for 12 months. On clinical examination, there was a hard mass, arising out of the pelvis, more to the right side. The provisional diagnosis was carcinoma of the ovary. Histological examination showed hyaline and cystic degeneration throughout the large tumour, and adenomyosis uteri, which may have accounted for the dysmenorrhoea.

330

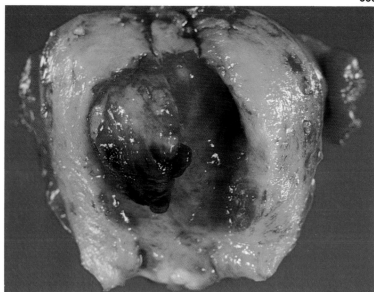

Plate 330 Haemorrhagic adenomyomatous uterine polyp in a 63-year-old patient who presented with heavy postmenopausal bleeding. A polyp protruding 3 cm through the cervix had been twisted off 7 months previously. Bleeding recurred and abdominal hysterectomy was performed. The specimen shows that only part of the polyp had been removed, its ulcerated tip being the source of bleeding. This case illustrates the possible value of hysteroscopy. Note the absence of the lower part of the cervix which had been amputated at a previous Manchester repair.

331

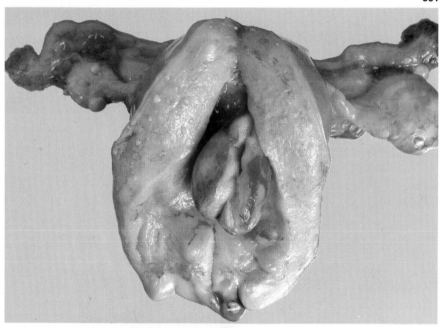

Plate 331 Fibromyomatous polyp. This uterus was removed from a 54-year-old patient who had complained of persistent vaginal bleeding for 3 months. Her haemoglobin value was 7.2 g/dl. After transfusion, a curettage was performed which revealed a degenerate and necrotic endometrium, but no evidence of cancer. The uterus has been incised posteriorly and shows the polyp in the enlarged cavity, together with smaller intramural fibromyomas and normal adnexa.

332

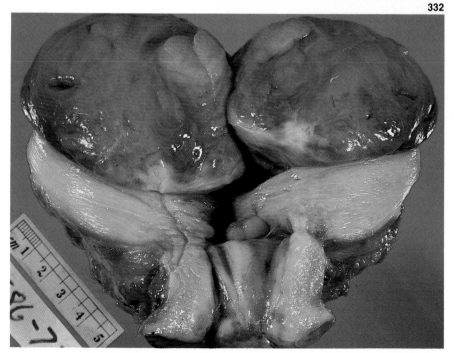

Plate 332 Red degeneration of a fundal fibromyoma (8 cm diameter) apparently caused by intrauterine infection associated with an intrauterine device. The patient was a 48-year-old para 3 who presented with menorrhagia, vomiting and severe abdominal pain of 9 days' duration. Hysterectomy was performed 8 days later when pain persisted in spite of intravenous fluids and antibiotic therapy after removal of the Grafenberg ring (see also plate 326).

333

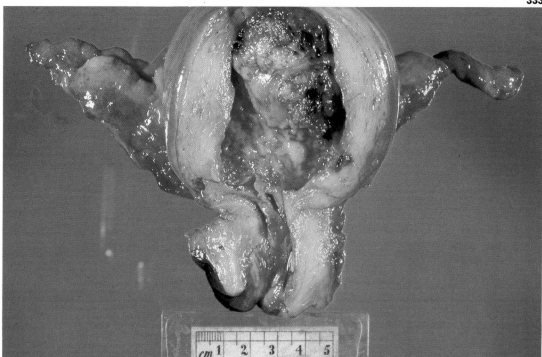

Plate 333 Adenocarcinoma of the endometrium in a 75-year-old para 1 who presented with vaginal bleeding of 4 days' duration. Chest radiography revealed multiple opacities and glucose tolerance testing showed diabetes. Total hysterectomy and bilateral salpingo-oophorectomy produced this 170 g specimen. The tumour (5 × 4 cm) infiltrated the posterior uterine wall and extended to the serosa. In spite of chemotherapy, the patient died 9 months later and at autopsy the pulmonary metastases showed no effect of the cytotoxic drug therapy. It is most unusual for the disease to be so advanced at the time postmenopausal bleeding is first noticed.

334

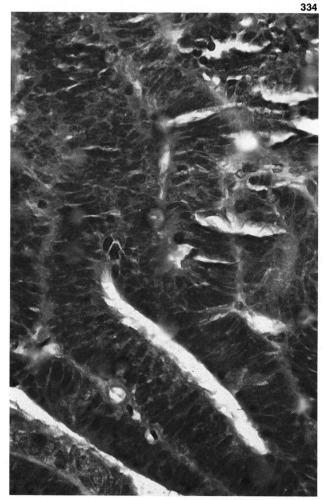

Plate 334 Adenocarcinoma of endometrium. The patient was a 51-year-old para 1 who presented because of irregular vaginal bleeding for 4 weeks. This photomicrograph of curettings shows irregular glands with nuclei arranged at various levels. There is marked basophilia of both cytoplasm (increased RNA) and nuclei (increased DNA and RNA), indicative of increased metabolic activity. (Magnification × 750).

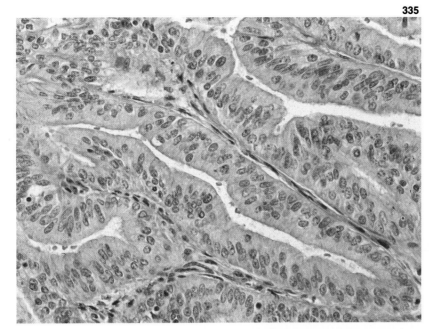

335

Plate 335 The patient was given Provera (medroxyprogesterone), 100 mg 6-hourly, and total hysterectomy and bilateral salpingo-oophorectomy was performed 7 days later. This section of tumour, stained by the same technique, shows a favourable response to progestogen. The glands have a more orderly pattern, with more uniform arrangement of cell nuclei and cytoplasm, more closely resembling that of endometrium in the secretory phase. (Magnification × 750).

336

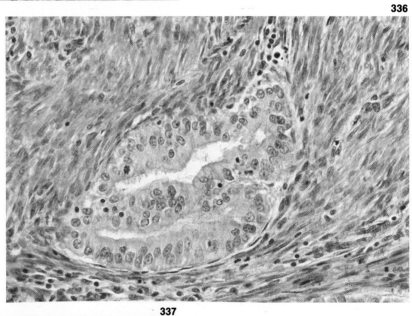

Plate 336 This section is from part of the tumour that had invaded the myometrium. It shows a similar progestogen effect on glandular and cytological characteristics. The patient has remained on Provera and is free of recurrence 3 years after hysterectomy. She had postoperative irradiation to the vagina to lessen the risk of vault recurrence. (Magnification × 750).

337

Plate 337 Choriocarcinoma recognized by demonstration of HCG production by the poorly differentiated cells in this section from a metastatic tumour of unknown origin. (Had the patient been alive, estimation of HCG in urine or plasma would have provided the diagnosis). The cytoplasmic content of beta HCG was shown by application of anti-beta HCG preparation labelled with peroxidase which has reacted to produce a dark brown colour. The tumour cells vary markedly in their capacity to produce HCG; in the midst of the dark-staining cell nest is one showing no HCG production. (Magnification × 1,500). (Courtesy of Dr John Hobbs).

338

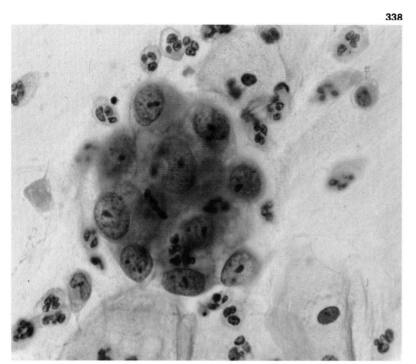

Plate 338 Papanicolaou smear of an adeno-carcinoma of the endometrium. There is a characteristic cluster of poorly differentiated cells with enlarged nuclei having a coarse chromatin pattern; nucleoli are prominent and sometimes multiple. Also shown are polymorphs and eosinophilic vaginal squames of intermediate or superficial type. Such squames in a postmenopausal patient not receiving oestrogen therapy are suggestive of carcinoma. The smear is positive in only 40-60% of all patients with endometrial carcinoma, and in such cases the lesion is often advanced (plates 273 and 274). (Magnification × 400).

Plate 339 Large carcinoma of the endometrium protruding into the uterine cavity as a broad-based polypoid mass showing areas of necrosis. The growth was a well differentiated papillary adenocarcinoma which invaded deeply into the myometrium. The patient was aged 56 years and presented with a history of postmenopausal bleeding for 12 months. She bled heavily at curettage. Treatment was total hysterectomy and bilateral salpingo-oophorectomy with postoperative megavoltage therapy to the pelvis, and Provera (medroxyprogesterone acetate) 100 mg twice daily. She has remained free of recurrence for 4 years (plate 20). **339**

Plate 340 Carcinoma of the endometrium shown as white tissue in this fixed hysterectomy specimen. The patient presented with postmenopausal bleeding and was treated by total hysterectomy and bilateral salpingo-oophorectomy 2 weeks after the diagnosis was established by curettage. The tumour infiltrates the uterine wall, especially anteriorly, where it comes to within 4 mm of the serosal surface. Histology showed an adenocarcinoma, poorly differentiated in areas of deep myometrial invasion, with other areas showing squamous metaplasia. Note that the ovaries are not attached to this specimen. They were resected before the hysterectomy, because they contain metastases in 10% of cases, and handling during the operation can cause peritoneal seeding of tumour cells. **340**

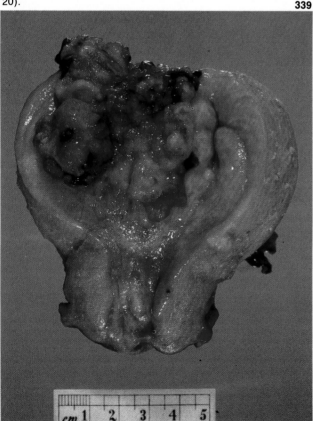

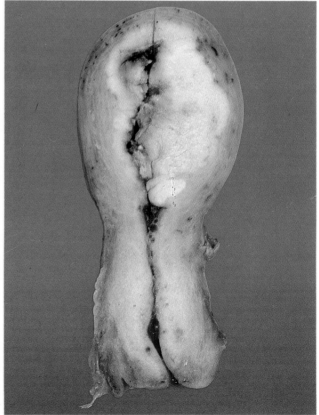

341

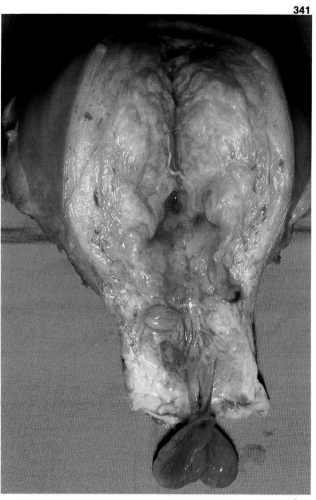

Plate 341 Enlarged uterus (10 × 10 × 7 cm) with thickened muscle wall (up to 5 cm), endometrial hyperplasia and benign endocervical polyp. The patient was a 62-year-old nulliparous widow. Postmenopausal bleeding had occurred intermittently for 16 years, had been regarded as haematuria, and multiple cystoscopies and open renal biopsy, all with negative findings, had been performed! Preoperative curettage was impossible due to a transverse high vaginal septum and so hysterectomy and bilateral salpingo-oophorectomy was performed.

Plate 342 Cystic glandular hyperplasia (Swiss-cheese endometrium) seen in a section of endometrium from the uterus shown in plate 341. Note the distinctive gland pattern with gland size ranging from small to large and cystic. The stroma also shows increased cellularity due to hyperplasia. Such endometrial hyperplasia (glands and stroma) is typical of prolonged stimulation with oestrogen, either endogenous or exogenous (see also plates 85, 86 and 91).

Plate 343 Although the ovaries were not enlarged (1 × 1.5 × 1 cm and 2 × 1 × 1 cm) one on section was found to contain a yellow nodule, 0.7 cm in diameter. Histology revealed a granulosa cell tumour which explained the origin of the oestrogen responsible for both the endometrial hyperplasia and postmenopausal bleeding. This section shows groups of granulosa cells, some arranged in typical rosettes around a central lumen, giving a resemblance to primordial follicles. There was no evidence of metastases and the patient has remained well. (Magnification × 400).

342

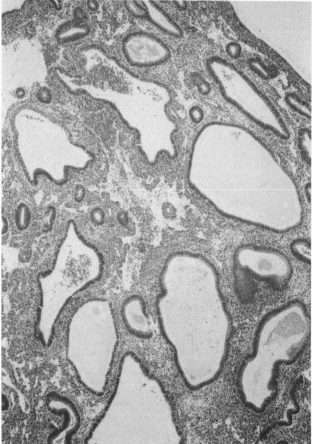

343

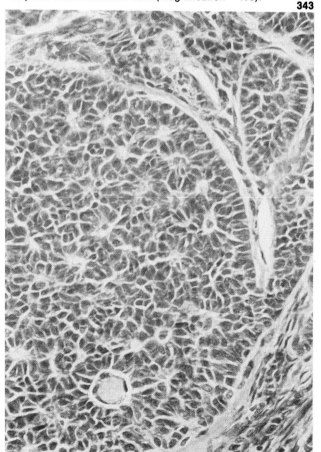

344

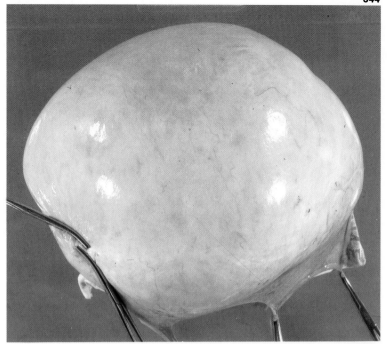

Plate 344 Benign cystic teratoma with typical thick, white glistening wall after enucleation (conservative ovarian cystectomy) from the left ovary of a 17-year-old girl. A continuous locking stitch obliterated the cavity and reconstituted the ovary which remained functional (producing ova and hormones). Although 20 cm in diameter, this tumour was asymptomatic. The patient presented because her sister had lost both ovaries due to torsion of cystic teratomas (see legend to plate 370).

Plate 345 Cystic teratoma of ovary containing hair and sebaceous material. The patient was aged 21 years and presented with abdominal pain due to torsion of the tumour. Treatment was ovarian cystectomy and wedge resection of the other ovary, which was polycystic, to exclude bilateral teratomas which occur in 20% of cases. Histology of tumour showed skin, cartilage, neural tissue and respiratory epithelium. Note characteristic thick smooth wall of tumour that renders enucleation, with conservation of the ovary, a simple bloodless procedure.

345

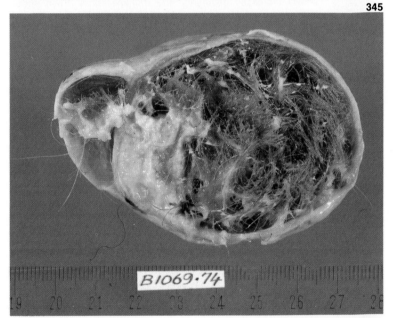

Plate 346 Fibroma of ovary (13 × 12 × 8 cm) from a 55-year-old woman who was found to have a firm, mobile adnexal mass on bimanual palpation at routine examination for cervical cytology. Total hysterectomy and bilateral salpingo-oophorectomy was performed (50% of all ovarian tumours in patients aged 50 years or more are malignant). There was no ascites. Section of the fibroma shows the typical whorled appearance. Occasionally ovarian fibromas, although benign, are associated with ascites and right-sided pleural effusion (Meig's syndrome).

Plate 347 Large theca cell tumour of ovary (830 g) from a 52-year-old woman who presented with abdominal pain due to torsion of the tumour. The uterus contained intramural and subserous fibromyomas. The endometrium was atrophic, showing no evidence that the tumour was secreting oestrogen. However, 15% of patients with oestrogen-producing tumours (thecoma, luteoma, granulosa cell tumour) have an associated carcinoma of the endometrium and this is the strongest evidence available that prolonged administration of unopposed oestrogen can cause cancer.

346

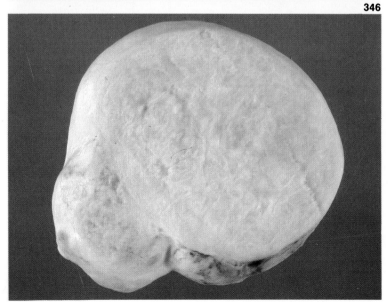

Plate 348 Granulosa-theca cell tumour of ovary and huge, oedematous, cystic endometrial polyp that fills the endometrial cavity and thins the expanded uterine wall. The patient was a 69-year-old para 9 who presented because of vaginal bleeding for 5 months. She was thought to have fibroids. Total hysterectomy and bilateral salpingo-oophorectomy was performed. Histology of the ovarian tumour showed both epithelial (granulosa cell) and connective tissue (theca cell) elements (plates 342 and 343).

Plate 349 Thecoma of right ovary (8 × 5 × 4 cm) removed from a 24-year-old nullipara who presented with 6 years' sterility and 12 months' amenorrhoea. The mass was noted on bimanual vaginal examination. Preoperative urinary hormone excretion was within the nonovulatory range (oestrogen 18ug/24 hours, pregnanediol 1.2 mg/24 hours). The tumour shows the typical yellow cut surface.

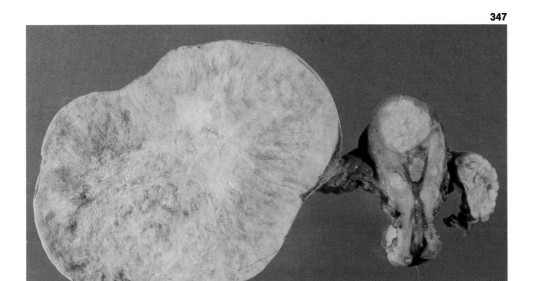

347

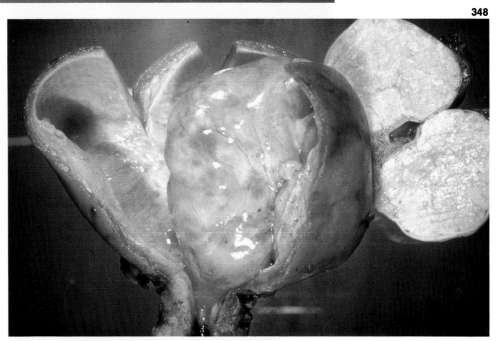

348

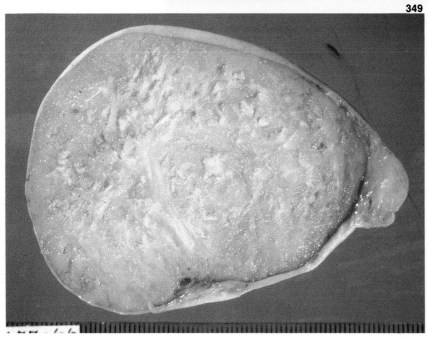

349

350

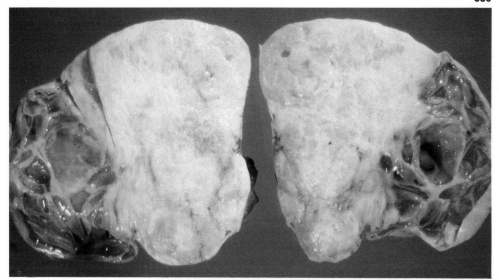

351

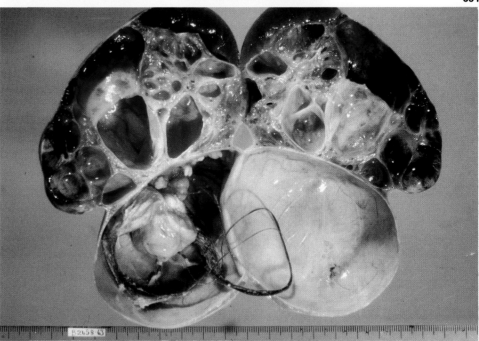

352

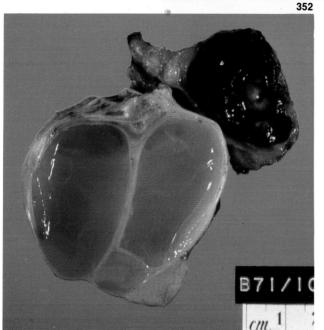

Plate 350 Brenner tumour of the ovary (12 × 10 × 8 cm) with an area of mucinous cystadenoma removed from a 65-year-old para 4 who presented with dysuria and was found to have a hard pelvic mass. Brenner tumours are almost always benign and have a similar cut surface to fibromas, although they contain epithelial cell nests. Brenner tumours and mucinous cystadenomas have a common origin from germinal epithelium of the ovary. However, some mucinous cystadenomas arise from teratomas with ectodermal and other endodermal tissues obliterated (plate 346).

Plate 351 Torsion of an ovarian tumour (12× 8 × 5 cm) comprising a haemorrhagic multilocular mucinous cystadenoma and cystic teratoma in which dermal papillae and hair are seen. The specimen illustrates the possible teratomatous origin of some mucinous cystadenomas as stated in legend to plate 350. The patient was a 20-year-old nullipara who presented with a 12-hour history of severe, colicky, lower abdominal pain. Treatment was ovarian cystectomy since the ovary was still viable.

Plate 352 Ovary removed from 19-year-old nullipara who presented because of progressive abdominal swelling for 3 years. At laparotomy, 10 litres of fluid was aspirated from a left ovarian cyst which was then removed (oophorectomy). The other ovary contained the cystic tumour (4 × 3 cm) shown here which was removed with preservation of the base of the ovary. Histology showed both tumours to be serous cystadenomas.

353

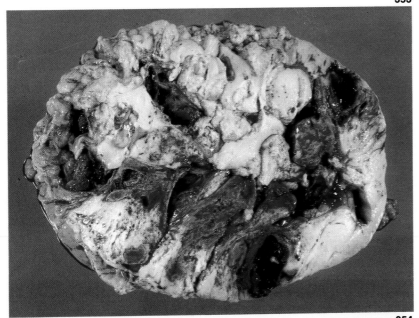

Plate 353 Granulosa cell tumour of ovary (18 × 13 × 8 cm) removed from a 71-year-old woman who had had a hysterectomy when aged 55 years (it is usual to advise prophylactic bilateral oophorectomy when performing hysterectomy in patients aged 45 years or more to avoid ovarian malignancy). This section shows firm, yellowish-pink nodular masses with patchy areas of haemorrhage. Urinary oestrogen excretion fell from 64 to 2.2 μg/24 hours after removal of the tumour. She returned 5 years later with an abdominal mass and distension, and oestrogen excretion was 43.4 μg/24 hours. Laparotomy revealed widespread metastases in bowel and liver; she died suddenly 30 days later (plates 343 and 348).

354

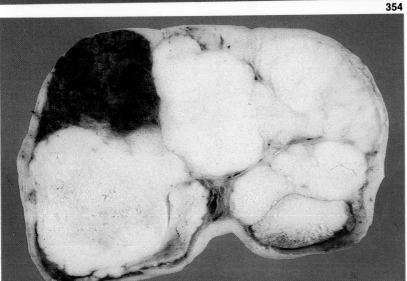

Plate 354 Dysgerminoma of the ovary (1,080 g) containing a primary haemorrhagic choriocarcinoma. The patient was aged 15 years and presented with a pelvic mass and positive pregnancy test. Pulmonary metastases became apparent 3 months after oophorectomy. She died 10 months after initial presentation in spite of chemotherapy. This specimen has been decolorized by formalin and so lacks the typical brain-like appearance shown in the tumour in plate 355.

355

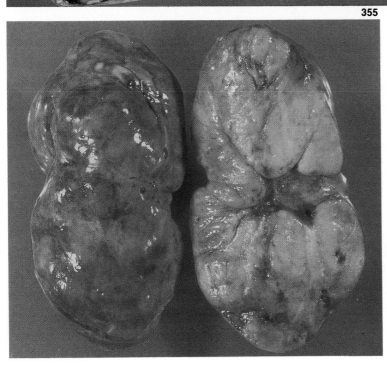

Plate 355 Dysgerminoma of the right ovary (23 × 9 × 11 cm, weight 1,370 g) showing the typical creamy-white, homogeneous (brain-like) cut surface with areas of haemorrhage and necrosis. The patient was an unmarried nullipara aged 30 years who presented 5 days after she noted an abdominal swelling. At laparotomy the mass was mobile, the tumour appeared encapsulated, and there was no evidence of lymph node enlargement or peritoneal matestases. Although the diagnosis of dysgerminoma was made on macroscopic appearance, the other ovary was not sectioned as it seemed normal. Two months later total hysterectomy and left oophorectomy was performed when the patient and her medical advisers had considered her prognosis and reproductive future. The remaining ovary had become enlarged and histology revealed the typical pattern of a dysgerminoma (uniform vesicular cells separated by fibrous septa infiltrated by lymphocytes). Radiotherapy was administered postoperatively and the patient remains in good health without evidence of residual disease. This tumour often affects young women and is sometimes bilateral. Hence the cruel decision regarding removal of the apparently normal ovary even though the tumour and its metastases are very radiosensitive.

356

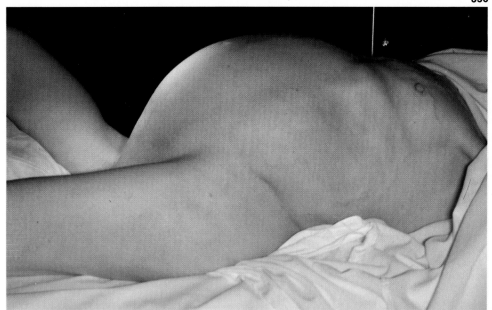

Plate 356 This 62-year-old nulliparous widow presented with a history of painless, progressive abdominal distension for 18 to 24 months. A physician aspirated her 'ascites' and pseudomyxoma peritonei was diagnosed when cytological examination of this greenish fluid showed atypical columnar cells. Note the distended veins in her abdominal wall.

357

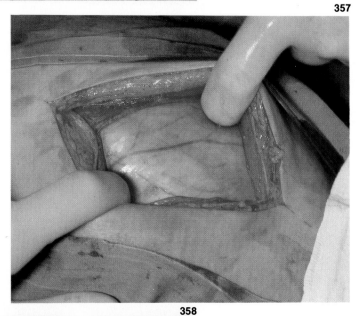

Plate 357 Through a subumbilical midline incision the thick smooth wall of a large mucinous cystadenoma was seen. The cyst was adherent to the parietal peritoneum of the abdominal wall and to the liver and was separated by digital pressure. This is an unusual finding even when a cyst has been present for years. There was no ascites.

Plate 358 The trocar and cannula was passed and the trocar withdrawn and 7,000 ml of fluid was aspirated by attaching the rubber tubing of the sucker to the cannula. Decompression of the bulk of the tumour allowed its removal through a relatively small incision. Spillage of fluid into the peritoneal cavity was carefully avoided.

358

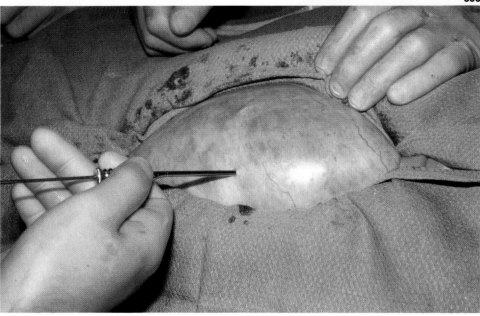

359

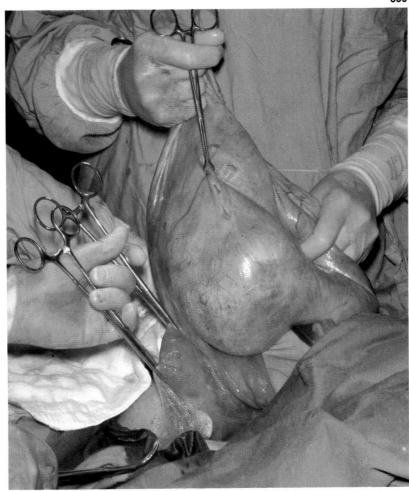

Plate 359 The cyst has been delivered from the abdominal cavity. Straight forceps are attached to the sides of the uterus which has been held forwards to show the normal left ovary. Total hysterectomy and bilateral salpingo-oophorectomy was performed. The mucinous cystadenoma showed a single layer of well differentiated columnar cells. The moral is that very big tumours are often benign; despite this, laparotomy should be undertaken as soon as possible (plate 366).

Plate 360 Benign mucinous cystadenoma in a 70-year-old para 6 alcoholic widow (weight 46 kg) who presented with a 12-month history of abdominal distension, increasing epigastric discomfort and vomiting. She was emaciated, but had swollen legs due to vena caval compression. A provisional diagnosis of ovarian tumour with malignant ascites was made. At laparotomy, 21 litres of mucinous, dark brown fluid was aspirated from the tumour which was adherent to anterior and posterior abdominal walls. There was no ascites. Total hysterectomy and bilateral salpingo-oophorectomy was performed and the abdomen closed with tension sutures.

360

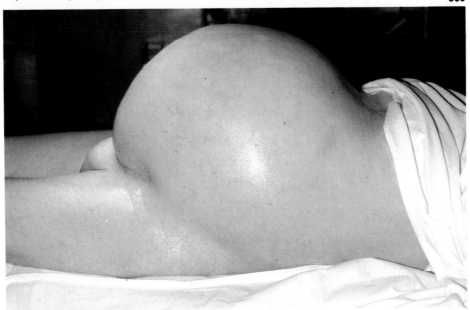

144

361

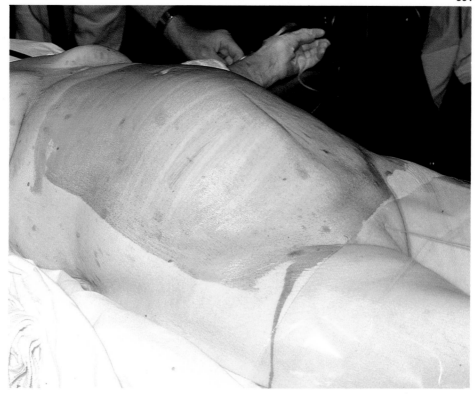

Plate 361 Huge ovarian cyst outlined preoperatively by antiseptic skin preparation of povidone iodine (1%). Note symmetrical enlargement of abdomen. The patient was aged 84 years and presented because her local practitioner noted the abdominal mass when she complained of weight loss. The mass was painless, ballottable and caused no pressure symptoms. The midline scar was that of a long past tubal ligation although the patient said she had had a hysterectomy!

Plate 362 Laparotomy revealed this huge, mobile, polycystic enlargement of the left ovary (28 × 18 × 13 cm) due to a benign mucinous cystadenoma. There was no ascites. The slightly enlarged uterus is held forward with clamps and the normal-sized atrophic right ovary is shown. Total hysterectomy and bilateral salpingo-oophorectomy was performed and the patient was discharged from hospital 8 days later.

362

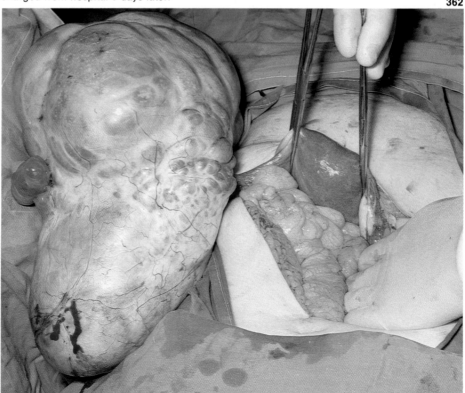

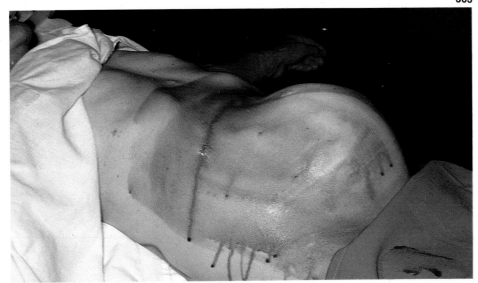

Plate 363 Large extraperitoneal ovarian cyst with limited mobility in a 66-year-old para 1 who had had abdominal hysterectomy performed for menorrhagia many years ago. Note that the abdominal distension is subumbilical and not generalized as in plate 361. When cysts or tumours develop in ovaries conserved at hysterectomy, they often grow into the broad ligament rather than the peritoneal cavity.

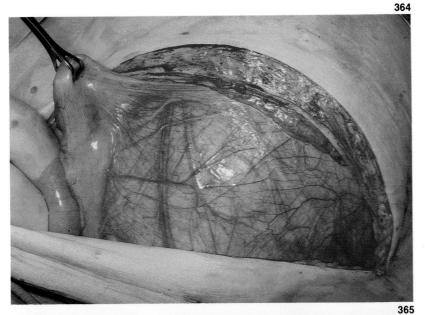

Plate 364 Same patient showing how the ovarian cyst had grown into sigmoid colon mesentery. The peritoneum was incised, avoiding blood vessels, and the cyst enucleated, at first with ease and then with difficulty because the ureter was adherent to its inferior aspect.

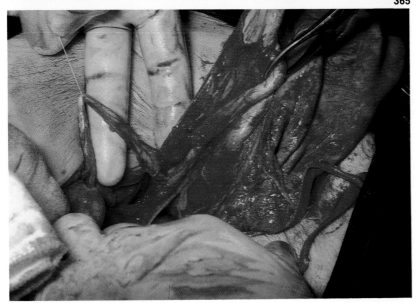

Plate 365 Ninety minutes later the benign cyst with ruptured fibrous wall (histologically no viable epithelium) has been removed after dissection of the left ureter shown by tissue forceps and catgut loop. Note the hole in the bladder 3 cm from the forceps which was closed in layers. The patient had an indwelling catheter for 8 days and was discharged 10 days after operation, following an uneventful convalescence. The moral is to be ready for a difficult dissection when an ovarian tumour develops in a patient who has had a hysterectomy. Preoperative barium enema and pyelography are useful investigations in such patients.

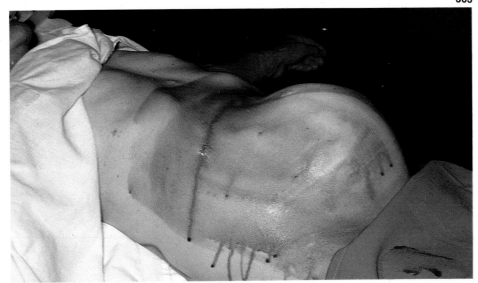

366

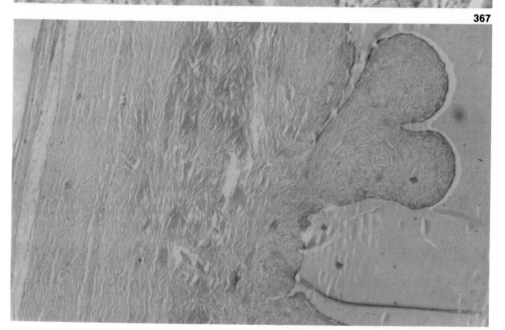

367

Plate 366 Section of benign mucinous cystadenoma of ovary showing characteristic tall columnar epithelium and basal nuclei. The patient was a 33-year-old para 3 diabetic who was found to have a huge ovarian tumour (cystadenoma with smaller serous and larger mucinous components) at elective Caesarean section. The stroma shows striking theca cell hyperplasia, presumably an effect of the hormones of pregnancy. (Magnification × 400).

Plate 367 Section of serous component from the same tumour shown in plate 366 illustrating characteristic papillae lined by cuboidal cells indicative of the origin from the germinal epithelium of ovary. Serous cystadenomas have a greater tendency to malignant change than the commoner mucinous cystadenomas. (Magnification × 40).

Plate 368 View at myomectomy performed for menorrhagia and secondary infertility in a 36-year-old para 1. Red degeneration of this fibroid caused acute abdominal pain at 19 weeks' gestation in her pregnancy 2 years previously. The fibroid was hard and pale and weighed 75 g when enucleated; histology showed extensive hyaline necrosis. An unexpected finding was the 5 cm diameter mucinous cystadenoma of the ovary. This cystic tumour was excised, but oophorectomy may have been wiser in view of the malignant potential of such lesions. Round ligament and tube are held with forceps to display how the fibroid distorted the interstitial portion of the tube (plates 326 and 332).

368

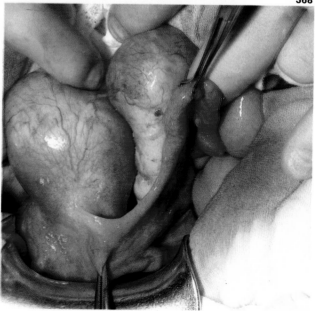

369

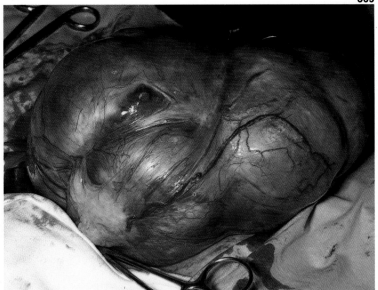

Plate 369 Huge (benign) serous cystadenoma of right ovary (2,365 g) in a 51-year-old para 2. The patient had hepatomegaly and chronic liver disease and paracentesis (6,000 ml) of 'ascites' had been performed 2 years previously, when her local practitioner referred her with a provisional diagnosis of advanced ovarian carcinoma. There were numerous adhesions of bowel to tumour. Note that large vessels coursing over a tumour are not positive evidence of malignancy. There was no free fluid in the peritoneal cavity. Total hysterectomy and bilateral salpingo-oophorectomy was performed. The patient then returned to her physician for continued care of hepatic insufficiency. The moral is that abdominal masses merit laparotomy not paracentesis. Ascites and large cystic ovarian tumours can be impossible to differentiate clinically. Ultrasonography is often very helpful.

370

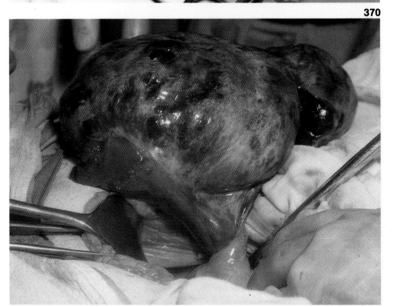

Plate 370 Torsion of benign cystic teratoma and tube in a 16-year-old girl who presented with increasing pain radiating from loin to groin for 2 days. A radiograph showed teeth within the tumour. Because of delay in presentation, the ovary was gangrenous and had to be removed. The pedicles upon which such a tumour twists are infundibulopelvic ligament laterally and ovarian ligament and Fallopian tube medially. Sadly this patient had lost her other ovary due to the same complication 5 years earlier. Such a case illustrates the rationale for bisection (and resuture) of the other ovary to exclude bilateral disease (20% of cases) (plate 344).

Plate 371 Huge (2,215 g) primary mucinous cystadenocarcinoma of the left ovary in a 49-year-old para 7 who presented with increasing abdominal distension, menorrhagia, anorexia and epigastric pain, all of 6 weeks' duration. She weighed 85 kg. At laparotomy, 12 litres of ascitic fluid was aspirated, the tumour (24 × 18 × 10 cm) was removed and hysterectomy with removal of right ovary and omentum was performed. The tumour had invaded the uterus and filled the endometrial cavity, thus accounting for the menorrhagia. Chlorambucil (5 mg/day) was prescribed for 6 months and intermittently thereafter. The patient is alive and apparently free of residual disease or recurrence (weight now 115 kg!) 7 years after operation.

371

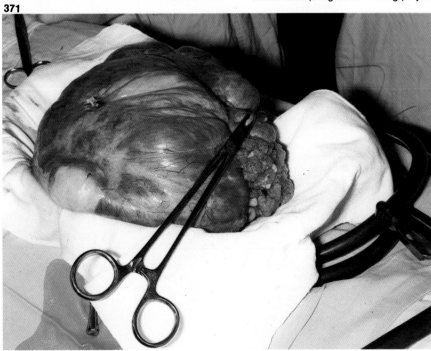

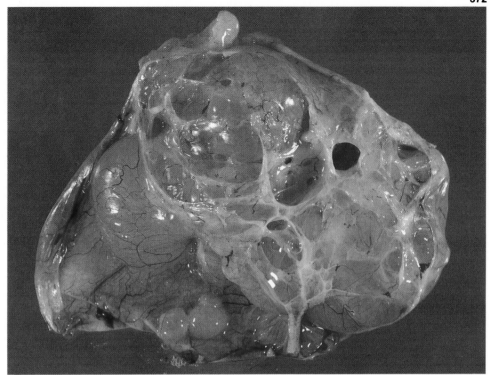

Plate 372 Mucinous cystadenoma (15 × 17 × 12 cm) of left ovary from a 52-year-old para 3 who presented 7 years after her menopause with a 'lump in the side'. Palpation revealed a central abdominal mass extending above the umbilicus. Treatment was total hysterectomy and bilateral salpingo-oophorectomy. Multilocular mucin-containing cysts are shown. These had the typical lining of a single layer of columnar cells (plate 366).

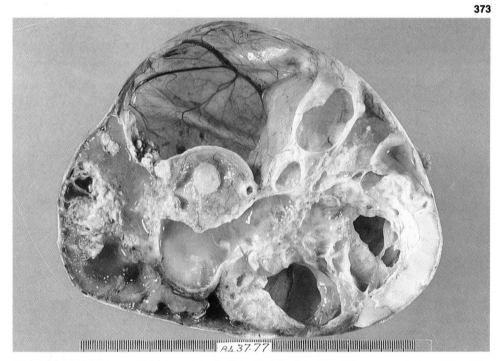

Plate 373 Mucinous cystadenocarcinoma (17 × 12 × 8 cm) of the left ovary weighing 800 g. The section shows solid areas of pinkish-white tumour and a smooth outer surface. The patient was aged 59 years and presented with acute abdominal pain due to spontaneous rupture of the tumour. Treatment was total hysterectomy and bilateral salpingo-oophorectomy and postoperative mega-voltage therapy. At operation there was no evidence of spread beyond the ovary. The patient returned 30 months later with bowel obstruction due to metastases and died 7 days later. Omentectomy is now routinely performed at the time of initial surgical management.

374

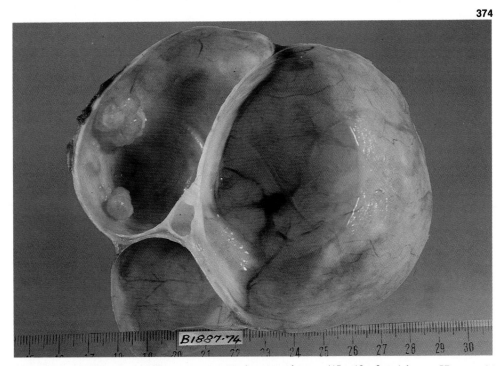

Plate 374 Multilocular papillary serous cystadenoma of ovary (15 × 13 × 9 cm) from a 57-year-old para 2 who had had a hysterectomy performed 15 years earlier for fibromyomas. This lesion was asymptomatic and was noted when the patient presented with a large cystocele. Ascites occasionally causes raised intraabdominal pressure and precipitates uterovaginal prolapse.

375

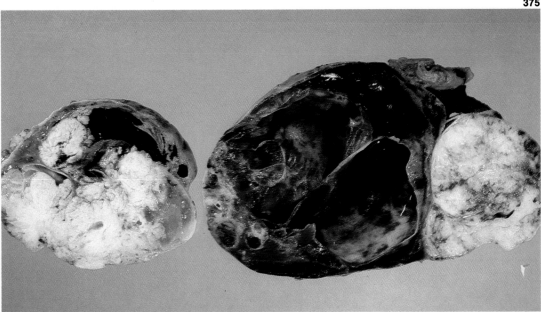

Plate 375 Bilateral ovarian serous cystadenocarcinomas (10 × 8 × 7 cm and 15 × 10 × 8 cm). Solid pinkish-white masses of tumour and multilocular cysts containing clotted blood are shown. The patient was a 54-year-old para 4 who presented with a 3-month history of increasing abdominal pain and distension. She had bled vaginally on one occasion 2 months earlier. Total hysterectomy and bilateral salpingo-oophorectomy was performed. There were seedling secondaries in the pouch of Douglas and 500 ml of ascitic fluid. Late presentation is the sad stigma of ovarian cancer.

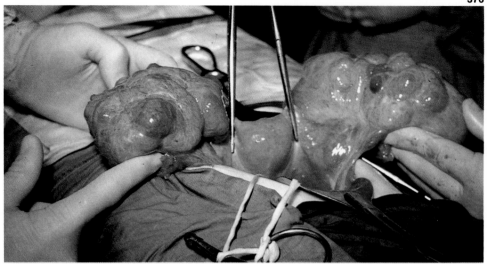

Plate 376 Krukenberg tumours of the ovary seen at laparotomy; the uterus is held forwards. These tumours are bilateral, firm, rapidly-growing and mobile, even when large. Almost invariably metastatic, the pathognomonic histological features are intracellular mucin secretion forming signet ring cells (nuclei displaced peripherally), and marked stromal reaction that may simulate the appearance of a sarcoma.

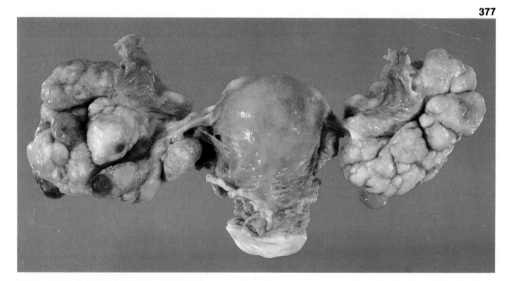

Plate 377 Krukenberg tumours and uterus removed from a 41-year-old patient who was due to have a gastrectomy performed for a gastric ulcer. These tumours comprise 4% of all ovarian secondary carcinomas, usually arise from the stomach (pylorus) and the primary can be small. The average time from diagnosis to death is 6 months. Note the striking similarity to the tumour in the patient shown in plate 376.

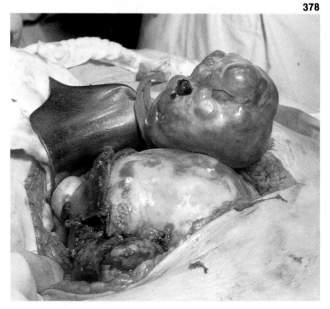

Plate 378 Bilateral, poorly differentiated, serous cystadenocarcinomas of ovaries, with primary well differentiated, papillary adenocarcinoma of the uterus in a 76-year-old woman who presented with an abdominal mass and palpable supraclavicular lymph gland. Histology of curettings and neck gland biopsy revealed adenocarcinomas of separate origin. Total hysterectomy and bilateral salpingo-oophorectomy was performed. About 20% of patients with gynaecological malignancy have 2 or more primary tumours.

379

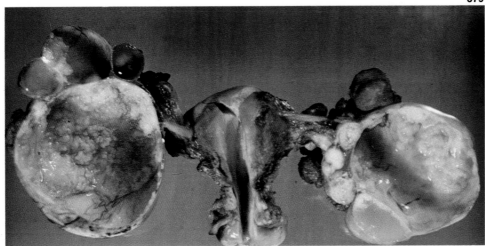

Plate 379 Bilateral papillary serous cystadenocarcinomas and uterus removed from a 42-year-old woman who presented (unfortunately too late) with menorrhagia and was found to have large pelvic masses. There was no ascites or evidence of peritoneal metastases, but the tumours recurred.

380

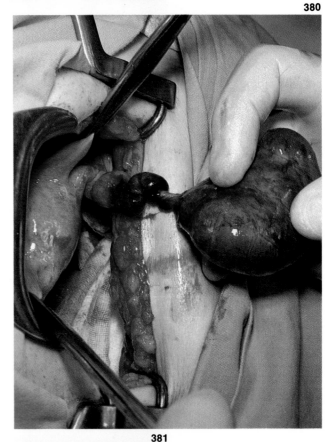

Plate 380 Torsion of a haemorrhagic Fallopian tube. The patient was a 37-year-old para 1 who presented with abdominal pain 7 days after removal of an intrauterine device. The initial diagnosis was pelvic inflammatory disease. Laparotomy was performed when pain persisted and the tubal mass, which was situated in the pouch of Douglas, was removed. The right ovary contained a corpus luteum. There was no evidence of a precipitating lesion such as a cyst or ectopic pregnancy.

Plate 381 Carcinoma of the left Fallopian tube in a 60-year-old woman who presented with postmenopausal bleeding. Hysterectomy and bilateral salpingo-oophorectomy was performed when friable white curettings indicated endometrial carcinoma. The primary adenocarcinoma of the tube was an incidental finding seen as a white mass bulging the fimbriated end of the tube. It did not penetrate through the tubal wall. The classical history of a clear, copious vaginal discharge precipitated by bimanual palpation was lacking. The upper part of the endometrial cavity shows the separate, primary, well differentiated carcinoma of endometrium.

381

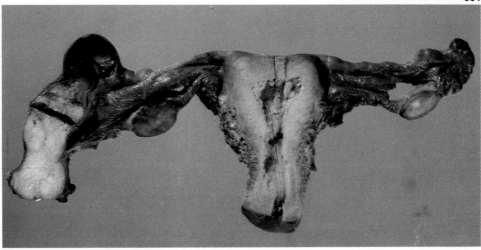

382

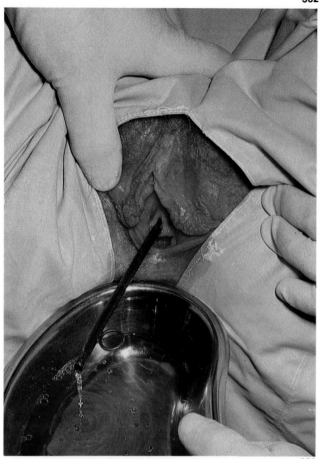

Plate 382 Dilatation and curettage, the commonest operation in medical practice, requires careful technique to avoid the serious complications of perforation, haemorrhage and damage to the cervix. After preparation and draping of the anaesthetized patient, the bladder was emptied, so that bimanual vaginal examination could outline the size and position of the uterus and check for adnexal pathology.

Plate 383 Having noted the position of the uterus (anteversion, midposition, retroversion), the cervix was grasped with a volsellum and steadied, while a uterine sound was introduced in the appropriate direction to measure the length of the uterine cavity, and thus the length of the dilator that could be introduced with safety.

Plate 384 The endocervical canal was dilated to 8 mm diameter using progressively wider dilators. In nulliparas and postmenopausal women, the cervix is often fibrous and resists dilatation. Narrow curettes must be available so that excessive dilatation can be avoided. Note that perforation of the uterus was prevented by the finger on the Hegar dilator limiting penetration to the uterine cavity.

383

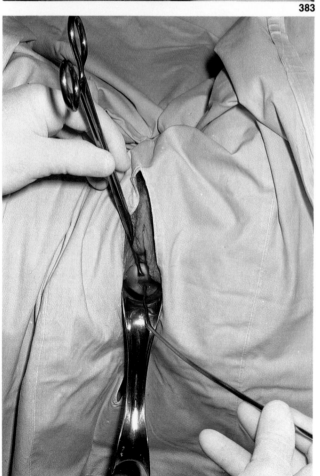

384

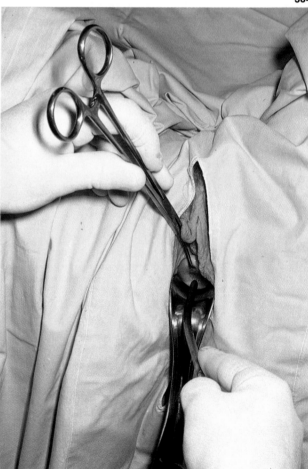

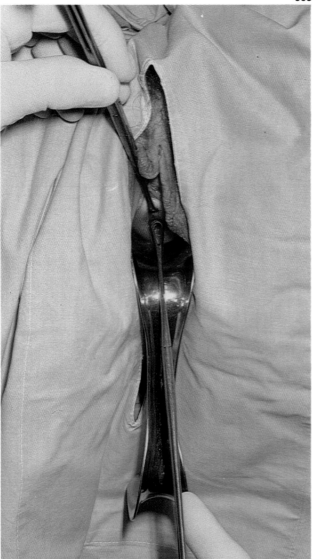

Plate 385 Small forceps are introduced prior to curettage to grasp polyps or intrauterine devices with missing tails. Polyps often evade the curette (plate 330) and hence the value of hysteroscopy in patients with abnormal uterine bleeding. When inside the uterus the forceps were opened, rotated 90 degrees, closed and withdrawn.

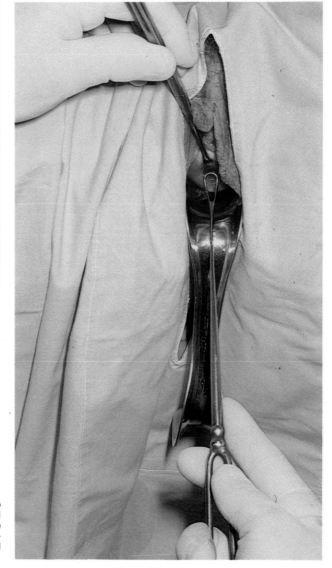

Plate 386 The curette, held as shown, and appropriate in size to the dilatation of the cervix, was introduced and the endometrial surface systematically scraped over. To obtain samples of the endometrium, curettes are introduced slowly and removed briskly. The curettings are best collected on a gauze swab placed beneath the cervix (plates 19 and 20).

387
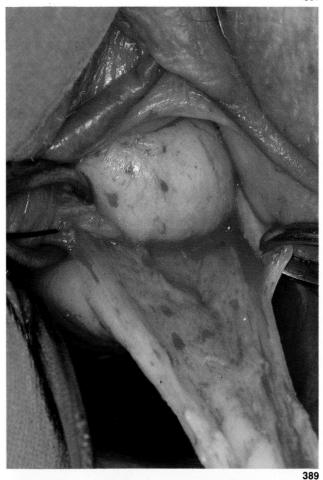

388
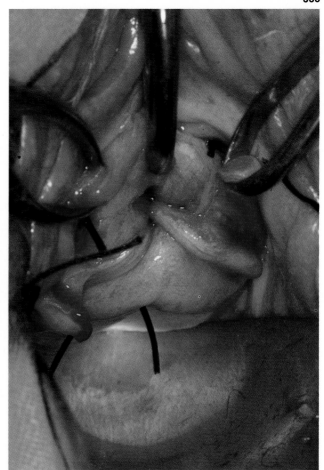

389
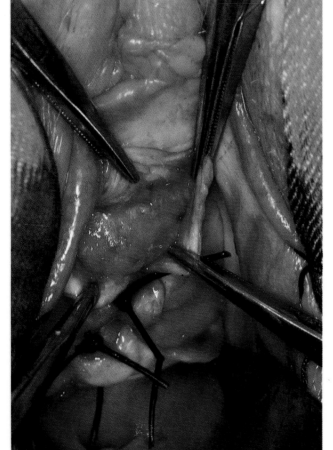

Plate 387 Manchester repair in a 78-year-old para 2 who had noted vulval discomfort due to a lump, and urinary frequency for 6 months. There was a second degree uterine prolapse, cystocele, small rectocele, but no enterocele. A triangular flap of epithelium has been dissected from the anterior vaginal wall and reveals the posterior wall of the bladder which is forming the cystocele; the cervix is seen below the bladder (see also plates 184 to 193).

Plate 388 The cardinal ligaments have been clamped, cut and ligated and the posterior Sturmdorf suture has been inserted, thereby covering the posterior aspect of the amputated cervix with vaginal epithelium. The tissue forceps hold the edges of vaginal epithelium which will be sutured together and attached to the cervix by the anterior Sturmdorf suture.

Plate 389 The cervical stump has been covered with epithelium and the artery forceps hold the cut edges of vagina preparatory to insertion of mattress sutures in the vaginal (pubocervical) fascia (plate 192).

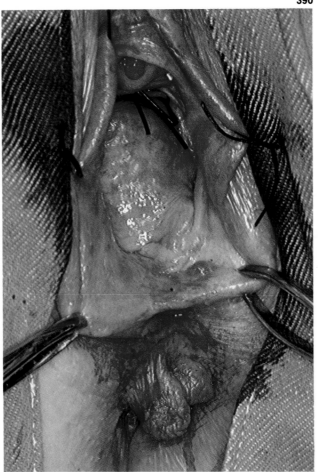

390

Plate 390 Tissue forceps display the perineal deficiency and outline the base of the triangular flap of epithelium to be removed from the posterior vaginal wall overlying the rectocele. The apex of the flap extends to the cervix to avoid missing a potential enterocele.

Plate 391 The defect in the posterior vaginal wall is being closed with a continuous locking suture beginning at the apex of the excision. At this stage a mattress suture was inserted in the levatores ani muscles to suture them together anterior to the rectum and anal canal (plate 414).

Plate 392 Appearance on completion of the posterior colpoperineorrhaphy. An indwelling urinary catheter and vaginal pack impregnated with an antiseptic cream were then inserted (plate 416).

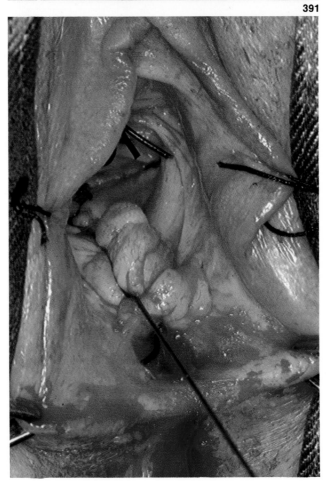

391

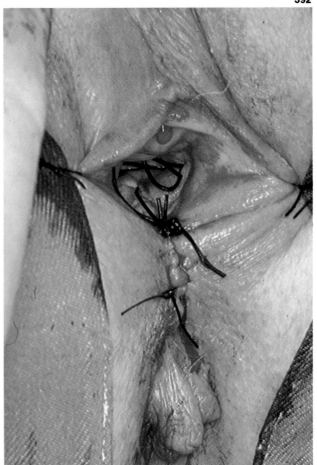

392

393

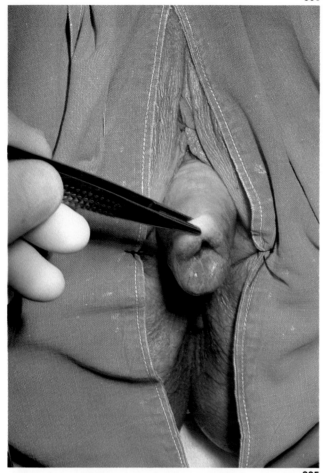

395

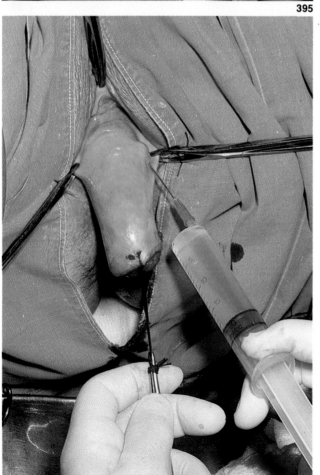

394

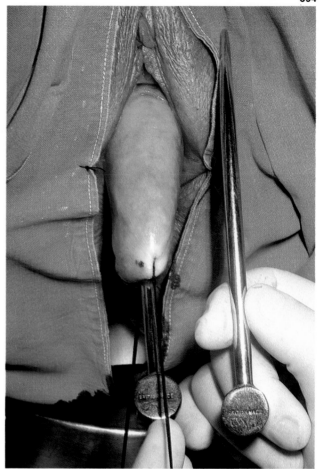

Plate 393 Vaginal hysterectomy and repair in a 79-year-old para 2 who presented with a vaginal lump of 12 months' duration. She stated that she had to push the lump back in order to void. It is difficult to understand how prolapse occurs suddenly in such elderly patients if the aetiology is postmenopausal atrophy of vaginal and uterine supports due to oestrogen deprivation. The hypertrophied cervix is shown, like a vaginal intussusception, with almost complete eversion of the vagina. Note the patulous external os and cervix reddened by abrasion from clothing.

Plate 394 Marked elongation of the cervix is shown, 11 cm of the Hegar dilator lying within the endocervical canal and uterine cavity; the uterus itself was small and retroverted.

Plate 395 Tissue forceps at the margins of the introitus mark the extent of the lateral aspect of the triangular flap of anterior vaginal epithelium to be excised (plates 175 and 185). A vaso-constrictor solution (ornipressin, 5 iu in 50 ml normal saline) was injected beneath the vaginal epithelium to reduce blood loss and facilitate dissection.

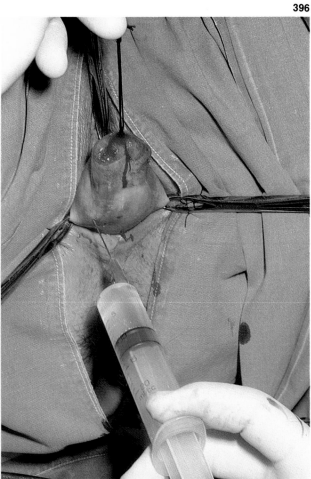

Plate 396   The solution was also injected in the proposed line of incision in the posterior vaginal wall. Note that because the vagina was almost completely everted the posterior vaginal wall was too short for a speculum to be inserted.

Plate 397   The anterior flap of vaginal epithelium has been reflected and the bladder pushed off the cervix to expose the vesicouterine fold of peritoneum. The stretched lateral cervical ligaments are displayed.

Plate 398   The incision in the vaginal epithelium was continued posteriorly so that the uterus and attached upper vaginal epithelium was mobilized and freed from the vaginal walls.

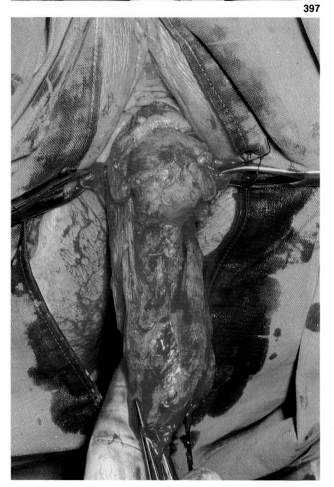

397

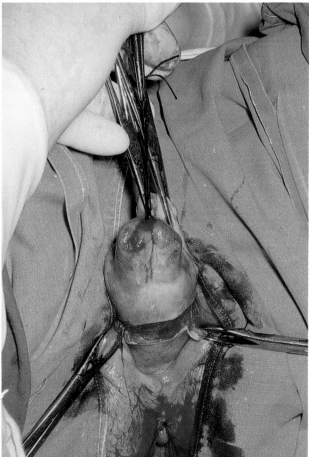

398

158

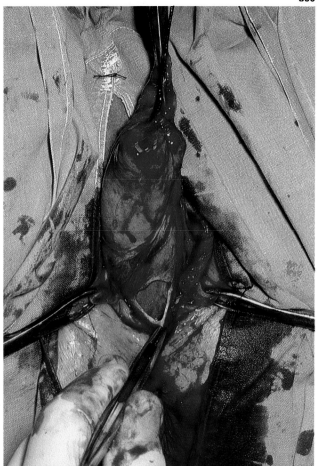

399

Plate 399 The peritoneal cavity has been entered by incision of the posterior fold of the pouch of Douglas; a moderate-sized enterocele is shown. Some surgeons first enter the peritoneal cavity via the anterior (vesicouterine) pouch, but we consider that the easiest and safest route from the vagina into the peritoneal cavity is through the posterior fornix.

Plate 400 With the bladder held safely away anteriorly, and the uterosacral and cardinal ligaments put on the stretch by traction on the uterus downwards and to the patient's right side, the left uterosacral and cardinal ligaments are clamped, cut and ligated. The hidden blade of the curved clamp was introduced via the peritoneal cavity.

Plate 401 Both uterosacral and lateral cervical ligaments have been clamped and cut. The suture holds the midline edge of the peritoneum posteriorly. The uterus has descended further having been freed from its major supports.

400

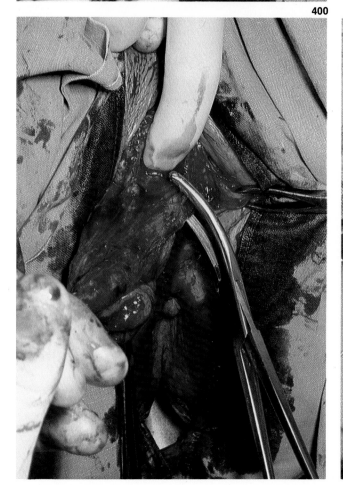

401

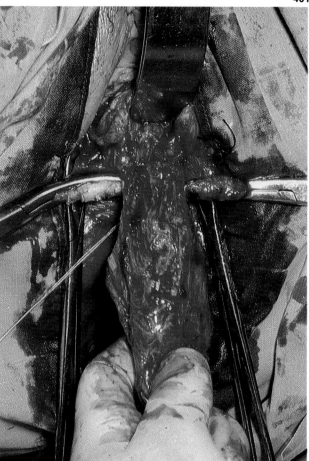

402

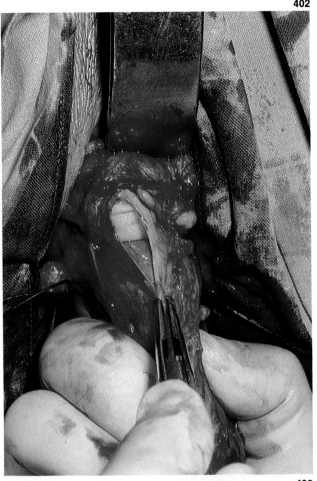

Plate 402 The bladder was held anteriorly by a retractor to prevent its injury as the anterior pouch of peritoneum was opened, the pouch having been displayed by the finger passing upwards over the uterine fundus.

Plate 403 The uterine arteries have been clamped and ligated on each side and the uterine fundus has prolapsed posteriorly.

Plate 404 The third and highest pedicle (Fallopian tube, round ligament, ovarian ligament) has been clamped on the right side, having been already clamped and divided on the left side. Note the degree of cervical hypertrophy by comparison of the length of the cervix with that of the uterine body.

403

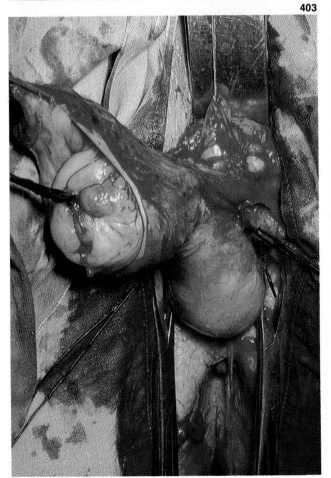

404

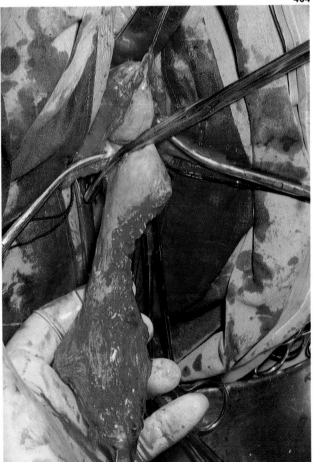

405

406

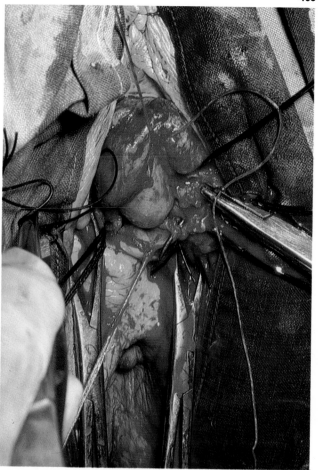

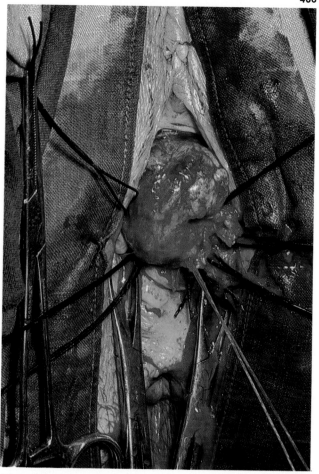

Plate 405   The uterus has been removed and the 3 pedicles on each side tied. The peritoneal cavity is now closed by a purse-string suture. This step is important to prevent prolapse of Fallopian tubes or bowel, especially if the vaginal vault is left open to prevent possible extraperitoneal haematoma formation.

Plate 406   The prolapsed bladder has flopped over the vaginal vault. The 3 pairs of ligatures on uterosacral and cardinal ligaments, uterine vessels and parametrium, and ovarian ligament, round ligament and Fallopian tube are shown. The 2 members of each pair will now be tied together to form a firm extraperitoneal keel at the vaginal vault (plate 407).

407

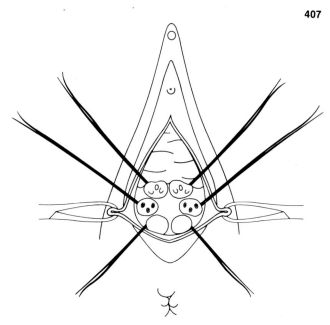

Plate 407   Diagram showing the 3 pairs of doubly-ligated pedicles. The lowermost pair of pedicles (uterosacral and cardinal ligament) are first tied together and this forms the apex of the new vaginal vault, eliminates the pouch of Douglas, and minimizes the risk of a posthysterectomy enterocele occurring. Next, the middle pedicles (containing the uterine vessels) are tied and finally the broad ligament pedicles (round and ovarian ligaments and Fallopian tubes).

408

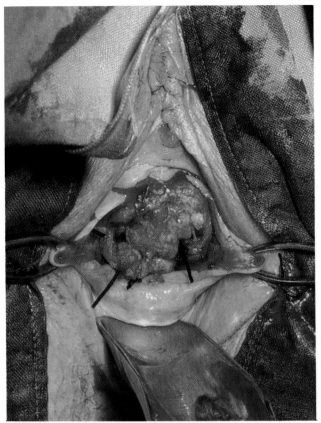

Plate 408 The vault pedicles have been tied and the cystocele partly reduced by mattress sutures placed in the pubovesical fascia inverting the bladder wall. The vaginal vault is displayed between the 2 tissue forceps that have remained in position throughout the operation (plate 395). The vault can be closed transversely or vertically. We prefer the latter since it is easier, and restores length to the posterior vaginal wall.

409

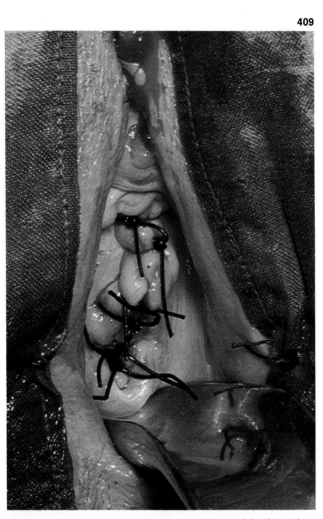

Plate 409 Mattress sutures have been inserted in the pubovesical vaginal fascia (plate 192) and the anterior vaginal wall closed with interrupted chromic catgut sutures. The Sims' speculum illustrates that the vaginal vault is well supported and adequate length restored to the posterior vaginal wall.

410

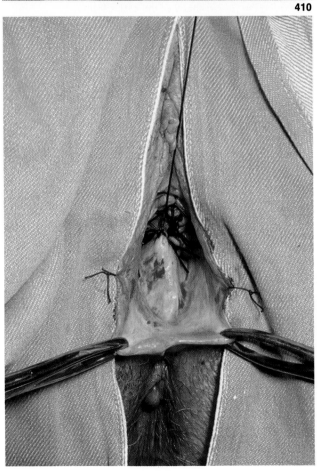

Plate 410 The posterior colpoperineorrhaphy begins with placement of a stitch at the top of the posterior vaginal wall leaving no gap between it and the recently reformed vaginal vault, where an enterocele could develop. The tissue forceps outline the extent of the epithelial edge of the introitus that will be excised; at the end of the operation, these 2 points will be sutured together, forming the new posterior fourchette.

162

411

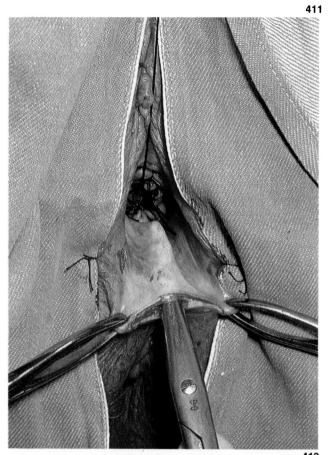

Plate 411 The epithelial edge has been excised with the curved Mayo scissors which are now used to separate the posterior vaginal wall from the rectum. Injury to the rectum is avoided by traction on the suture at the top of the vagina to tense the posterior wall, and by directing the scissors anteriorly, as they are opened to separate the fascial rectovaginal septum from the posterior vaginal wall. On conclusion of the posterior colporrhaphy, the incision at the introitus is closed vertically, to restore the perineal body between the anal canal and vagina, and narrow the introitus to a normal calibre.

Plate 412 The vaginal wall has been incised in the midline to the vaginal vault, exposing the rectum and the levatores ani muscles which lie laterally. In this patient there was no need, as is often the case, to excise any posterior vaginal wall epithelium. To do so could have caused an hour-glass shaped vagina with a constriction in the middle (plate 237). The incision allows the torn prerectal fascia (which lies between the rectum and vagina) to be sutured, thus repairing the rectocele.

Plate 413 There is no need to undermine the edges of the vagina in order to place sutures in the fascia between the rectum and vagina to repair a rectocele. Mattress sutures are inserted by the technique described in the legend to plate 192, care being taken not to narrow the vagina excessively. The continuous locking stitch has been advanced half-way down the vagina; the first mattress stitch in the prerectal fascia has been inserted. A mattress suture is now placed in the levatores ani muscles bringing them together anterior to the anal canal, thereby restoring the wedge shape of the perineal body.

412

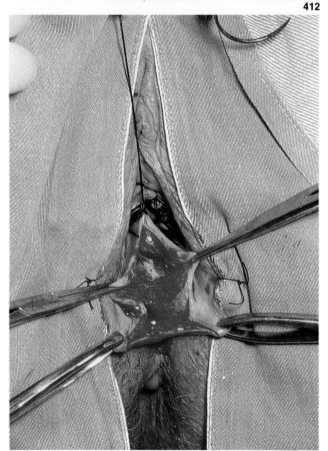

413

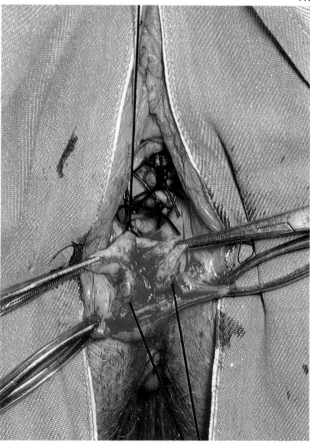

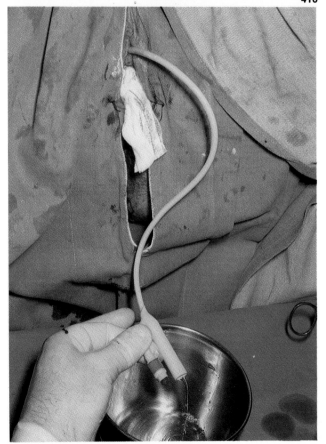
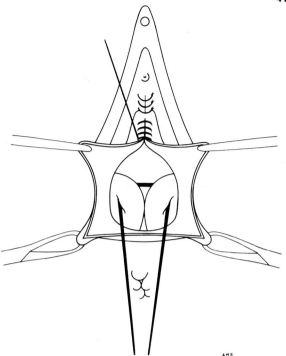
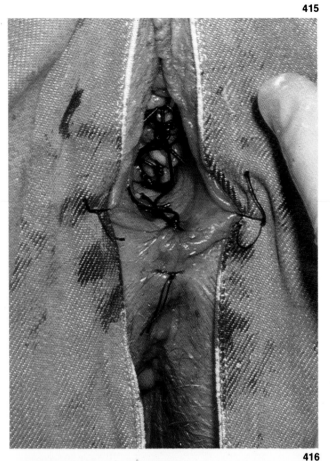

414

415

416

Plate 414 The suture in levatores ani muscles is illustrated. Some surgeons prefer to undermine the cut edges of vagina to expose the muscle more extensively. We prefer the simpler technique outlined above. Excessive suturing of the levatores ani anterior to the anal canal and rectum causes superficial dyspareunia.

Plate 415 Appearance on completion of the vaginal hysterectomy with anterior and posterior colporrhaphy. A single non-absorbable suture has been inserted in the perineum and will be removed 6 days later. The chromic catgut sutures dissolve during the following 10-20 days.

Plate 416 An indwelling, size 14 Foley catheter has been inserted. This will drain continuously for 3-5 days, then be removed, and residual urine volume tested by catheterization after voiding 4-6 hours later. The bladder is functioning adequately if residual urine volume is less than 60-100 ml. The vaginal pack prevents venous oozing and adhesion of suture lines on the anterior and posterior vaginal walls. It is removed after 24 hours. Before the patient is discharged from hospital, gentle digital examination is performed to break down any adhesions between anterior and posterior vaginal walls.

164

417

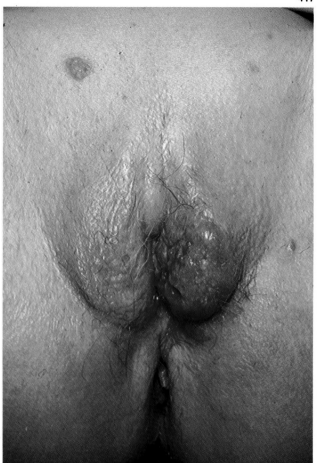

Plate 417 Carcinoma replacing left labium majus in a vague 86-year-old woman who was noted to be bleeding from the vulva by the nursing staff when in hospital for excision and grafting of a squamous cell carcinoma of the arm. Biopsy showed a well differentiated keratinized squamous cell carcinoma. The mass was not fixed to deep tissues and inguinal lymph glands were not enlarged.

Plate 418 Simple vulvectomy was performed. The oval incision extends to deep fascia, includes labia majora, and ends posteriorly at the fourchette. A second circular incision is made around the introitus, sparing the external urinary meatus.

Plate 419 The cut edges of skin were readily approximated (an advantage of loose skin folds around the vulva) after securing haemostasis. Note that the vulval skin is sutured to the circumferential incision around the introitus. The indwelling catheter allows the dressing on the wound (sofra-tulle and gauze) to be undisturbed. Histology revealed a large fungating, ulcerating growth (3.5 × 3 cm) invading to the depth of the excision. The patient was discharged to a nursing home 6 weeks later with healing of the wound almost complete. Subsequently, a small granuloma persisted but radiotherapy was deferred. She died peacefully in her sleep 6 months after the vulvectomy.

418

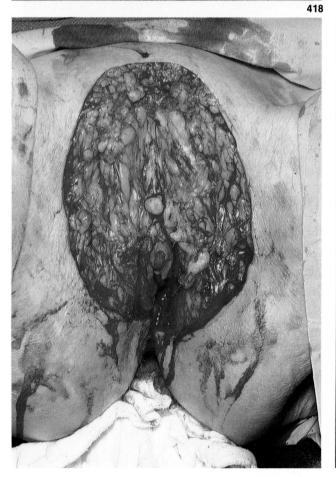

419

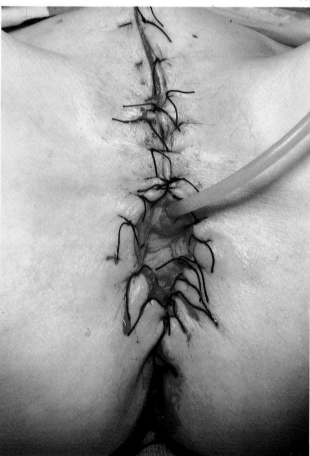

420

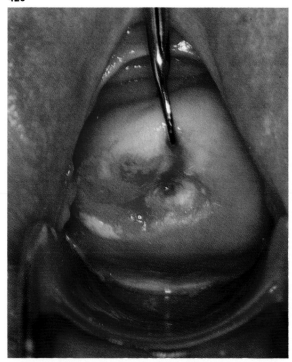

Plate 420 Leukoplakia of the cervix in an asymptomatic 54-year-old para 0 diabetic who presented for routine cytology. The initial smear was indicative of dysplasia and the second smear suggested invasive carcinoma. Colposcopy indicated invasive carcinoma, but target biopsy from the anterior lip of cervix was inconclusive because insufficient depth of stroma was obtained. The bleeding site of the target biopsy is shown.

422

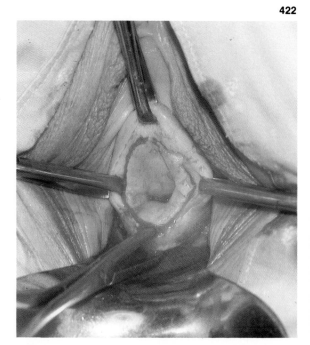

Plate 422 Cone biopsy was performed in this patient who had a positive smear because the area of abnormality extended into the endocervical canal beyond the range of the colposcope. After excision of the cone, haemorrhage was controlled by 2 nylon sutures that were removed 6 weeks later. The indication for cone biopsy was to exclude invasive cancer when colposcopy was unable to do so.

421

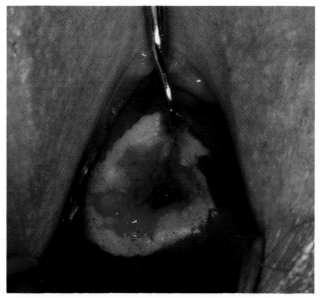

Plate 421 The cervix was painted with 2½% iodine solution and the area outlined by the circle of macroscopic leukoplakia failed to stain. Biopsy showed stromal invasion by squamous carcinoma exceeding 5 mm in depth and involving lymphatic vessels. Subsequent treatment was radiotherapy and radical hysterectomy with pelvic lymphadenectomy. Colposcopy is of more value in excluding invasive carcinoma than in assessment of the degree of invasion. It has reduced the need for diagnostic cone biopsy by 90%. Under colposcopic control, local treatment of noninvasive cervical lesions (dysplasia, intraepithelial carcinoma) can be carried out by electrocoagulation diathermy, cryosurgery or carbon dioxide laser.

Plate 423 Cervical incompetence in a 32-year-old nullipara at 25 weeks' gestation. Cone biopsy had been performed 4 years previously when cervical cytology and colposcopy indicated intraepithelial carcinoma. Although the operculum has fallen out, exposing the endocervical canal and fetal membranes, the patient had not experienced the typical profuse serosanguineous vaginal discharge. The diagnosis was made when routine inspection revealed the bluish fetal membrane, suggesting that the outer (white) chorionic layer had ruptured. A McDonald cervical purse-string suture (Mersilk) was inserted and the pregnancy proceeded. Normal delivery of a surviving male infant occurred after spontaneous labour began at 37 weeks, when the suture was removed. Note that although incompetent, the cervix is symmetrical, without the lateral laceration seen in many patients with this condition. Cervical incompetence may be diagnosed earlier by careful palpation of the internal os at the beginning of the second trimester.

423

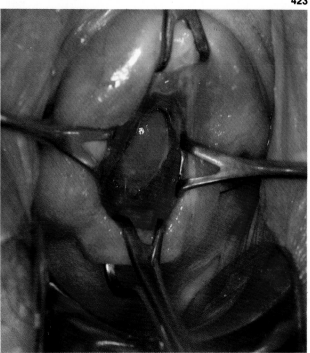

166

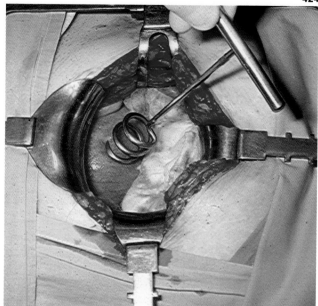

Plate 424 Devine's frame, popular with many Australian gynaecologists because it provides excellent exposure, can be used in median, paramedian or transverse incisions as in this 48-year-old para 2 who presented with irregular menses and severe dysmenorrhoea. She had uniform enlargement of the uterus to the size of a pregnancy of 24 weeks' maturity. Although still menstruating, the patient complained of hot flushes and sweating attacks which suggested an organic cause of the bleeding. Pregnancy should be excluded (ultrasonography, urinary HCG or oestrogen excretion) when there is such regular uterine enlargement.

Plate 425 This large corkscrew is a marvellous instrument for bloodless mobilization of a fibromyomatous uterus impacted in the pelvis. During hysterectomy the uterus must be pulled up for safe access to infundibulo-pelvic ligaments, uterine vessels and transverse cervical ligaments. This uterus weighed 450 g and contained an intramural fibromyoma 8 cm in diameter. There was extensive adenomyosis which explained the secondary dysmenorrhoea. The right ovary contained a corpus luteum which makes the flushes and sweating difficult to explain! However, episodic ovulation occurs during the climacteric, causing fluctuation in hormone levels.

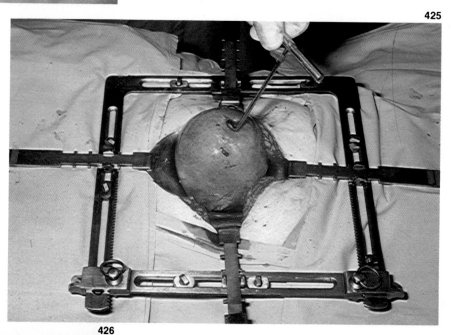

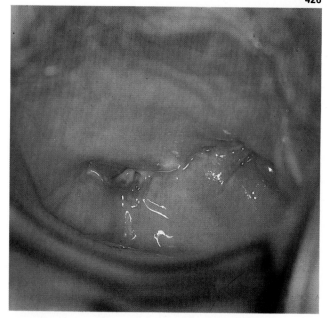

Plate 426 Vaginal vault showing incomplete healing 41 days after total abdominal hysterectomy in a 41-year-old para 3 whose ovaries were conserved. Postoperative recovery had been uneventful and afebrile. She had not noticed any vaginal discharge, although this is common for 2-3 weeks after surgery as catgut sutures in the vaginal vault dissolve. There was minimal induration on bimanual vaginal examination.

427

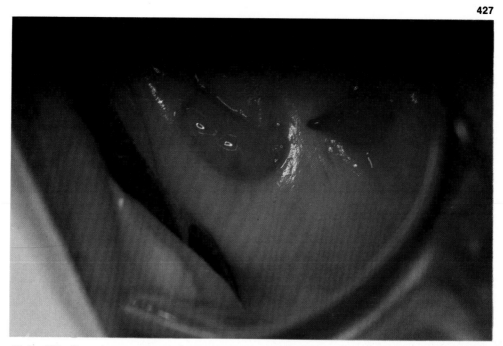

Plate 427 Granulomas at the vaginal vault marking sites of incomplete healing seen 4 months after total abdominal hysterectomy performed for carcinoma in situ in the 32-year-old para 2 shown in plates 4 and 5. The patient complained of postcoital bleeding and deep dyspareunia. These lesions had persisted in spite of application of silver nitrate; electrocautery resulted in complete healing. Granulomas are common after any vaginal surgery, especially in postmenopausal patients and usually resolve spontaneously within 3 months. It is wise to arrange a second routine postoperative visit at this time to check that healing is complete and coital function satisfactory.

Plate 428 Wound dehiscence imminent and inevitable. The patient was an obese (86 kg) 36-year-old para 3 diabetic who felt 'something go in her stitches' during a fit of coughing 3 days after Caesarean section. She then developed the copious, pink watery discharge from the sinus between stitches that is pathognomonic of a dehiscence of the deep wound layers.

428

Plate 429 The patient was taken back to theatre 7 days after Caesarean section. After the skin sutures were removed the wound literally fell apart. Note how bowel and omentum were lying under skin, ready to pop out, the continuous stitch (1 plain catgut) in the peritoneum having broken. The wound was resutured in a single layer with nylon tension sutures and convalescence thereafter was uneventful. Occasionally the skin remains intact after incomplete dehiscence, resulting in a large incisional hernia.

429

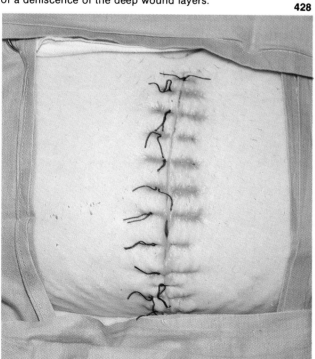

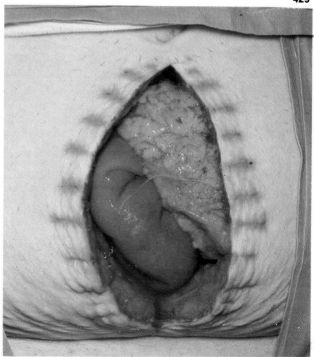

430

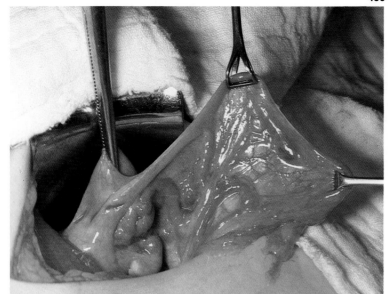

Plate 430 Fallopian tube vascular architecture seen at the time of tubal ligation in a 28-year-old para 3. Anteriorly, the round ligament is held by forceps and the mesosalpinx is displayed by 2 Babcock's forceps. The ovary lies behind the tube and is partly hidden by numerous dilated ovarian veins in the medial end of the infundibulopelvic ligament.

431

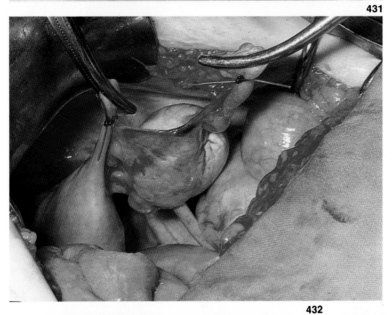

Plate 431 The Fallopian tube has been divided between artery forceps clamped across it in an area of the isthmus selected for its avascularity (Pomeroy technique). Care is taken not to tear the mesosalpinx and damage a blood vessel. Since about 1 in 200 patients request reversal of sterilization, it is important to destroy as small a segment of the tube as possible. Technically, the isthmus is the most favourable area for reanastomosis.

Plate 432 Sterilization by electrocoagulation diathermy. The following 6 photographs were taken at laparotomy because those taken through the laparoscope lack clarity.

Plate 433 Note that unipolar electrocoagulation necrosis has involved most of the tube and extended into the mesosalpinx. Use of a bipolar lead allows greater control, with reduction of the length of tube destroyed and carries a lesser risk of accidental electrical burns to bowel or adjacent structures. The tube can be divided or partly resected via the laparoscope after electrocoagulation.

432

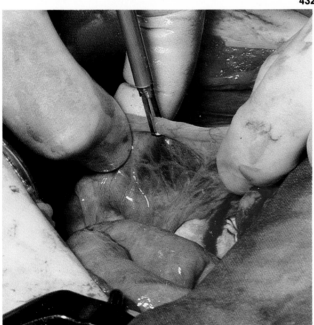

433

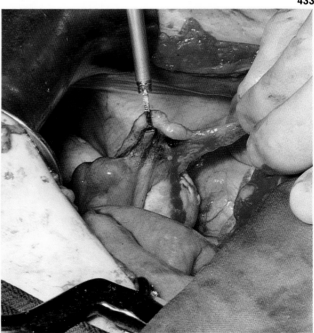

434

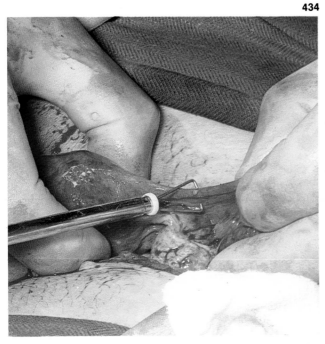

Plate 434 Application of the silicone rubber Falope ring to the isthmus of the tube. This method of sterilization destroys approximately 2 cm of tube (comparable to the Pomeroy technique or careful electrocauterization using the bipolar electrode).

435

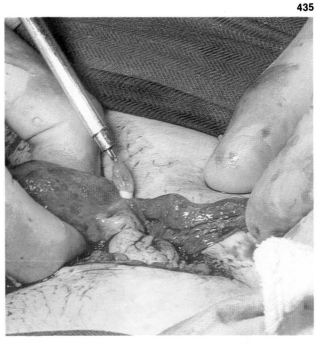

Plate 435 The jaws of the applicator grasp the Fallopian tube, a loop of which is then drawn gently up into its hollow sleeve. The rubber ring is then rolled off the instrument to occlude the loop of tube as shown in the photograph.

436

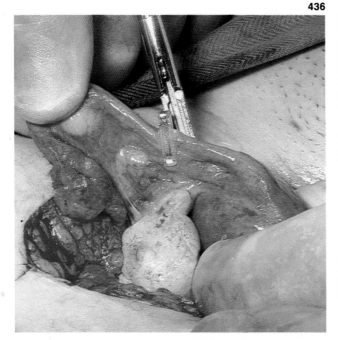

Plate 436 The plastic Hulka clip has a metallic spring and is about to be applied to the isthmus of the tube. Only a 3 mm length of tube is destroyed. Before application of the clip at laparoscopy, both medial and fimbrial ends of the tube are inspected, to ensure that the round ligament is not mistaken for the Fallopian tube. (Courtesy of Professor John Leeton)

437

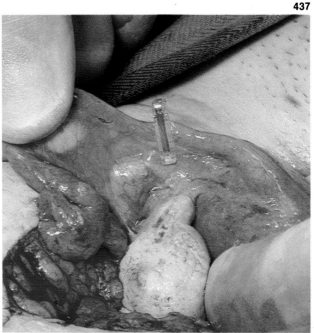

Plate 437 The failure rate with this method is less than 1%. The success rate of tubal reanastomosis after sterilization ranges from 0-75% in reported series, according to the technique of sterilization used and the selection of patients. Microsurgery appears to provide the best chance of success (patency rate 90%, pregnancy rate 75%). Minilaparotomy sterilization using a small suprapubic incision does not require special surgical skills or extensive training and has a failure rate and surgical complication rate that compares favourably with laparoscopic techniques.

Examination Questions and Answers

1. Q. **What are the chief indications for catheterization in gynaecological practice?**

    A. As a routine preoperatively, for urinary retention, and to test for residual urine after operations for urinary incontinence or where bladder innervation can be affected (radical hysterectomy).

2. Q. **What are the causes of acute urinary retention in women?**

    A. Abdominal or perineal pain postoperatively or postpartum, incarceration of the gravid uterus, fibromyomas impacted in the pelvis, carcinomatous infiltration and hysteria (plates 169, 208, 215).

3. Q. **Why is catheterization a routine preoperative practice in gynaecology?**

    A. In abdominal procedures to avoid injury to the bladder when the peritoneal cavity is opened and to prevent the distended bladder obscuring the operative field. The bladder must be empty before examination under anaesthesia or curettage to allow accurate bimanual palpation (plate 382).

4. Q. **What information is sought during bimanual vaginal examination?**

    A. The position of the uterus (anteversion, retroversion) and its size, shape, consistency and mobility; also the presence of adnexal masses (ovaries of normal size are seldom palpable in the conscious patient).

5. Q. **What are the indications for ordering a glucose tolerance test in gynaecology?**

    A. (a) Persistent monilial vaginitis or vulvitis.
       (b) Glycosuria detected on routine urine test at the first visit.
       (c) Brick-red vulva with or without pruritus vulvae (plate 209).
       (d) Age over 45 years (5% incidence of diabetes).
       (e) Obesity
       (f) Carcinoma of the uterine body (plate 20).

6. Q. **When does bleeding occur from cervical lesions?**

    A. After intercourse, or trauma due to bimanual examination, taking a Papanicolaou smear, or biopsy (plates 36, 39).

7. Q. **What are the types and causes of postoperative haemorrhage?**

    A. Reactionary haemorrhage occurs within 24 hours of operation and is due to inadequate ligation of an artery; secondary haemorrhage occurs more than 24 hours after operation, usually 8-10 days later, and is due to infection (plate 117). (Primary haemorrhage is defined as that occurring during an operation).

8. Q. **What is the typical macroscopic appearance of curettings when the patient has carcinoma of the uterine body?**

    A. White or yellow, friable, usually copious tissue (plate 20).

9. Q. **What are the commonest findings at curettage when performed for postmenopausal bleeding?**

    A. Usually there are no curettings unless that patient has been receiving oestrogen therapy; often a small amount of mucus is obtained (plates 92, 93).

10. Q. **What is the treatment of secondary haemorrhage from the cervix 8 days after cone biopsy?**

    A. Admit the patient to hospital, give morphine 10 mg or pethidine 100 mg IM and commence chemotherapy after taking a swab for bacteriological investigation. If the bleeding continues pack the vagina and give a blood transfusion if necessary. Further measures (exploration and ligation of bleeding vessels under anaesthesia) are seldom required.

11. Q. **How do you distinguish between an enterocele and rectocele?**

A. When viewed with a Sims' speculum, a rectocele bulges the middle third of the posterior vaginal wall forwards whereas an enterocele bulges the upper third. A finger in the rectum will help determine if the bulge is all rectocele. Often a high rectocele cannot be distinguished from an enterocele until the pouch of Douglas is opened at operation (plates 177, 178).

12. Q. **What criteria should be satisfied before myomectomy or surgery for endometriosis in patients with infertility?**

A. The patient should have evidence of patent Fallopian tubes, ovulatory menstruation and her husband a normal seminal analysis (plate 368).

13. Q. **What is the nature of conservative surgery for endometriosis?**

A. Mobilization of ovaries and Fallopian tubes by freeing adhesions, excision of ovarian cysts, excision or cauterization of peritoneal nodules and shortening of round ligaments to correct retroversion and dyspareunia (plates 130-133).

14. Q. **What is the incidence of successful pregnancy after conservative surgery when endometriosis is associated with infertility?**

A. Approximately 30% which is similar to the results after myomectomy in infertile patients.

15. Q. **What level of urinary excretion of oestrogen per 24 hours is indicative of pregnancy?**

A. Above 100 ug.

16. Q. **What features suggest that an infertile patient has ovulatory menstrual cycles?**

A. (a) Presence of primary dysmenorrhoea.
(b) Midcycle change in cervical mucus.
(c) Midcycle lower abdominal pain.
(d) Biphasic basal temperature chart.
(e) Presence of secretory change in a premenstrual endometrial biopsy (plates 12, 16-18).
(f) Level of urinary excretion of pregnanediol above 2 mg/24 hours or plasma progesterone above 5 ng/ml.

17. Q. **What symptom is most suspicious of cervical carcinoma?**

A. Postcoital bleeding in a middle-aged multipara; bleeding is often spontaneous in the older woman (plate 305).

18. Q. **How do you decide when genital prolapse warrants surgery?**

A. (a) If the prolapse (uterus or vagina) is of a major degree (visible at the vulva) (plates 168-170).
(b) If the symptoms cause distress to the patient — pain, presence of a lump, interference with urinary, bowel or coital function (plate 169).
(c) Presence of associated pathology — ulceration of exposed cervix or vagina, urinary infection due to retention of urine (plate 171).

19. Q. **When and why is uterine prolapse associated with pain?**

A. During the early stage of development when the pelvic peritoneum and uterosacral ligaments are dragged upon as the uterus descends. Ironically, the largest prolapses are usually painless and the patient (often over 70 years of age) may refuse surgery (plates 170, 172).

20. Q. **What are the indications for conservative treatment of uterovaginal prolapse?**

A. (a) Patient refuses surgery — when the patient is old and immobile, even a large prolapse may cause her little discomfort.
(b) Patient unfit for anaesthesia and/or surgery due to severe medical or orthopaedic disease.
(c) Pregnancy or the puerperium.
(d) Patient wanting more children — the Manchester repair markedly reduces fertility.
(e) Symptoms of prolapse are tolerable. Prolapse is rarely a threat to life and so the patient, not the doctor, decides when symptoms warrant surgery.

21. Q. **What methods of conservative treatment of prolapse are available?**

A. Perineal exercises, vaginal pessary.

172

22. Q. **By what mechanism does a pessary relieve symptoms due to genital prolapse?**

A. Usually a malleable, non-irritating plastic ring pessary (no offensive discharge) of appropriate size is used. The pessary is placed above the levatores ani muscles which hold the pessary and hence the uterus in position.

23. Q. **How do you distinguish between a vesicovaginal and a ureterovaginal fistula?**

A. Put a dry gauze swab in the vagina and inject methylene blue into the bladder through a catheter. If the swab is wet but not blue, a ureterovaginal fistula is likely. A wet blue swab indicates that the fluid has come from a vesicovaginal fistula. Rarely, dye can reflux from the bladder and reach the swab via a ureterovaginal fistula! (plates 194, 195).

24. Q. **What is the usual cause of menorrhagia in the adolescent?**

A. Anovulation associated with prolonged menstrual cycles with overgrowth of endometrium (cystic glandular hyperplasia), the irregular shedding of which results in prolonged and heavy bleeding (plates 85, 86).

25. Q. **What is the treatment of menorrhagia in the adolescent female?**

A. (a) Full blood examination to exclude anaemia and rare haematological causes (leukaemia, idiopathic thrombocytopenic purpura).
(b) Prescribe iron tablets; also hormone therapy (a minipill or norethisterone 5 mg per day from day 15-25 of the cycle) is given if the symptom is significant.
(c) If bleeding is persistent and heavy then local examination to exclude cervical and vaginal pathology is necessary (this is usually impossible without anaesthesia).
(d) Control by curettage is avoided if possible because of the risk of causing cervical damage (cervical incompetence) (plate 423).

26. Q. **What happens to a woman's temperature after ovulation and in pregnancy?**

A. (a) After ovulation the temperature rises 0.4°C or more as a result of the thermogenic effect of progesterone. The elevation remains until 2-3 days before menstruation when the corpus luteum ceases to produce progesterone.
(b) In pregnancy the luteal phase temperature elevation persists since corpus luteum function continues due to stimulation by chorionic gonadotrophic hormone from the trophoblastic cells of the recently implanted embryo.

27. Q. **How do you decide at laparotomy that an ovarian tumour is malignant?**

A. (a) If the ovarian tumour is immobile and involves adjacent tissues or has friable papilliferous outgrowths (plates 371, 378)).
(b) Presence of nodules on peritoneum, bowel and/or omentum.
(c) Ascites, especially if blood-stained.
(d) Involvement of the contralateral ovary is suggestive but this can occur with benign tumours (plate 376).

28. Q. **How do you find out if a patient has residual urine after a vaginal repair?**

A. Pass a urinary catheter after she has voided. A residual volume of 100 ml or less is acceptable.

29. Q. **What are the causes of pyometra?**

A. Obstruction of the endocervical canal and associated infection results in collection of pus within the uterine cavity.
The usual causes of obstruction are:—
(a) Cervical stenosis following trauma (cone biopsy, cautery, or Manchester repair (cervical amputation)).
(b) Carcinoma of the cervix (plate 312).
(c) Carcinoma of the endometrium (plate 166).
(d) Postmenopausal atrophy (plates 144, 145).

30. Q. **What are the site and symptoms of a Bartholin's cyst.**

A. (a) The cyst is situated at the posterolateral aspect of the introitus. Obstruction to Bartholin's duct results in formation of the cyst which need not involve the gland it drains (plate 211).
(b) There may be no symptoms until the cyst becomes infected when the patient complains of tenderness,

pain and discharge if the resultant abscess bursts as it often does before the patient seeks medical attention.

31. Q. **What conditions are associated with secondary dysmenorrhoea?**

A. Endometriosis, adenomyosis, chronic pelvic infection and submucous polyps (endometrial or fibromyomatous) (plates 90, 130-139).

32. Q. **How do polyps cause dysmenorrhoea?**

A. The uterus attempts to expel the pedunculated mass and hence painful spasms occur, particularly at the time of menstruation (plates 165, 252).

33. Q. **How does endometriosis cause dysmenorrhoea?**

A. (a) Irritation of peritoneum by blood shed from ectopic endometrial tissue.
(b) Pain due to increasing pressure as 'menstruation' occurs into cystic lesions in ovaries, uterine wall (adenomyosis), and other involved structures (plate 90).
(c) Release of prostaglandins into the uterus and peritoneal cavity.

34. Q. **What values are indicative of a normal seminal analysis?**

A. (a) Abnormal forms of spermatozoa less than 20%.
(b) Sperm count above 20-40 million per ml.
(c) Motility approximately 70%.
(d) Volume of ejaculate 2-5 ml.

35. Q. **What are the commonest primary ovarian neoplasms?**

A. (a) Mucinous and serous cystadenomas and cystadenocarcinomas (plates 372-375).
(b) Cystic teratoma (plates 344, 345).
(c) Sex cord tumours (granulosa and theca cell tumours) (plates 347-349).

36. Q. **What is the differential diagnosis of an ovarian tumour felt on bimanual examination?**

A. (a) Pregnancy — the cervix is thought to be the entire uterus and the fundus is the tumour!
(b) Pedunculated subserous fibromyoma (plate 329).
(c) Tubal pathology — ectopic pregnancy, hydrosalpinx.
(d) Nearby gut — caecum on the right, sigmoid on the left.

37. Q. **What is a Krukenberg tumour?**

A. A secondary ovarian tumour, usually bilateral, mobile and with microscopic features of signet-ring cells and myxomatous stroma. The primary growth usually arises in the gastrointestinal tract or breast, and can be clinically silent at the time the ovarian lesion is diagnosed (plates 376, 377).

38. Q. **How can you distinguish between an ovarian cyst and a broad ligament (mesonephric) cyst?**

A. The cyst in the broad ligament will displace the uterus towards the opposite side; at laparotomy it will be seen not to be connected to the uterus by the uteroovarian ligament.

39. Q. **How can you distinguish between a large ovarian cyst and a fibromyomatous uterine enlargement on clinical examination?**

A. Pass a sound into the uterus — a large fibromyomatous uterus usually has a greatly enlarged endometrial cavity (plate 324).

40. Q. **What is the treatment of decubitus ulceration of the cervix?**

A. After taking a Papanicolaou smear replace the prolapsed uterus and insert a vaginal pack (plus oestrogen or antibiotic cream). Suspect malignant ulceration if healing is not complete within 10 days. Treat the genital prolapse by vaginal hysterectomy and repair or by a Manchester repair (plate 171).

41. Q. **What is a Manchester repair?**

A. Devised by Fothergill and Donald from Manchester the operation consists of:—
(a) Dilatation and curettage — to exclude endometrial pathology and allow resuturing of vaginal epithelium to cervix after (b).
(b) Amputation of the cervix.

174

(c) Anterior colporrhaphy and suturing of the transverse cervical (cardinal) ligaments anterior to the remaining cervical stump (plates 184-193).
(d) Posterior colpoperineorrhaphy (plates 387-392).

42. Q. **What are the common indications for hysterectomy?**
A. (a) Uterine enlargement (fibromyomas, adenomyosis) with associated menorrhagia (plates 323-329).
(b) Menorrhagia plus uterovaginal prolapse requiring surgery.
(c) Menorrhagia in a multipara aged 35 years or more especially if hormone therapy has failed (plates 2, 3).
(d) Second or third degree uterine prolapse (plates 168-174, 180-183).
(e) As an alternative to tubal ligation for sterilization when the patient has an enlarged uterus and/or menorrhagia.
(f) Life-threatening indications (carcinoma of cervix or endometrium, uncontrollable haemorrhage) are relatively uncommon (plate 117).

43. Q. **What is the incidence of hysterectomy in western affluent societies?**
A. About 30% of women in Australia, Canada, United Kingdom and United States can expect to undergo hysterectomy.

44. Q. **What are the complications of dilatation and curettage?**
A. (a) Cervical incompetence (plate 423).
(b) Perforation of the uterus with sound, dilator, curette or suction cannula causing damage to uterine vessels, ureters, bowel, omentum or Fallopian tubes.
(c) Infection if placental tissue is left after termination of pregnancy.
(d) Menstrual abnormalities — common after diagnostic curettage.
(e) Asherman's syndrome (oligo-amenorrhoea and infertility due to partial or total removal of the endometrium).

45. Q. **What is the treatment if the uterus is perforated with a sound?**
A. (a) Conservative (observe pulse rate and blood pressure, since usually there is no haemorrhage — i.e., vaginal bleeding or abdominal tenderness).
(b) Laparoscopy can be undertaken if there is thought to be damage to the uterus and/or abdominal viscera. Occasionally it is necessary to suture the perforation site or ligate the uterine artery to control haemorrhage. Hysterectomy can be necessary if there is lateral perforation involving the uterine vessels causing a broad ligament haematoma.

46. Q. **What are the physiological causes of secondary amenorrhoea?**
A. Pregnancy, lactation and the menopause.

47. Q. **What are the surgical causes of secondary amenorrhoea?**
A. Hysterectomy, bilateral oophorectomy, removal of endometrium at curettage (Asherman's syndrome), hypophysectomy.

48. Q. **What is the first sign of puberty in girls?**
A. Breast bud development (thelarche) which precedes the first period (menarche) by an average of 2 years (range 6 months — 6 years).

49. Q. **What causes the onset of puberty?**
A. Production of oestrogens by ovarian follicles responding to follicle stimulating hormone from the anterior lobe of the pituitary gland. The pituitary is activated by the hypothalamus which also stimulates the adrenal production of androgens (pubic and axillary hair) at this time.

50. Q. **What is the incidence of infertility and what are the results of treatment?**
A. Infertility affects 10-15% of couples and pregnancy occurs in more than 50% after evaluation and treatment.

51. Q. **What are the causes of infertility?**

A. Anovulation, tubal disease and abnormalities in the male partner are equally common and together account for about 60% of cases. In 20% no cause is apparent but cervical and immunological factors (postcoital and sperm antibody tests), corpus luteum defect, hyperprolactinaemia and disorders of thyroid or adrenal glands should be excluded.

52. Q. **What studies are carried out in the investigation of the infertile couple?**

A. (a) Seminal analysis (see question 34).
(b) Tests for ovulation (see question 16).
(c) Hysterosalpingogram to test tubal patency and exclude uterine abnormalities.
(d) Laparoscopy to detect endometriosis, pelvic inflammatory disease, tubal patency and peritubal adhesions.
(e) Postcoital and sperm antibody tests.

53. Q. **What are the symptoms and signs of tubal ectopic pregnancy?**

A. Amenorrhoea (75%), vaginal bleeding (75%), abdominal pain and/or tenderness on moving the cervix (95%), mass in lateral fornix (60%) or posterior fornix (15%); 25% of patients are in a state of shock and 10% are sent home only to return later (plates 107-116).

54. Q. **What is the differential diagnosis of ectopic pregnancy?**

A. (a) When there is a pelvic mass (subacute variety) consider appendicitis with abscess, ovarian cyst complication (rupture, haemorrhage or torsion), tuboovarian abscess, uterine abortion with palpable corpus luteum.
(b) With acute rupture tenderness is extreme and usually no mass is palpable, so consider appendicitis with peritonitis, acute salpingitis, perforation of ulcer or gall bladder, haemorrhage from ruptured ovarian or follicular cyst or spleen.

55. Q. **What is the differential diagnosis of uterine abortion?**

A. (a) Irregular menstruation, dysfunctional uterine bleeding, ectopic pregnancy, hydatidiform mole, cervical carcinoma (plate 106).
(b) If there is pain without bleeding and the patient is pregnant consider round ligament strain, appendicitis, complication of an ovarian cyst, pyelonephritis, salpingitis, red degeneration of a fibromyoma.

56. Q. **How do hormone tablets produce their contraceptive effect?**

A. (a) Cause anovulation by suppression of FSH (oestrogen effect) or LH midcycle peak (progesterone effect) i.e., negative feedback inhibition of the hypothalamus and pituitary gland.
(b) Changes endometrial glands and stroma which affects implantation of the fertilized ovum.
(c) Changes the quality of cervical mucus which affects fertilization.

57. Q. **What is the mode of action of intrauterine devices?**

A. (a) Tubal motility increased and fertilized ovum propelled too rapidly to allow implantation.
(b) Local effect on endometrium of devices containing progestogens or copper.
(c) Abortifacient action by evoking endometrial inflammatory reaction. Phagocytosis of fertilized ovum (plate 325).

58. Q. **What are the complications of oral contraceptives?**

A. (a) Death from pulmonary and cerebral thromboembolism; also hypertension and cardiovascular disease are increased by a factor of 3, an effect which is related to smoking and age over 35 years.
(b) Nausea, leucorrhoea, menorrhagia, chloasma, breast fullness, migraine, moniliasis (oestrogen effects).
(c) Weight gain, mastalgia, breakthrough bleeding, amenorrhoea, acne, loss of libido, depression, chloasma (progestogen effects).
(d) Anovulation and amenorrhoea after ceasing therapy.

59. Q. **What are the complications of intrauterine devices?**

A. (a) Bleeding (menorrhagia, metrorrhagia) and dysmenorrhoea which necessitate removal in 15% (plate 325).
(b) Expulsion.

(c) Pregnancy in 2-4% with a relative increase in ectopic sites.
(d) Salpingitis and peritonitis resulting in sterility (tubal occlusion) in 2-4%.
(e) Tuboovarian abscess.
(f) Perforation of uterus during insertion or removal (plate 96).

60. Q. **What are the contraindications to oral contraceptives?**

A. (a) Hypertension, cardiovascular disease, previous thrombosis or bad varicose veins.
(b) Cholestatic jaundice or history of recurrent pruritus in pregnancy.
(c) Oestrogen-containing pills are contraindicated during lactation or if the patient has had carcinoma of the breast.

61. Q. **Where are swabs taken from to establish a diagnosis of gonorrhoea?**

A. From endocervix, urethra and rectum (and perhaps pharynx) because the gonococcus attacks columnar epithelium. Vaginal swabs are less useful since the vagina is lined by squamous epithelium and has no glands (plates 31, 32).

62. Q. **What is the key anatomical relationship of cervix, ureter and uterine artery?**

A. The ureter passes 1 cm lateral to the cervix as it approaches the trigone of the bladder and the uterine artery crosses it anteriorly as it runs medially towards the cervix.

63. Q. **What is the mode of death in untreated cervical carcinoma?**

A. (a) Uraemia due to obstruction of nearby ureters (often without extension of the disease outside the pelvis) (plate 321).
(b) Haemorrhage (plate 322).
(c) Vesicovaginal fistula plus sepsis (plate 320).
(d) Metastatic disease (plate 319).

64. Q. **From where do you take the biopsy in a patient with an ulcerated lesion of the cervix suspicious of cancer?**

A. From the junction with macroscopically normal tissue; a histological or cytological diagnosis may not be possible if the central necrotic area is sampled (plates 307, 308).

65. Q. **What is the management of an abnormal cervical smear indicative of severe dysplasia or carcinoma in situ?**

A. (a) Repeat the smear after treatment of associated infection.
(b) Biopsy of any suspicious area on the cervix. If the cervix appears normal, colposcopy and target biopsy is indicated. Staining with iodine solution (Schiller test) can delineate an abnormal area (fails to stain due to lack of glycogen in epithelium) (plates 292, 302, 304, 421).
(c) Cone biopsy is indicated if the abnormal area extends beyond the range of the colposcope (plates 290, 420-423).
(d) Definitive treatment by electrocautery, laser, cryotherapy, conization or hysterectomy according to the patient's age, parity and preference (plates 4, 37, 422).

66. Q. **Why is cone biopsy performed in the investigation of an abnormal smear?**

A. To exclude invasive carcinoma. Once done the lesser lesion (intraepithelial cancer) is usually cured and cytology becomes normal; i.e., the procedure often serves as definitive treatment of intraepithelial cancer but that is not the reason the cone biopsy was performed (plate 290).

67. Q. **What are the branches of the internal iliac artery?**

A. (a) Posterior division divides into iliolumbar, lateral sacral and superior gluteal (3 branches).
(b) Anterior division mainly supplies pelvic viscera — superior and inferior vesical, vaginal, uterine (arises from hypogastric which becomes the obliterated umbilical after giving off the superior vesical), obturator, internal pudendal and inferior gluteal (7 branches).

68. Q. **What is the lymphatic drainage of the cervix?**

A. (a) Anterolaterally to external iliac and obturator nodes.
(b) Posterolaterally to internal iliac nodes and thence common iliac and paraaortic nodes.
(c) Posteriorly to presacral and pararectal nodes.

69. Q. **What is the lymphatic drainage of the uterine body?**

A. (a) Mainly via the infundibulopelvic ligament to paraaortic nodes.
   (b) Lower uterine body drains as for the cervix.
   (c) Along the round ligament to the inguinal nodes.

70. Q. **What is the lymphatic drainage of the ovary?**

A. To the paraaortic nodes. Most carcinomas of ovary spread locally in the peritoneal cavity. Dysgerminomas typically spread via lymphatics and are very radiosensitive.

71. Q. **How do you distinguish between Stage 2 and Stage 3 carcinoma of the cervix?**

A. In Stage 3 the growth has extended to the lateral pelvic wall or to the lower one-third of the vagina. Parametrial infiltration is diagnosed best by combined vaginal and rectal examination (plates 306, 308, 310).

72. Q. **How do you know that you have perforated the uterus with a sound, dilator or curette?**

A. When the instrument passes further than the length of the uterus, as previously assessed by bimanual examination.

73. Q. **When is perforation of the uterus more likely to occur?**

A. When the uterine wall is softened due to pregancy, infection (postabortal or puerperal), carcinoma or postmenopausal atrophy, or when there is unrecognized retroversion.

74. Q. **When would you perform an endometrial sampling to check if a patient has secretory endometrium if she has irregular cycles (3-8 weeks)?**

A. As soon as the period begins because the endometrial histology can still be discerned.

75. Q. **Why are curettings sent for histological examination after curettage for incomplete abortion?**

A. To exclude neoplastic disease of the trophoblast (hydatidiform mole, choriocarcinoma) or unexpected uterine pathology (adenocarcinoma) if the cause of bleeding was not due to a complication of pregnancy.

76. Q. **When is surgery indicated for stress incontinence of urine?**

A. When the patient considers that the inconvenience and embarrassment warrant major surgery, and there are no contraindications (pregnancy, severe respiratory disease, heavy smoking, gross obesity).

77. Q. **When does stress incontinence improve spontaneously?**

A. After pregnancy.

78. Q. **What is the success rate of operations for cure of stress incontinence of urine?**

A. About 85%.

79. Q. **How do you decide when to treat a cervical 'erosion'?**

A. The presence of symptoms (discharge, postcoital bleeding, dyspareunia), macroscopic suspicion of malignancy, or a smear indicative of dysplasia or worse (plates 36-39).

80. Q. **List the usual postoperative orders after a Manchester repair or vaginal hysterectomy.**

A. (a) Routine observations of conscious state, pulse rate, temperature, blood pressure, urinary output.
   (b) Vaginal pack, if used, to be removed in 24 hours (plate 416).
   (c) Remove catheter after continuous drainage for 3-5 days and test for residual urine after voiding 4-6 hours later.
   (d) Pethidine (meperidine) 100 mg 4-hourly as required for pain.
   (e) Ampicillin trihydrate 250 mg 6-hourly orally.
   (f) Heparin, 2,500 units 12-hourly, by subcutaneous injection.
   (g) Metronidazole 200 mg 8-hourly orally for 7 days.
   (h) Early ambulation to avoid deep venous thrombosis.
   (i) Orders for intravenous infusion and blood transfusion if necessary.

81. Q. **What are the postoperative complications after abdominal hysterectomy?**

A. (a) Infection of vaginal vault or abdominal wound, respiratory tract, or bladder if catheterization is required (plates 427, 428).
   (b) Reactionary or secondary haemorrhage.
   (c) Paralytic ileus.
   (d) Superficial or deep venous thrombosis, pulmonary thromboembolism.
   (e) Wound dehiscence (plates 428, 429).
   (f) Psychosexual problems.
   (g) Incisional hernia.

82. Q. **What would make you suspect that a patient had uterine fibromyomas?**

A. An irregular, firm, nontender, midline abdominal mass, arising from the pelvis and which on bimanual examination is mobile and continuous with the uterus. Often there is associated menorrhagia. When speculum examination shows a cervix held high in the vagina, suspect that it is continuous with a mass (fibromyoma) too large to enter the pelvis (plates 323-329).

83. Q. **What urinary symptoms may a patient with uterovaginal prolapse complain of?**

A. (a) Often none at all.
   (b) Difficulty in initiating micturition unless the mass is replaced.
   (c) Stress incontinence of urine.
   (d) Frequency due to associated cystitis.

84. Q. **What are the usual preoperative investigations before major gynaecological surgery?**

A. (a) Blood group and Rh type.
   (b) Haemoglobin estimation.
   (c) Chest radiograph and electrocardiograph if the patient is elderly, hypertensive or has reduced exercise tolerance.
   (d) Glucose tolerance if the patient is obese and over 40 years of age.
   (e) Renal function tests (creatinine clearance, intravenous pyelogram) if there is a procidentia or large abdominal mass since these lesions may obstruct the ureters.
   (f) Barium enema when there is a large abdominal mass to exclude primary bowel pathology (carcinoma of the colon, diverticulitis).

85. Q. **What is the treatment of recurrent postmenopausal bleeding when curettage reveals no uterine pathology?**

A. (a) Cystoscopy and sigmoidoscopy to exclude carcinoma of bladder or bowel — an elderly patient may mistake the orifice of exit of the blood.
   (b) Hysterectomy and bilateral salpingo-oophorectomy because of the possibility of a small carcinoma missed by the curette (plate 330), or present in the ovary or tube.

86. Q. **How do you decide the site to biopsy when an elderly patient has an extensive area of chronic vulvitis that resists the usual treatment?**

A. Radioactive phosphorus uptake and/or colposcopy indicate the areas most likely to be malignant (plates 218-220). Failure of an area of vulval epithelium to stain with toluidine blue (Collin's test) is also used to select biopsy sites.

87. Q. **What are the indications for treatment of a urethral caruncle?**

A. When it is causing symptoms (bleeding, dysuria, dyspareunia) (plate 200).

88. Q. **What is the differential diagnosis of a urethral caruncle?**

A. (a) Patulous external urinary meatus with exposure of the posterior urethral mucosa.
   (b) Carcinoma of the urethra or of the adjacent squamous epithelium (plate 204).
   (c) Prolapsed urethra (plates 202, 203).

89. Q. **What is a missed abortion?**

A. The fetus has died but the cervix remains closed. The conceptus may be entirely absorbed or shed piecemeal when spontaneous abortion eventually occurs. Missed abortion is usually preceded by an episode of bleeding (threatened abortion).

90. Q. **What are the principles in the treatment of a patient with an incomplete abortion?**
   A. (a) Stop the bleeding by administration of ergometrine (ergonovine) 0.5 mg by intravenous or intramuscular injection.
   (b) Resuscitation with intravenous fluid or blood if the patient is shocked.
   (c) With the patient in the left lateral or dorsal position a speculum is passed and clotted blood and placental tissue are removed from the vagina and cervix with sponge-holding forceps (plates 102-105).
   (d) Chemotherapy to cover both aerobic and anaerobic bacteria (penicillin and metronidazole) is commenced (after taking a cervical swab for bacteriological examination) if there is evidence of infection.
   (e) Curettage is performed to remove remaining placental tissue.

91. Q. **What are the causes of spontaneous first trimester abortion?**
   A. (a) Usually there is death or development failure of the fetus. The cause of this is usually not known, although chromosomal abnormalities are present in about 30% of cases. This is nature's method for rejection of the imperfect. Usually no fetus is present in first trimester abortions.
   (b) Infection of the fetus (rubella); pyrexia due to maternal infection (influenza, hepatitis or pyelonephritis); infection of the birth canal.
   (c) Defective corpus luteum.
   (d) Uterine malformation (plate 60).
   (e) Physical or emotional trauma.

92. Q. **What is the probable cause of an offensive, yellow vaginal discharge associated with pruritus vulvae?**
   A. Trichomonal vaginitis.

93. Q. **What is the typical appearance of monilial vaginitis as seen during speculum examination?**
   A. The vaginal epithelium is oedematous and has white patches like curds, which when dislodged leave reddened areas. The appearance is similar to thrush in a baby's mouth and the same fungus is the cause of both conditions (plates 25-28, 143).

94. Q. **What is the treatment of monilial vaginitis?**
   A. Application with a cotton wool swab of gentian violet 1% aqueous solution, after cleansing with 2% solution of acetic acid. The other effective method is the use of nystatin or a similar type of vaginal pessary (miconazole, econazole), 1 being inserted each night, for 2 weeks.

95. Q. **What is the typical appearance of trichomonal vaginitis as seen during speculum examination?**
   A. There is a frothy, greenish-yellow, offensive discharge which tends to collect in the posterior fornix. The vagina has many small, red 'strawberry' spots (plates 29, 30, 140-142).

96. Q. **What is the treatment of trichomonal vaginitis?**
   A. Metronidazole (Flagyl) tablets (200 mg) by mouth, 3 times daily for 1 week, or tinidazole (Fasigyn) tablets (500 mg) by mouth, 4 tablets being given as a single dose.

97. Q. **Why do vaginal infections recur after treatment?**
   A. Reinfection from the husband who should be treated at the same time as his wife if infection recurs, or if he has symptoms. Another possibility in monilial infections is that the patient may have a predisposing cause such as diabetes mellitus, which is excluded by performing a glucose tolerance test. Systemic (oral) treatment may be necessary.

98. Q. **What symptoms may the husband have when his wife has trichomonal or monilial vaginitis?**
   A. Penile and scrotal rash with intolerable itching. Red papular rash with oedematous foreskin is typical of monilial infection. He is prescribed metronidazole (or tinidazole), nystatin cream or gentian violet solution according to the cause of his symptoms.

99. Q. **What are condylomata?**
   A. They are warts which differ in size and are usually multiple; they are found in the vagina and on the vulva and perineum. Small multiple vaginal nodules are usually diagnosed by palpation rather than inspection during speculum examination (plates 146-149).

100. Q. **What are the causes of condylomata?**

A. The common variety are condylomata acuminata which are due to a papilloma virus infection, but occur in association with vaginitis due to trichomonas or monilia. Condylomata lata are due to syphilis which should always be excluded in patients with genital warts. Pregnancy predisposes to the rapid growth of condylomata acuminata (plates 159, 210).

101. Q. **What pelvic masses can show calcification in a plain radiograph?**

A. Ovarian cystic teratoma (25% contain teeth), uterine fibromyomas, lithopaedion (plate 370).

102. Q. **What is the advantage of local therapy with oestrogen cream or pessaries?**

A. Relief of burning, discharge, dyspareunia and urinary symptoms (postmenopausal vaginitis and bladder problems) with a relatively small dose of oestrogen.

103. Q. **What are the disadvantages of pessary treatment for uterovaginal prolapse?**

A. The need to review and change the pessary periodically and the risks of infection, ulceration and carcinoma (rare). Also the pessary may fail (levator ani atrophy) and operation may be required when the patient is even older and less fit.

104. Q. **What type of vaginal bleeding occurs in a patient with a ruptured tubal ectopic pregnancy?**

A. There may be no bleeding but usually there is a small loss of dark blood. If the bleeding is copious the diagnosis is more likely to be incomplete uterine abortion.

105. Q. **Why does vaginal bleeding occur in ruptured tubal pregnancy?**

A. Because tubal haemorrhage results in placental death and withdrawal of oestrogen and progesterone and so the endometrium is shed as in menstruation.

106. Q. **How can you distinguish between an enlarged abdomen due to ascites and one due to an ovarian tumour?**

A. Shifting dullness is characteristic of ascites, but the sign is often not helpful and in any case ascites can coexist with an ovarian tumour. Ultrasonography can also be misleading. Laparotomy is required; do not perform paracentesis since cells may be disseminated from a malignant ovarian cyst (plates 356-363).

107. Q. **What predisposes to torsion of an ovarian cyst?**

A. (a) Changes in size, weight, mobility, position (plates 82, 351).
(b) Uterine enlargement in pregnancy by pulling the ovarian mass out of the pelvis.
(c) Exercise (including coitus).

108. Q. **What are the pedicles upon which ovarian tumours twist?**

A. The infundibulopelvic and ovarian ligaments with the Fallopian tube also involved (plates 4, 370).

109. Q. **What is the treatment of condylomata acuminata?**

A. (a) Small multiple lesions usually disappear when the irritating discharge (often due to trichomonads or monilia) responds to treatment (plate 146).
(b) Large lesions (vulval and perianal skin) often require electrocoagulation diathermy or laser therapy (plates 147, 148).
(c) Application of podophyllin 20%, salicylic acid 25%.

110. Q. **How can gonorrhoea present?**

A. (a) Frequency, scalding and purulent discharge from the cervix or urethra.
(b) Vulval pain (superficial dyspareunia) due to infection of Bartholin's gland.
(c) Acute or chronic pelvic inflammatory disease (plates 31, 164).
(d) Acute conjunctivitis in the newborn may indicate infection acquired from the mother during delivery.
(e) Acute symptoms in the male (dysuria and penile discharge) after infection acquired from an asymptomatic carrier.

111. Q. **How is the diagnosis of gonorrhoea confirmed bacteriologically?**

A. (a) Gram-negative intracellular diplococci seen on a stained smear obtained from the cervix or from

secretion expressed from the urethra or rectum (plate 32).
  (b) Culture on Thayer-Martin medium under increased carbon dioxide tension.

112. Q. **What are the causes of a retroverted uterus?**

A. (a) It is the normal position in 20-30% of women in most of whom there is no associated pathology.
    (b) If the retroverted uterus is immobile, likely causes are endometriosis, chronic pelvic inflammatory disease or advanced carcinoma.

113. Q. **When is surgical treatment of a retroverted uterus indicated?**

A. (a) If associated deep dyspareunia is relieved by trial of pessary (Smith Hodge).
    (b) At the time of conservative surgical treatment of endometriosis (plates 130-133).
    (c) Possibly as a last resort in treatment of infertility when all tests of husband and wife are normal.

114. Q. **What are the causes of an abnormally-shaped uterus?**

A. Fibromyomas, congenital abnormalities (bicornuate, unicornuate) and attached adnexal masses (plates 34, 60, 323, 329).

115. Q. **What observations are made routinely during speculum examination?**

A. (a) The vulva and perineum are inspected for varicosities, neoplastic and inflammatory disease as the instrument is introduced.
    (b) The presence of uterovaginal prolapse is assessed, enterocele and rectocele being excluded with the patient bearing down as the speculum is withdrawn.
    (c) The vagina is inspected for hormonal state (colour and thickness, presence of rugae) and evidence of infection (plates 26, 29, 61).
    (d) The cervix is inspected for hypertrophy and ulceration (plates 1, 2, 174).

116. Q. **What may be the sequelae of cervical stenosis?**

A. (a) Secondary dysmenorrhoea.
    (b) Amenorrhoea (cryptomenorrhoea), haematometra and haematosalpinges.
    (c) Infertility.
    (d) Pyometra, mainly in postmenopausal patients (plates 145, 166, 312).

117. Q. **What is the treatment of a ruptured ectopic pregnancy?**

A. (a) Begin resuscitation (intravenous saline while blood is being cross-matched) and perform laparotomy to control haemorrhage.
    (b) Before clamping the ruptured or bleeding Fallopian tube check that the other tube is normal. If the patient wants more children, conservative surgery to the involved tube may be possible.
    (c) Remove blood from the peritoneal cavity.

118. Q. **Why does the patient lose small spurts not floods of urine when she has stress incontinence?**

A. When she feels the loss of urine she contracts her external urinary sphincter (voluntary muscle) and stems the flow; this is less likely with bladder dyssynergia when the bladder is actively contracting.

119. Q. **What are the postoperative complications after vaginal repair or vaginal hysterectomy?**

A. (a) Reactionary or secondary haemorrhage from the vagina.
    (b) Haemorrhage into the broad ligament causing a large haematoma (later palpable abdominally) which produces severe lower abdominal pain and signs of shock.
    (c) Urinary infection and inability to void or empty the bladder adequately (residual urine less than 100 ml) after the catheter is removed.
    (d) Anaesthetic complications.
    (e) Venous thrombosis, pulmonary thromboembolism.
    (f) Dyspareunia or apareunia if the vagina is excessively narrowed (plates 237-239).
    (g) Vault prolapse due to enterocele if posterior repair is inadequate (plates 177, 179).

120. Q. **What is the value of cytology in gynaecology?**

A. (a) Detects cervical dysplasia, intraepithelial and invasive carcinoma and about 40% of corpus carcinomas (plates 259, 260, 262, 265-274).
    (b) Diagnosis of vaginal and cervical infection — trichomonas, monilia, herpes, wart virus disease and bacterial infections (plates 25, 27, 30, 140, 152, 153, 275-280).

(c) Cellular pattern indicates phase of menstrual cycle and whether ovulation has occurred (plates 21, 22).

(d) Special application is cytology of jet washings of endometrial cavity for diagnosis of endometrial hyperplasia and carcinoma.

(e) Vulval cytology (scalpel scrape) can identify neoplasia and infecting organism in cases of chronic vulval dystrophy.

(f) Diagnosis and staging of pelvic cancer from peritoneal fluid.

121. **Q. What is the treatment of endometriosis?**

A. (a) Conservative treatment with progestogens or surgery (see question 13) is indicated if the patient wishes to conceive. Presacral neurectomy is rarely performed to control severe pain (plates 130-133).

(b) No treatment may be required if there are no symptoms such as dysmenorrhoea, dyspareunia and infertility.

(c) If symptoms are severe, relief by surgery requires removal of all ovarian tissue (total hysterectomy and bilateral salpingo-oophorectomy) (plate 135).

122. **Q. What is the mechanism of amenorrhoea when taking an oral contraceptive pill?**

A. (a) Atrophic endometrium that does not shed. This is the extreme form of hypomenorrhoea which is common in pill takers. Amenorrhoea whilst taking the pill does not imply an increased risk of secondary amenorrhoea when the pill is ceased.

(b) Pregnancy!

123. **Q. What is the proper advice to give an infertile couple re the timing of intercourse?**

A. (a) Concentrate on days 8-18 in a regular 28 day cycle (ovulation ± 4 days).

(b) Mid-cycle pain (mittelschmerz) or bleeding may indicate ovulation — pain can otherwise dissuade from coitus at this time.

(c) Peak flow of preovulatory mucus (like raw egg-white) is a useful guide; ovulation usually occurs 30-40 hours later.

(d) The mid-cycle rise in temperature (basal temperature chart) allows anticipation of the time of ovulation in subsequent cycles if these are regular. The lowest point on the temperature graph usually coincides with ovulation.

124. **Q. What is the cause of flushes and sweating during the climacteric?**

A. Reduced secretion of oestrogen from the ovary with resultant increased pulsatile release of gonadotrophin releasing hormone, causing increased secretion of FSH from the pituitary gland. Oestrogen therapy controls these symptoms by feedback suppression of the hypothalamus.

125. **Q. What steps are taken to avoid postoperative deep venous thrombosis and pulmonary thromboembolism?**

A. (a) Preoperative physiotherapy and correction of anaemia, sepsis, obesity and heavy smoking.

(b) Calf muscle stimulation during operation.

(c) Avoidance of pressure on calves by padding them when in lithotomy position and placing rubber under the heels when the patient is supine.

(d) Postoperative physiotherapy.

(e) Elevation of the foot of the bed 10-20 cm.

(f) Early ambulation after operation plus routine anticoagulation (heparin 2,500 — 5,000 IU 12-hourly by subcutaneous injection).

126. **Q. What is the transformation zone of the cervix?**

A. It is the area between the original squamocolumnar junction and the upper (cranial) limit of columnar epithelium undergoing squamous metaplasia. The squamocolumnar junction can be situated in the endocervical canal, at the external os, or on the ectocervix, the latter giving the appearance of an 'erosion' (ectropion, ectopy), because blood vessels are visible through the single layer of columnar cells.

In the neonate the junction can extend onto the vagina. Hormonal influences at puberty, first pregnancy and the climacteric change the bulk of the cervix and cause the squamocolumnar junction to advance (puberty, pregnancy) or retreat (climacteric) in relation to the endocervical canal (plates 36, 38, 39, 282-285, 298).

127. **Q. What are Nabothian follicles?**

A. They are retention cysts on the cervix containing mucus secreted by imprisoned columnar epithelial cells covered by epithelium which has undergone squamous metaplasia (plates 40, 41, 88, 89, 281).

128. Q. **What is the treatment of cystic glandular hyperplasia of the endometrium?**

A. (a) The curettage that provided the endometrial tissue for diagnosis may cure the associated menorrhagia (plates 85, 86, 91).

(b) A progestogen (e.g. norethisterone 5 mg 1-3 times daily from day 15-25 of the cycle) often controls excessive bleeding. A high dose progestogen contraceptive pill is an alternative regimen and is more likely to cause scanty periods.

(c) Follow-up (plus sampling of endometrium by Mi-Mark plastic spiral, jet washer or curettage) is necessary to exclude progression to atypical hyperplasia or carcinoma.

(d) Hysterectomy according to age and parity and response to above measures (plates 341-343).

129. Q. **What are the types of intrauterine polyp?**

A. (a) Endometrial (proliferative, atypical, hyperplasia, carcinoma, sarcoma) (plates 84, 87, 246-249, 253-258).

(b) Fibromyomatous (plates 252, 331).

(c) Adenomyomatous (plate 330).

(d) Placental (benign or malignant) (plate 117).

130. Q. **What is the treatment of postmenopausal bleeding?**

A. (a) Examine vulva, vagina and cervix and perform cervical cytology and curettage.

(b) If no curettings, consider possibility of origin of blood from bladder or rectum; also consider possibility of carcinoma of the ovary or tube (plate 381).

(c) Presence of a caruncle or benign pathology (senile vaginitis) does not remove the need for curettage to exclude endocervical or endometrial carcinoma (which are present in 20% of patients with postmenopausal bleeding) (plates 92-94, 169, 200).

131. Q. **What is the treatment of senile vaginitis?**

A. Oestrogen vaginal cream inserted each evening for 1 week, then at decreasing intervals according to response. Oral oestrogen with progestin 7-10 days each month may be a safer alternative (no increased risk of endometrial carcinoma) (plates 92-94).

132. Q. **What is a fractional curettage?**

A. Stepwise curettage of endocervical canal, lower one-half of uterine body then fundus with separate collection of curettings in patients suspected of having carcinoma to determine if the growth extends to lower uterus or cervix — in which case treatment involves radical rather than simple hysterectomy. Hysteroscopy is more accurate in determining if the growth extends to involve cervix.

133. Q. **How do fibromyomas cause menorrhagia?**

A. (a) The uterus and endometrial cavity are larger with an increased area to bleed from (plates 323, 325, 327).

(b) Submucous lesions are prone to ulceration and cause heavy bleeding during and between the periods (plates 252, 331).

(c) Multiple fibromyomas may impair uterine contraction and haemostasis.

(d) Associated anovulation with endometrial hyperplasia.

(e) Blood vessels in relation to the neoplasm are often abnormal.

134. Q. **What is the reason for cervical mucus ferning on an air-dried glass slide?**

A. It is due to a certain ratio of sodium chloride to proteins in cervical secretion and is an oestrogenic effect (preovulation). Change to a cellular pattern without crystals indicates that ovulation has occurred (progesterone effect).

135. Q. **What are the gynaecological causes of a haemoperitoneum?**

A. Ruptured tubal pregnancy or ovarian cyst. Retrograde menstruation. Bleeding can also occur from the ovary at ovulation or from endometriotic lesions and cause pain out of proportion to blood loss. Rarer causes include malignant disease of the uterus or ovary (plates 107-116).

136. Q. **What are the gynaecological causes of lower abdominal rebound tenderness?**

A. Salpingitis, ruptured ectopic pregnancy, torsion or rupture of an ovarian cyst, ovulation bleeding, red degeneration of a fibromyoma, septic abortion, uterine perforation if recent curettage; also consider appendicitis and pyelonephritis (plates 82, 326, 332, 351, 370, 380).

137. Q. **What conditions are identifiable by hysterosalpingography?**

A. Uterine abnormalities (unicornuate, bicornuate, didelphys), intrauterine polyps, adhesions (Asherman's syndrome), tubal occlusion and site of blockage, hydrosalpinges.

138. Q. **What advantage has laparoscopy over hysterosalpingography in the investigation of an infertile female?**

A. Laparoscopy detects endometriosis and peritubal adhesions that warrant surgery even when the tubes are patent (as seen by emergence of methylene blue-coloured saline from fimbrial ends after injection through the cervix).

139. Q. **What structures are attached to the uterus?**

A. (a) At the fundus are the round ligament, Fallopian tube and ovarian ligament in order from anterior to posterior (plates 4, 33, 43).
(b) Anterior and posterior peritoneum of broad ligament (plate 45).
(c) The important uterine supports (transverse cervical, uterosacral and pubocervical ligaments) attach to the supravaginal cervix (plate 47).
(d) The vagina.

140. Q. **What types of ulcer occur on the vulva?**

A. Carcinoma, herpes simplex, traumatic due to scratching (pruritus vulvae), secondary syphilis (plates 150, 151, 159, 219, 222-231).

141. Q. **What is Huhner's test?**

A. Postcoital smear from the endocervix and vaginal pool taken soon after coitus to detect the density of motile spermatozoa. The test is performed to assess cervical hostility (local inflammation, immunological reaction by cervical secretion) as a cause of infertility.

Advanced Questions and Answers

1. Q. **What causes postcoital bleeding 6 weeks after an abdominal or vaginal hysterectomy?**

   A. Granulomas where stitches were inserted to close the vaginal vault (plate 427).

2. Q. **What symptoms are characteristic of a cystocele?**

   A. A vaginal lump and perhaps difficulty in initiating micturition and emptying the bladder completely unless the lump is pushed upwards (plates 3, 168-170, 173, 180, 184, 387, 397).

3. Q. **What factors predispose to recurrent monilial vaginitis?**

   A. Diabetes mellitus, pregnancy, oral contraceptives, corticosteroids and failure to treat the male partner. Broad-spectrum antibiotic therapy (eradication of bacterial flora allows overgrowth of fungus) and excessive perspiration with chafing due to tight clothing (pantyhose) are common predisposing factors (plates 25-28).

4. Q. **What are the complications of cone biopsy of the cervix?**

   A. Primary and especially secondary haemorrhage, broad ligament haematoma, cervical stenosis or incompetence, dysmenorrhoea and pyometra (plate 423).

5. Q. **How does the lymphatic drainage of the cervix and body of uterus determine the different surgical treatment of primary carcinoma in these sites?**

   A. The body drains mainly upwards along the infundibulopelvic ligaments to paraaortic nodes, whereas the cervix drains laterally to iliac and obturator nodes; thus cervical carcinoma requires wide lateral excision (radical hysterectomy ± lymphadenectomy), whereas body carcinoma requires total hysterectomy and bilateral salpingo-oophorectomy (plates 320-322).

6. Q. **When should carcinoma of the uterine body be treated by radical surgery as for cervix?**

   A. When the growth extends to the cervix and thus drains as does cervix and the patient's general condition allows this treatment regimen.

7. Q. **What causes a fetus to differentiate as a male?**

   A. (a) The Y chromosomes (H-Y antigen) in primitive germ cells induce tubular formation of gonadal cells.
   (b) Leydig cells in the Y-organized testis then produce testosterone which induces differentiation of Wolffian ducts into the male reproductive tract, and urogenital sinus into the scrotum and phallus into the penis.
   (c) These changes occur between 10 and 18 weeks' gestation.

8. Q. **What cysts occur in the vagina?**

   A. Cysts of Gartner's (mesonephric) duct which are always anterolateral and usually in the upper third of the vagina; inclusion cysts from squamous epithelium buried at the site of an episiotomy wound, repair or vaginal laceration; cysts of Bartholin's gland or duct which can bulge into the vagina posterolaterally just inside the introitus; endometriotic cysts occasionally occur at the vaginal vault, the disease having extended from the pouch of Douglas (plates 61, 167, 201, 206, 211, 240).

9. Q. **What are the types of urinary incontinence?**

   A. Stress (mechanical bladder neck problem), urge (infection or dyssynergia), overflow (neurological), true (fistula or ectopic ureter), or mixed (plates 194, 195, 198, 199).

10. Q. **What is the common cause of urinary incontinence where the patient is wet all the time and wears an absorbent napkin?**

A. Old age often associated with senility and cerebrovascular disease. These patients are also likely to have frequency and precipitancy of micturition.

11. Q. **What is the treatment of such patients (question 10) in the absence of genital prolapse?**

A. Oestrogen cream inserted digitally or by applicator into the vagina, propantheline bromide (Probanthine) 15 mg 3 times daily and imipramine hydrochloride (Tofranil) 25 mg 3 times daily.

12. Q. **What is the infundibulopelvic ligament?**

A. The fold of broad ligament peritoneum running from where the infundibulum of the Fallopian tube embraces the ovary, to the lateral pelvic wall. It contains ovarian artery, veins and lymphatics and crosses the pelvic brim where the ureter overlies the bifurcation of the common iliac artery (plates 4, 5, 43).

13. Q. **How may surgical damage to a ureter be recognized postoperatively?**

A. Anuria if both are involved, or when paralytic ileus develops followed by urinary incontinence 8-10 days after operation due to development of a ureterovaginal fistula.

14. Q. **What complication of endometriosis typically presents after the menopause?**

A. Bowel obstruction, since fibrosis occurs in annular endometriotic lesions of the intestine (usually sigmoid colon) after ovarian failure.

15. Q. **How do you distinguish between stress and urge incontinence?**

A. From the history. Stress incontinence is caused by sneezing, coughing, laughing, jumping and the loss of spurts not floods of urine, for the patient contracts her external urinary sphincter when she notes what has happened. Urge is due to infection — the irritable bladder must empty, often frequently, and the patient cannot control the flow (plate 199).

16. Q. **What are the 3 histological criteria for the diagnosis of a hydatidiform mole?**

A. The chorionic villi are avascular, hydropic and show trophoblastic proliferation.

17. Q. **What is the aetiology of urethral caruncle?**

A. Oestrogen deprivation, perhaps with infection of the exposed urethral mucosa. Hence it occurs only in postmenopausal women (plates 169, 200).

18. Q. **How do you distinguish between endometriosis and chronic pelvic infection in a patient with a fixed retroverted uterus and tender adnexal masses?**

A. A history of infection (postabortal, puerperal, gonococcal) and the presence of a yellow vaginal discharge indicate pelvic infection; thickened uterosacral ligaments, palpable rectally, suggest endometriosis (plates 135-139).

19. Q. **If an infertile patient has a short luteal phase, how can function of the corpus luteum be prolonged?**

A. By administration of human chorionic gonadotrophin in small doses (1,000-1,500 IU IM) during the luteal phase on days 16, 18 and 20.

20. Q. **What is the best time in a regular 28-day cycle to order oestrogen and progesterone assays to assess ovarian function in an infertile patient?**

A. On day 21 since both hormones are at peak levels of excretion.

21. Q. **What is the treatment of red degeneration of a fibromyoma?**

A. Conservative — analgesia for pain and avoidance of laparotomy, especially during pregnancy when myomectomy is contraindicated (plates 326, 332).

22. Q. **How can adenomyosis be diagnosed?**

A. Clinically the association of secondary dysmenorrhoea with regular uterine enlargement; section of the uterus after hysterectomy shows a thickened myometrium with dark spots which indicate areas of ectopic endometrium with retained menstrual blood (plate 90).

23. Q. **How do you account for the appearance of pubic and axillary hair in patients with ovarian agenesis?**

A. Hormonal activity of the adrenal gland (androgens) triggered by hypothalamic-pituitary activity.

24. Q. **Why is a pack inserted into the vagina at the conclusion of a vaginal repair operation?**

A. To control venous oozing by pressure and to prevent the anterior and posterior vaginal walls becoming adherent by apposition of the 2 sutured midline incisions (plate 416).

25. Q. **How is the diagnosis of a defective corpus luteum established?**

A. (a) Shortened luteal phase and failure to sustain the temperature rise after ovulation as seen in a basal temperature chart.
(b) Patchy secretory change in a premenstrual endometrial biopsy or secretory change less advanced than expected for the day of the luteal phase that the biopsy was taken.

26. Q. **What are the possible causes of copious clear fluid discharge from the vaginal vault 3-4 weeks after a vaginal hysterectomy?**

A. (a) Vesicovaginal or ureterovaginal fistula (plate 194).
(b) Leakage of fluid from the Fallopian tube which has prolapsed through the suture line at the vault.

27. Q. **What contraindicates the vaginal route for hysterectomy?**

A. (a) Uterine size bigger than the pelvic cavity (size of 10-12 weeks' pregnancy).
(b) Absence of uterine prolapse — no prolapse means much traction and suturing under tension which increases the risk of haemorrhage.
(c) Previous pelvic surgery, inflammatory disease, or significant endometriosis.
(d) Carcinoma of the endometrium. Here the ovaries must be removed (10% contain metastases) and they are not readily accessible for safe removal by the vaginal route.

28. Q. **What are the advantages of marsupialization compared with excision of a Bartholin's cyst?**

A. (a) The operation is quicker, easier and associated with less haemorrhage and less postoperative pain.
(b) Marsupialization retains the gland and its function. The same can be achieved by dilatation of the opening of the duct where it enters the vagina (plates 211-216).

29. Q. **What is the significance of a 1 cm dilated internal cervical os in a nonpregnant patient?**

A. The patient is likely to have an incompetent cervix or a large endometrial or fibromyomatous polyp that the uterus is trying to expel; associated uterine enlargement or menorrhagia would support the latter diagnosis (plates 246-249).

30. Q. **What is the differential diagnosis of a large ovarian tumour?**

A. (a) Ascites.
(b) Pregnancy especially with polyhydramnios.
(c) Obesity — a large abdomen can wobble and seem cystic!
(d) Distended bladder.
(e) Fibromyomas are often impossible to distinguish from an ovarian tumour which extends into the pouch of Douglas and seems to arise from the pelvis.
(f) Any large tumour of kidney, pancreas or intestines. A large lower abdominal mass in a postmenopausal women is most likely to be ovarian and as more than 50% are malignant, laparotomy should be performed without delay (plates 356-365).

31. Q. **What hormones are produced by ovarian neoplasms?**

A. (a) Oestrogens are classically produced by granulosa cell tumours and thecomas, but also by some of the epithelial tumours both benign and malignant (plates 341-343, 347-349).
(b) Androgen is produced by Sertoli-Leydig cell tumours (androblastomas) and arrhenoblastomas.
(c) Chorionic gonadotrophic hormone and thyrotrophic hormone from the rare primary ovarian choriocarcinoma (plate 354).

(d) Thyroxine is produced by thyroid tissue in a cystic teratoma. Other ectopic hormones can also be produced by ovarian cancers.

32. Q. **What conditions are associated with theca-lutein cysts?**
   A. (a) Hydatidiform mole, invasive mole, choriocarcinoma (plate 121).
   (b) Conditions where the placenta is large and produces excessive chorionic gonadotrophic hormone — multiple pregnancy, erythroblastosis, diabetes, very large fetus.
   (c) Overstimulation of the ovaries with clomiphene citrate or follicle stimulating hormone in the treatment of anovulation can also produce a similar picture.

33. Q. **What experiments of nature indicate that prolonged exposure to oestrogen can produce endometrial carcinoma?**
   A. (a) A 15% incidence of endometrial carcinoma in patients with granulosa cell tumours (plates 341-343).
   (b) The occurrence of endometrial carcinoma in patients with the Stein-Leventhal syndrome and in sex chromosome mosaics whose gonads produce oestrogens.

34. Q. **What is Meigs' syndrome?**
   A. Association of a benign ovarian tumour, usually a fibroma, with ascites and a right-sided hydrothorax. The message is that ascites plus tumour does not always indicate metastatic carcinoma.

35. Q. **What is the Stein-Leventhal syndrome?**
   A. Bilateral polycystic ovaries with a thickened germinal epithelium associated with infertility, obesity, hirsutes and oligomenorrhoea (plates 82, 83, 127, 128).

36. Q. **What are theca-lutein cysts?**
   A. Atretic follicles in the ovaries stimulated by abnormally high blood levels of chorionic gonadotrophic hormone. The ovaries are polycystic and up to 15 cm in diameter (plate 121).

37. Q. **What drug can be prescribed to relieve menopausal symptoms when oestrogen therapy is contraindicated?**
   A. Clonidine hydrochloride (Dixarit) 25 μg twice daily. This drug is also used in much larger doses (Catapres) for treatment of hypertension.

38. Q. **What are the advantages of administration of oestrogens to all postmenopausal women?**
   A. (a) Prevention of menopausal symptoms of flushes, sweating and dyspareunia (due to genital atrophy and dryness).
   (b) Prevention of osteoporosis; 50% of women have crush fractures of the vertebrae by 75 years of age.
   (c) Avoidance of the wrinkled old prune appearance of the skin typical of ovarian failure.

39. Q. **What are the disadvantages of 'oestrogen forever' therapy in postmenopausal patients?**
   A. (a) Incidence of endometrial carcinoma trebled to approximately 1%.
   (b) Risk of hypertension and venous thromboembolism.

40. Q. **How can the risk of development of endometrial carcinoma be minimized when long-term oestrogen therapy is required for climacteric symptoms?**
   A. (a) Avoid continuous dosage — prescribe the drug for the first 21 days of each month or 5 days each week.
   (b) Use the smallest dose necessary.
   (c) Prescribe a progestogen for 7-10 days at the end of each month with the oestrogen to ensure that the proliferative effect of oestrogen is 'switched off'. This can cause cyclical bleeding which creates the problem of needing to exclude carcinoma as the cause.
   (d) Perform a hysterectomy.

41. Q. **What are the indications for hysterectomy in obstetric practice?**
   A. (a) Rupture of the uterus.
   (b) Uncontrollable primary or secondary postpartum haemorrhage (includes haemorrhage at Caesarean section).
   (c) Morbidly adherent placenta (accreta, increta, percreta) (plate 117).
   (d) Hydatidiform mole in a parous patient aged 40 years or more (plates 120, 121).

(e) Carcinoma of the cervix (plate 306).
(f) Caesarean hysterectomy as a method of sterilization — not advocated by the authors.
(g) Uterine gangrene due to Clostridium welchii infection (plates 154, 155).

42. Q. **What are the advantages of Billings' mucus observation method of natural birth control?**
A. (a) No risk of impairment of fertility as with the contraceptive pill (secondary amenorrhoea) or intra-uterine device (blocked tubes due to salpingitis).
(b) Recognition of preovulatory safe days which cannot be identified by the basal temperature chart.
(c) Equally effective during lactation and in patients with prolonged or irregular menstrual cycles.

43. Q. **What are the main causes of primary amenorrhoea?**
A. (a) Chromosome abnormalities (Turner syndrome and mosaic XY female) (25%).
(b) Delayed menarche (15%).
(c) Pituitary lesions (15%).
(d) Anatomical lesions (congenital absence of uterus, gonads or vagina) (10%) (plate 62).
(e) Imperforate vaginal septum (cryptomenorrhoea) (plates 58, 234-236).

44. Q. **What are the main nonphysiological, nonsurgical causes of secondary amenorrhoea?**
A. (a) After use of the contraceptive pill (10-15%).
(b) Premature menopause (5%).
(c) Anorexia nervosa (5%).
(d) Polycystic ovary (Stein-Leventhal syndrome) (5%) (plate 128).
(e) Stress (psychological).
(f) Sheehan's syndrome.
Unlike primary amenorrhoea, no cause is found in the majority of patients. Approximately 20% of patients with secondary amenorrhoea have hyperprolactinaemia and about 20% of these have demonstrable pituitary tumours.

45. Q. **What proportion of patients with primary amenorrhoea are potentially fertile?**
A. About 60%; with oestrogen therapy most of the remainder can lead normal, sexually active lives.

46. Q. **What are the methods of ovulation induction in infertile women after exclusion of thyroid and adrenal disease?**
A. (a) Ovulation commonly returns spontaneously without treatment or with appropriate diet or placebo therapy.
(b) Clomiphene citrate (Clomid) 50 mg or more orally for 5 days from day 5 of menstrual cycle. Success rate — ovulation 75%, pregnancy 40%.
(c) Follicle stimulating hormone and chorionic gonadotrophic hormone. Method applicable to about 10%; success rate — ovulation 90%, pregnancy 80%.
(d) Bromocriptine (Parlodel) if patient has hyperprolactinaemia.
(e) Wedge resection of polycystic ovaries (plate 83).

47. Q. **What complications can result from overstimulation with gonadotrophins?**
A. (a) Multiple pregnancy.
(b) Rapid follicular enlargement causing ovarian pain or an acute abdomen due to rupture or haemorrhage from the cysts.

48. Q. **What treatment is possible for male infertility?**
A. (a) Quantity and quality of sperm can be improved by administration of gonadotrophins, clomiphene citrate or bromocriptine.
(b) Surgical correction of occluded vas deferens (vasectomy or inflammatory disease).
(c) Correction of varicocele can improve sperm count.
(d) Periodic abstinence can improve sperm count — coitus only at likely time of ovulation.
(e) Artificial insemination using the husband's split ejaculate.
(f) Artifical insemination donor.

49. Q. **In what circumstances does an ectopic pregnancy rupture late (10-18 weeks)?**
A. When the containing muscle wall is thick as in an interstitial or cornual pregnancy, or when there is implantation in a rudimentary uterine horn.

50. Q. **What congenital anomaly is often associated with a unicornuate uterus?**

A. Absence of the kidney on the contralateral side because the Mullerian (paramesonephric) system is close to the mesonephric system as it arises lateral to it from the urogenital ridge on the dorsal body wall. The ovary develops from the medial aspect of the urogenital ridge and is not involved.

51. Q. **What clinical features would lead you to suspect the diagnosis of a hydatidiform mole?**

A. Hyperemesis usually in the second trimester associated with excessive uterine size, hypertension and proteinuria; usually there is vaginal bleeding and at presentation 30% of patients are passing vesicles.

52. Q. **How would you confirm the diagnosis of hydatidiform mole if the patient had not passed vesicles?**

A. (a) Ultrasonographic appearance of a snowstorm of echoes.
    (b) Low urinary oestrogen and pregnanediol and high HCG excretion (over 300,000 IU HCG/24 hours excludes a normal pregnancy).

53. Q. **What is the important differential diagnosis of hydatidiform mole?**

A. Multiple pregnancy.

54. Q. **What is the treatment of the patient with an intact hydatidiform mole?**

A. (a) Suction curettage plus oxytocin infusion with cross-matched blood available in case of excessive bleeding.
    (b) Primary hysterectomy if aged 35 and para 3 or more because of the greater risk of invasive mole or choriocarcinoma (plates 120, 121).
    (c) Follow-up for 1-2 years with chest radiography and serial urinary (or plasma) HCG estimations until the level has fallen to and remained below 100 IU/24 hours for 1 year (plate 122, 123).

55. Q. **What are the indications for chemotherapy in a patient following evacuation of a hydatidiform mole?**

A. (a) Presence of metastases, usually in lungs or vagina, with or without histological verification of the diagnosis.
    (b) Beta HCG titre remaining positive after 60 days from evacuation of the uterus or rising after an initial fall (a new pregnancy having been excluded).
    (c) Prophylactic chemotherapy is not favoured because toxicity can be severe and malignant sequelae may not be prevented.

56. Q. **Why is evacuation of an intact hydatidiform mole by induction of abortion with an oxytocic infusion not favoured?**

A. (a) Risk of pulmonary molar embolization causing acute heart failure.
    (b) Incidence of malignant sequelae said to be increased to about 20%.
    (c) Suction curettage is safer, with significantly less blood loss.

57. Q. **What are the indications for vulvectomy?**

A. (a) Invasive carcinoma or malignant melanoma of the vulva (plates 225-233).
    (b) Intractable pruritus vulvae.
    (c) Chronic skin disease of the vulva when biopsy shows intraepithelial carcinoma (including Bowen's and Paget's diseases).

58. Q. **What are the causes of vesicovaginal fistulas?**

A. (a) Gynaecological surgery (hysterectomy or vaginal repair) (plate 194).
    (b) Irradiation of cervical carcinoma.
    (c) Obstetrical trauma or neglected obstructed labour (plate 195).

59. Q. **What is the management of severe haemorrhage from a cervical carcinoma during treatment by external irradiation?**

A. (a) Vaginal packing, blood transfusion and chemotherapy to treat associated infection usually controls the haemorrhage.
    (b) Cautery of the bleeding area or ligation of cervical branches of the uterine artery per vaginam are occasionally needed.
    (c) Abdominal hysterectomy and/or ligation of uterine or internal iliac arteries.

60. Q. **What is the treatment when a patient is bleeding vaginally at the conclusion of an abdominal hysterectomy?**

A. Put the patient (still anaesthetized) in the lithotomy position, locate the bleeding point (usually the unsutured lateral angle of the vaginal vault) and ligate it. If the source of bleeding cannot be located the abdomen must be reopened.

61. Q. **What is the mechanism for cessation of menstrual bleeding each cycle?**

A. Increase in secretion of oestrogen as a result of gonadotrophin releasing factor stimulating FSH production and thus follicle development.

62. Q. **In which clinical situations may hysteroscopy be of value?**

A. (a) Investigation of infertility (intrauterine adhesions), habitual abortion (bicornuate uterus, endometrial polyp).
(b) When curettage has failed to reveal the cause of postmenopausal bleeding (small polyp — benign or malignant) (plate 330).
(c) Staging of cancer of the uterine body.

63. Q. **What clinical signs are characteristic of Clostridium welchii infection in a patient with a septic abortion?**

A. (a) Jaundice and 'port wine' urine due to intravascular haemolysis; oliguria.
(b) Extreme uterine tenderness or crepitus; this indicates uterine gangrene and the need for hysterectomy (plates 154, 155).

64. Q. **How do you explain the presence of climacteric symptoms (flushes, sweating) in a patient who still menstruates?**

A. (a) The symptoms are due to waning ovarian function with inadequate production of oestrogen by the ovarian follicle although there is still sufficient to induce an endometrial response.
(b) Carcinoma of the cervix or endometrium can be the cause of the bleeding, especially if the menses are irregular.

65. Q. **Why does a patient not menstruate at the time of the first missed period and so abort the recently implanted embryo?**

A. Because the trophoblastic cells have produced sufficient chorionic gonadotrophic hormone to maintain the corpus luteum in the mother's ovary. The corpus luteum therefore continues to produce oestrogen and progesterone which sustain the endometrium. Normally, menstruation occurs because the corpus luteum regresses towards the end of the cycle.

66. Q. **How would you decide whether to use clomiphene citrate or FSH and chorionic gonadotrophic hormone to treat infertility in a patient with secondary amenorrhoea?**

A. Estimation of the 24-hour urinary excretion of oestrogen; less than 10 μg indicates ovarian inactivity and FSH and HCG would be preferred; clomiphene citrate is more likely to be effective if the oestrogen excretion exceeds 10 μg/24 hours (which is the minimum normal value).

67. Q. **How can you distinguish pelvic peritonitis from pelvic cellulitis on bimanual vaginal examination?**

A. Pelvic peritonitis would be associated with extreme pain on movement of the cervix, but there may be no adnexal mass palpable; with pelvic cellulitis there is less pain and the uterus is immobile and continuous with brawny swellings extending to the lateral pelvic walls.

68. Q. **How does carcinoma of the vulva kill the patient?**

A. (a) Haemorrhage from the femoral artery or vein due to neoplastic or inflammatory ulceration.
(b) Sepsis.
(c) Metastases to vital organs.

69. Q. **What complications occur after a simple vulvectomy?**

A. (a) Remarkably few; when the patient is young enough she can subsequently have spontaneous vaginal deliveries.
(b) Dyspareunia.
(c) Recurrence on the new vulval skin of the lesion that necessitated the vulvectomy.

70. **Q. When tubal insufflation is performed (Rubin test) how is it known that the tube(s) are patent?**

A. (a) The kymograph will show a fall in pressure and the patient (if conscious) will experience shoulder tip pain when she sits up (irritation of the diaphragm by carbon dioxide which was passed through the tubes).

(b) When the patient is anaesthetized the gas (carbon dioxide not air because of the risk of embolism) is heard bubbling through the Fallopian tube by a stethoscope placed on the abdomen suprapubically, or the dye (5 drops of methylene blue in 50 ml of normal saline) is seen flowing from the fimbriated end of the tube at laparoscopy.

71. **Q. What is the place of laparoscopy in gynaecological practice?**

A. (a) For diagnosis when there is pelvic pain (ectopic pregnancy, pelvic inflammatory disease, endometriosis) or infertility (confirm tubal patency by hydrotubation; tubal pathology warranting surgery can be present even when the tubes are patent).

(b) As an alternative to laparotomy for sterilization by tubal occlusion (clips and rings are less risky than cautery), biopsy of ovaries, ovum collection for in vitro fertilization, division of peritubal adhesions, recovery of intrauterine devices that have penetrated the uterus (plates 432-437).

72. **Q. What are the modes of presentation of ovarian cysts and tumours?**

A. (a) Incidental abdominal or vaginal bimanual examination. The tragedy of ovarian cancer is the lack of early symptoms.

(b) Vague abdominal discomfort, indigestion.

(c) Abdominal mass or distension (plates 356-365).

(d) Symptoms due to a complication (torsion, rupture, haemorrhage) (plates 82, 370).

(e) Incidental finding at laparotomy (e.g., Caesarean section).

(f) Pressure effects on veins, bowel or diaphragm.

(g) Effects of hormones (precocious puberty, postmenopausal bleeding, masculinization).

73. **Q. How does herpes infection of the female genitalia present?**

A. (a) Acute vulvovaginitis often with secondary bacterial infection. There is severe pain and sometimes acute retention of urine (plate 164).

(b) Vesicular lesions or ulcers on vulva or vagina. There is often a history of recurrent attacks (plate 150).

(c) Routine cervical cytology may show typical inclusion bodies in desquamated cells (plates 275, 276).

(d) Culture may be performed when indicated by herpes infection in the male partner or neonate, the patient herself being asymptomatic.

74. **Q. What are the causes of dyspareunia?**

A. (a) Pain at attempted penetration is due to anatomical or inflammatory lesions of the vulva (posterior colporrhaphy, episiotomy, intact hymen, trichomonas, monilia) or narrowing due to postmenopausal disuse atrophy or radical radiotherapy; or to psychosexual problems (levatores ani spasm) (plates 237-239).

(b) Deep pelvic pain is likely to be due to endometriosis, adenomyosis, pelvic inflammatory disease, prolapsed ovaries or pelvic congestion (soft, tender, enlarged uterus).

75. **Q. What are the incubation periods for herpes genitalis, gonorrhoea and syphilis?**

A. (a) Itching, burning and pain precede appearance of vesicles 3-5 days after infection with herpesvirus (90% of below the waist lesions are due to type 2 virus) (plate 150).

(b) Dysuria and discharge appear about 7 days after infection with the gonococcus (plates 31, 32).

(c) The primary chancre of syphilis appears about 21 days after exposure (plate 156).

76. **Q. Why do some women pass through the menopause without having hot flushes and episodes of sweating?**

A. (a) There must be an individual response to alteration of oestrogen levels or the woman may be insensitive to excessive activity of the hypothalamic – hyophyseal system (raised levels of FSH).

(b) Alteration of adrenal function as the ovary retires from the endocrine orchestra may result in oestrogen production sufficient to control symptoms of oestrogen deficiency.

(c) Sufficient peripheral production of oestrone may occur in fat depots.

77. **Q. How would you investigate a patient presenting with secondary amenorrhoea?**

A. (a) Exclude physiological causes — pregnancy, lactation, menopause (history, clinical examination, urinary or plasma HCG, plasma FSH).

(b) Exclude surgical causes (hysterectomy, oophorectomy), hormone (postcontraceptive pill) and drug therapy.

(c) Consider emotional factors and gross weight changes (anorexia nervosa, obesity).

(d) Exclude thyroid, adrenal and pituitary disease (thyroid function tests, plasma testosterone, urinary cortisol, serum prolactin and radiography of pituitary fossa).

(e) Assess ovarian activity (plasma or urinary oestrogen, ovarian biopsy for presence of primary follicles if plasma FSH elevated).

78. Q. **What are the stigmata of Turner's syndrome (ovarian agenesis) (karotype 45,XO) (streak gonad syndrome)?**

A. Short stature, female phenotype, primary amenorrhoea, webbing of the neck, infantile breast status, sparse pubic and axillary hair, infantile external genitalia and vagina, atrophic vaginal smear, immature uterus, high levels of serum FSH, low oestrogen levels, retarded ossification, osteoporosis, coarctation of the aorta.

79. Q. **Why is the cervix amputated in the Manchester repair operation?**

A. (a) The transverse cervical ligaments become more accessible for suturing together anterior to the cervical stump (plates 187-189).

(b) Many patients who require a vaginal repair have an elongated cervix and unless it is amputated the patient will continue to complain of a 'lump' vaginally (plate 174).

80. Q. **What is the treatment of an imperforate hymen or transverse vaginal septum that occludes the vagina?**

A. (a) Excision, hopefully before retained menses has resulted in haematosalpinges and tubal occlusion (plates 58, 59, 234-236).

(b) Intravenous pyelogram to exclude associated abnormality of the urinary tract.

81. Q. **When is stress incontinence of urine most likely to begin?**

A. During pregnancy.

82. Q. **What is the management of the catheter after a vaginal repair?**

A. (a) If a suprapubic indwelling catheter is used it is clamped after 3-5 days and removed if the patient is able to void and has a residual urine volume below 100 ml. If she cannot void the catheter is left in until she can void satisfactorily.

(b) An indwelling urethral catheter is removed after continuous drainage for 3-5 days and residual urine volume is measured (by catheterization) after voiding 4-6 hours later. Only if the residual urine volume is more than 100 ml is further testing (in 1-2 days) performed. If the patient cannot void the catheter is replaced for 48 hours and the urine is cultured to exclude infection (plate 416).

83. Q. **What is Bonney's test?**

A. Elevation of the bladder neck (restoration of the posterior urethrovesical angle) with fingers or open sponge forceps (without occluding urethra) to see if stress incontinence of urine is controlled — if it is, the test indicates that buttressing of the bladder neck area at anterior colporrhaphy is likely to cure the symptom. By pushing up the bladder neck above the pelvic diaphragm it indicates equally that elevation of the area by an abdominal operation (Marshall-Marchetti-Kranz) will be successful.

84. Q. **What is a cervical erosion?**

A. Erosion suggests ulceration, but the pink or red velvety appearance commonly seen on the ectocervix is due to the presence of endocervical-type epithelium (single layer) that shows the underlying vessels. Downward movement of the squamocolumnar junction is a physiological process influenced by oestrogen (puberty, oral contraceptive pill, first pregnancy). Passage of a speculum and particularly the opening of a bivalve speculum causes eversion of the cervix and exposure of the endocervical epithelium which can be mistaken for an erosion (ectropion) (plates 36, 38, 39, 284).

85. Q. **How is the appropriate operation for uterovaginal prolapse selected?**

A. (a) If there is second or third degree uterine prolapse or another indication for hysterectomy (menorrhagia), vaginal hysterectomy is preferred to Manchester repair (plates 168-174).

(b) Cystocele/rectocele without uterine prolapse may require only anterior/posterior colporrhaphy.

(c) Presence of stress incontinence determines need for buttressing of urethra or bladder neck suspension.

(d) A large enterocele may require an abdominal approach if cure is to be achieved without loss of calibre of the vagina; desire for continued coital function can determine the technique to be employed (plate 177).

86. Q. **What is the character of menstruation in the patient with anovular cycles?**

A. (a) The menses (usually painless) may occur regularly, presumably due to ovarian follicle decay similar to that of the corpus luteum.
(b) Often the cycles are irregular and bleeding can occur from the hypertrophied endometrium (cystic glandular hyperplasia) seemingly having outgrown its blood supply; minor fluctuations in oestrogen level can trigger the endometrial breakdown (plate 85).

87. Q. **What is decubital ulceration of the cervix or vagina?**

A. When there is gross prolapse, the cervix is traumatized when the woman sits or walks causing ulceration with discharge and haemorrhage (plate 171).

88. Q. **What arteries are tied during abdominal hysterectomy?**

A. (a) Ovarian and uterine arteries on both sides (plates 33, 44-46).
(b) The descending branch of the uterine artery can require separate ligation.

89. Q. **What are the principles of anterior and posterior colporrhaphy?**

A. (a) In anterior colporrhaphy the prolapsed bladder and urethra are replaced and supported by sutures in the torn pubovesical (or bladder) fascia (plates 184-192).
(b) In posterior colporrhaphy the enterocele, rectocele, and relaxed introitus are repaired by sutures in the uterosacral ligaments, rectal fascia and levatores ani muscles (plates 410-416).

90. Q. **What are the indications for therapeutic curettage?**

A. (a) To control bleeding and risk of sepsis in incomplete abortion (all cases) (plates 102-105).
(b) To control bleeding and remove retained placental tissue when secondary postpartum haemorrhage is heavy or persistent.
(c) Menorrhagia — removal of hypertrophied endometrium often controls the symptom as well as providing tissue for histology (anovulation, cystic glandular hyperplasia, carcinoma) (plates 19, 20).
(d) Termination of pregnancy.

91. Q. **What are the complications of tubal ligation?**

A. (a) Usually none, although if the patient is young and her marriage fails, and especially when the operation is carried out postpartum, she may change her mind and request reversal, or show psychological sequelae.
(b) Complications of the anaesthetic and incision.
(c) Menorrhagia. After tubal ligation at least 20% of women have a hysterectomy performed, usually for abnormal bleeding. Periods may previously have been modified by an oral contraceptive pill.
(d) Ectopic pregnancy.
(e) Hydrosalpinges which can undergo torsion.

92. Q. **What conditions should be excluded in a patient with a history of habitual abortion?**

A. (a) Incompetent cervix — history of painless second trimester abortion preceded by copious serosanguineous or mucoid discharge.
(b) Uterine abnormality (unicornuate, bicornuate, didelphys).
(c) Deficient corpus luteum.
(d) Submucous fibromyomas or polyps.
(e) Chromosome abnormalities.
(f) Chronic infection in the uterus or cervix.

93. Q. **What malignant diseases can cross the placenta?**

A. (a) Choriocarcinoma.
(b) Hodgkin's disease.
(c) Malignant melanoma and lymphoma.
(d) Leukaemia.

94. Q. **What are the criteria for removal of fibromyomas?**

A. (a) Size — if large there is always the possibility of misdiagnosis of a (malignant) ovarian tumour. Large tumours are more likely to give pressure symptoms (plates 323-329).
(b) Associated menorrhagia or infertility — more likely when submucous in position.
(c) Uterine pain and rapid increase in size suggesting possibility of malignant change (sarcoma).

95. Q. **What are the indications for anticancer chemotherapy in gynaecology?**

A. (a) Malignant trophoblastic disease. Methotrexate or actinomycin D alone or combined with cyclophosphamide for special cases.
(b) Carcinoma of ovary. All adenocarcinomas and most malignant germ cell tumours (malignant teratoma, endodermal sinus tumour, embryonal carcinoma) except Stage 1(a) lesions without capsule rupture.
(c) Carcinoma of endometrium when there are metastases or deep invasion of myometrium. Agents used are progestogen (medroxy progesterone acetate), antioestrogen (Tamoxifen) or cytotoxic agents if no response to hormones.
(d) Carcinoma of the cervix with disseminated disease. Intraarterial perfusion to the pelvis when irradiation has failed to control local disease. Progestogens may be of benefit if the lesion is an adenocarcinoma.
(e) Carcinoma of vulva when surgery ± irradiation has failed or if disseminated disease is evident. Topical 5-fluorouracil can cure preinvasive disease.
(f) Sarcoma of the uterus or vagina and malignant melanoma warrant trial of cytotoxic drug therapy.

96. Q. **When is hysterectomy performed after cone biopsy of the cervix?**

A. (a) If the cone showed invasive carcinoma, hysterectomy (simple or radical) ± irradiation is indicated (plate 422).
(b) If the cone revealed carcinoma in situ/severe dysplasia to the edge of the specimen or if cytology remained positive and the patient elected to lose her uterus rather than continue conservative treatment.

97. Q. **What causes the changes in the vaginal pH during a woman's reproductive years?**

A. Oestrogen results in a build-up of glycogen within vaginal squamous cells upon which Doderlein's bacillus lives and produces lactic acid that provides defence against bacterial infection. Vaginal acidity favours monilial infection. The vagina becomes more alkaline at the time of menstruation and coitus and this facilitates infection with trichomonads.

Index

All figures in italics refer to page numbers
All figures in bold type refer to plate numbers
Q denotes question number